TEXT AND ATLAS ON
CORNEAL PIGMENTATION

TEXT AND ATLAS ON
CORNEAL PIGMENTATION

Editor

Jorge L Alió MD PhD
Professor and Chairman
Department of Ophthalmology
Miguel Hernandez University, Medical School
President, VISSUM Corporation
Alicante, Spain

Associate Editors

María Alejandra Amesty MD
Adnexal Fellow
Moorfields Eye Hospital
City Road, London, UK

Alejandra Rodríguez MSc
Senior Biologist/Microbiologist
Research, Development and
Innovation (RDI) Department
VISSUM Corporation
Alicante, Spain

Mohamed El Bahrawy MD
Senior Clinical Research Fellow
VISSUM-Instituto Oftalmologico
Miguel Hernandez University
Alicante, Spain

This work has been supported in part by a grant from the Spanish Ministry of Science and Innovation, Centro para el Desarrollo Tecnológico Industrial (CDTI), CENIT: "Customized Eye Care", CeyeC (CEN-20091021)

JAYPEE The Health Sciences Publisher
New Delhi | London | Philadelphia | Panama

Jaypee Brothers Medical Publishers (P) Ltd.

Headquarters
Jaypee Brothers Medical Publishers (P) Ltd.
4838/24, Ansari Road, Daryaganj
New Delhi 110 002, India
Phone: +91-11-43574357
Fax: +91-11-43574314
E-mail: jaypee@jaypeebrothers.com

Overseas Offices

J.P. Medical Ltd.
83, Victoria Street, London
SW1H 0HW (UK)
Phone: +44-20 3170 8910
Fax: +44(0) 20 3008 6180
E-mail: info@jpmedpub.com

Jaypee-Highlights Medical Publishers Inc.
City of Knowledge, Bld. 237, Clayton
Panama City, Panama
Phone: +1 507-301-0496
Fax: +1 507-301-0499
E-mail: cservice@jphmedical.com

Jaypee Medical Inc.
The Bourse
111, South Independence Mall East
Suite 835, Philadelphia
PA 19106, USA
Phone: +1 267-519-9789
E-mail: jpmed.us@gmail.com

Jaypee Brothers Medical Publishers (P) Ltd.
17/1-B, Babar Road, Block-B
Shaymali, Mohammadpur
Dhaka-1207, Bangladesh
Mobile: +08801912003485
E-mail: jaypeedhaka@gmail.com

Jaypee Brothers Medical Publishers (P) Ltd.
Bhotahity, Kathmandu, Nepal
Phone: +977-9741283608
E-mail: kathmandu@jaypeebrothers.com

Website: www.jaypeebrothers.com
Website: www.jaypeedigital.com

Inquiries for bulk sales may be solicited at: jaypee@jaypeebrothers.com

Text and Atlas on Corneal Pigmentation

First Edition: **2015**

ISBN: 978-93-5152-906-4

Printed at Replika Press Pvt. Ltd.

Dedicated to

Our patients, who gave us the motive
to develop and innovate in the art and science of keratopigmentation.
Knowing that, we may contribute even in a small way to improve their quality of life
through giving them a better cosmetic appearance, a higher quality of vision or
simply increasing their self-esteem with a desired eye color.

Contributors

Jorge L Alió MD PhD
Professor and Chairman
Department of Ophthalmology
Miguel Hernandez University
Medical School
President, VISSUM Corporation
Alicante, Spain

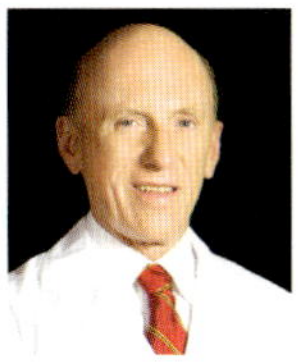

Alejandra Rodríguez MSc
Senior Biologist/Microbiologist
Research, Development and Innovation (RDI)
Department
VISSUM Corporation
Alicante, Spain

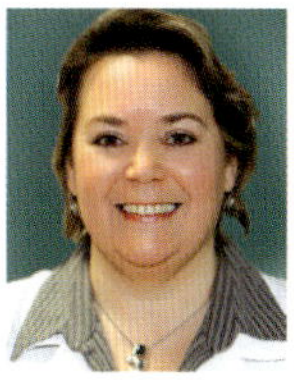

María Alejandra Amesty MD
Adnexal Fellow
Moorfields Eye Hospital
City Road, London, UK

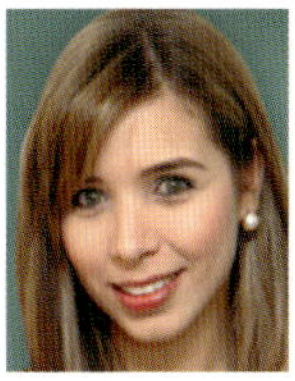

Mohamed El Bahrawy MD
Senior Clinical Research Fellow
VISSUM Instituto Oftalmologico
Miguel Hernandez University
Alicante, Spain

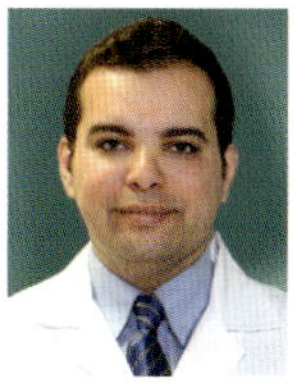

Preface

Even though it is true that since Galen's time pigmentation has been known, it is not until recently that keratopigmentation has become feasible with new tools, new pigments, and especially new knowledge about corneal behavior and tolerance to these pigments. The book tries to gather together all the scientific information available on this topic to offer ophthalmologists and in particular corneal surgeons, the possibility of using this technique for many patients who will benefit from its cosmetic therapeutic applications (leukomas and blind eyes, phthisical eyes with deformations as an alternative to evisceration and prosthesis), functional therapeutic applications (aniridic patients, colobomas, traumatic iris losses) or even purely cosmetic applications (changing the color of the eye on a voluntary basis). All these applications are possible and are presented in the book in a scientific way.

We have now 10 years of experience in keratopigmentation since we did the first case. We have always been attracted by the idea of avoiding losing the anatomies of young people affected by trauma and with cosmetically unacceptable appearances. Cosmetics is important today, just as it has always been, but in our modern environment, a cosmetic defect in the eye is unacceptable and limits the quality of life of many patients. Based on this idea, we have developed a systematic approach over the last 10 years in the field, creating and building up science on a topic that has always been empirical. So far, nobody has reported such a systematic approach, and we hope that we have done so adequately for the purpose of dissemination of this technique.

The clinical atlas will show clearly the evolution of this technique in our hands over the years and how perfect the outcomes are today with the adequate techniques and selected pigments. In the experimental atlas, we describe the methods that we have been using for the purpose of these investigations and indeed the outstanding knowledge that is obtained from the experimental model that we have used.

The reader will find in experimental atlas the evolution of the technique and also the very important changes that happen with very different or similar pigments when they are used at the surface or intrastromally inside the cornea.

The experimental use of pigments has taught us a lot about the performance and the optimal use of the pigments and also how the quality and character of their composition should be. It is the experimental model, where we have learnt and tested the secondary effects and the potential toxicity of the pigments as demonstrated in the reports that we have published.

We are sure that the readers will find the experimental part a tremendously interesting topic as from the experimental animal model to the human use keratopigmentation has reached maturity nowadays by using the adequate pigments and the adequate techniques.

Clinical atlas of keratopigmentation cases offer the readers the real facts and possibilities that corneal pigmentation may give our patients for therapeutic, cosmetic functional or purely cosmetic purposes. The cases have been selected from the many ones we have to indicate the evolution of the procedure. The initial cases performed by us show more variability in colors, while all cases have proven to be effective and stable depending on the quality of the colors used.

Corneal pigmentation is to be approached by adequate pigments and instruments. The pigments are essential as some metals and micronized pigments might induce chemical reactions with opacities and neovascularization. Adequately selected pigments do behave excellently over time and are stable.

The readers will enjoy these clinical cases as most of them have been selected for therapeutic purposes while some of them are really truly cosmetic and open a new perspective on the use of pigments to change the apparent color of the eye.

In Appendices, we demonstrate the presentations about keratopigmentation in different congresses and conferences since 2008, also some of the papers, we published about the methodology and outcomes of our keratopigmentation experience in world class peer-reviewed journals, such as Journal of Cataract and Refractive Surgery and Cornea journal.

Also, a screenshot of our updated website: *www.coloreyetattoo.com*, is a great tool for both patient and professional education.

Keratopigmentation was an art and is now an art and a science. We hope that all our colleagues who read the book will find useful advice and convenient descriptions of this technique for the benefit of their patients.

Instructive surgical videos are available on our official website: *www.coloreyetattoo.com.*

Jorge L Alió
María Alejandra Amesty
Alejandra Rodríguez
Mohamed El Bahrawy

Acknowledgments

In more than a decade of developments in the field of keratopigmentation, our team has cooperated with many scientists and enterprises, to ensure that highest levels of quality and safety in terms of surgical techniques and pigments, we would like to acknowledge the efforts of Dr Bader Toffaha; former Clinical Research Fellow, VISSUM-Instituto Oftalmologico de Alicante, for his investigative contributions through our team, which was utilized through a number of publications and congress presentations. We acknowledge the clinical efforts and expertise of Dr Sabat K Abu-Mostafa, Ahmadi Hospital, Kuwait. Finally, due thanks to the team of Epsilon, Irvine, California, as their professional and state-of-the-art technology was the reason for the development of the successive generation of surgical tools used in keratopigmentation procedures.

Contents

SECTION 1 : Keratopigmentation

Editors: Jorge L Alió, María Alejandra Amesty

SECTION 2 : Experimental Atlas of Keratopigmentation

Editors: Jorge L Alió, Alejandra Rodríguez

SECTION 3 : Clinical Atlas of Keratopigmentation

Editors: Jorge L Alió, Mohamed El Bahrawy

Section 1

Keratopigmentation

Editors: Jorge L Alió, María Alejandra Amesty

1

History of Keratopigmentation

The practice of corneal tattooing or keratopigmentation is by no means a new surgical technique. In fact, it was practiced in a very rudimentary way in ancient times and it was sporadically used to treat corneal opacities.[1,2]

HISTORY OF CORNEAL TATTOOING

The history of corneal tattooing can be divided in different periods. The Galen period (150 AD), Louis Von Wecker period (1869–1870) and then other authors are going to be mentioned (1870–1900).

Galen and Aetius Period (131–450 AD)

The famous Roman physician and philosopher Galen of Pergamum (131–210 AD), was the first to performed corneal tattooing and he is considered the first physician who pigmented a human cornea (Figure 1.1).[2,3]

Tattooing of the opaque cornea was practiced in a crude way by the ancients, the procedure first being described by Galen (150 AD) and later by Aetius (450 AD), both of whom attempted to cover-up leukomatous opacities by cauterizing the surface with a heated stylet and applying powdered nutgalls and iron (ferric tannate) or pulverized pomegranate bark mixed with a copper salt.[4,5] These procedures were probably performed only in patients with an unsightly corneal scarring.[6]

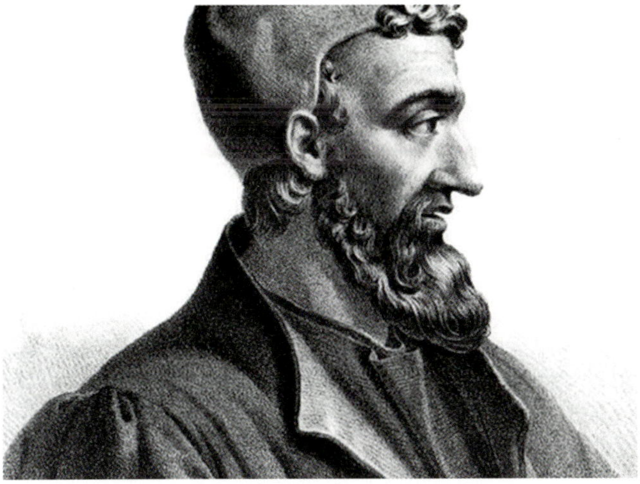

Fig. 1.1: Galen

Louis Von Wecker Period (1869–1870)

After Galen, the practice of corneal tattooing is not mentioned in the literature until 1869, when Louis Von Wecker an oculoplastic surgeon introduced a new method.[7] Fourteen centuries passed until Wecker designed, devise and put into practice the modern keratopigmentation method of procedure. It was also the first to use black ink, also called India ink. The author applied cocaine to anesthetize the eye surface, then covered the cornea with a thick ink solution and inserted the pigment with a needle.[5] This method has influenced all subsequent methods since then (Figure 1.2).

He acknowledged that the suggestion came from a simple inquiry in regard to the possible treatment of a clinical case, made by his then student, Abadie, but stated emphatically that the revival of this procedure and the details of technique were wholly his own. The details of his technique and procedures were published by the head of the clinic, Pomier of Pau in 1870.[8] Years later, in 1872, the author reintroduced the same principle but with the application of India ink.[4]

Other Authors (1870–1900)

Keratopigmentation gained popularity and many authors in the late 1870s and early 1900s suggested different indications and the use of a variety of dyes, several devices were designed and different techniques of application were proposed.[2]

These earlier trials were limited to the use of black or India ink, which was employed to fill in the pupillary area, to outline the iris circle, and occasionally to stipple the iris radiations.[4] During the succeeding decade, tattooing with multicolor pigments to imitate the natural iris stroma was attempted with considerable success by Dunnage,[9] Taylor,[10] Woinow,[11] Hasner,[12] and Archer [13] in Europe and by Levis,[14] Williams,[15] Thomson,[16] and Mathewson[17] in America.

Taylor's contribution attracted more attention than others chiefly because he advocated the use of a bundle of needles, which de Wecker on trial found to be more practical and efficient than his own single grooved needle, and so promptly adopted Taylor's suggestion (Figures 1.3 and 1.4).[10]

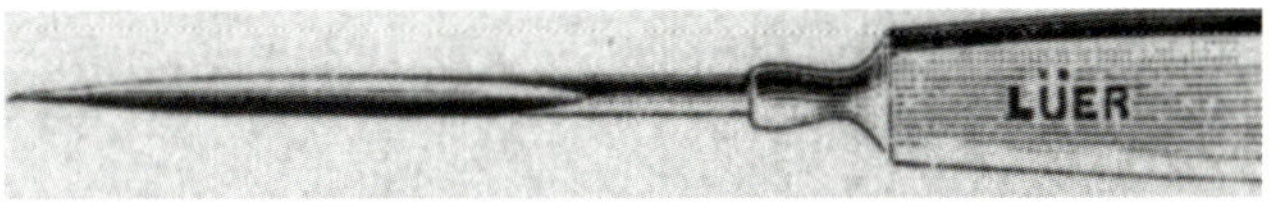

Fig. 1.2: Wecker's needle (Ziegler)

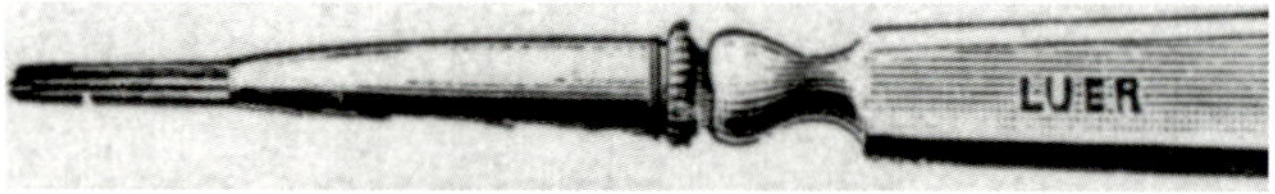

Fig. 1.3: Taylor's needle (Ziegler)

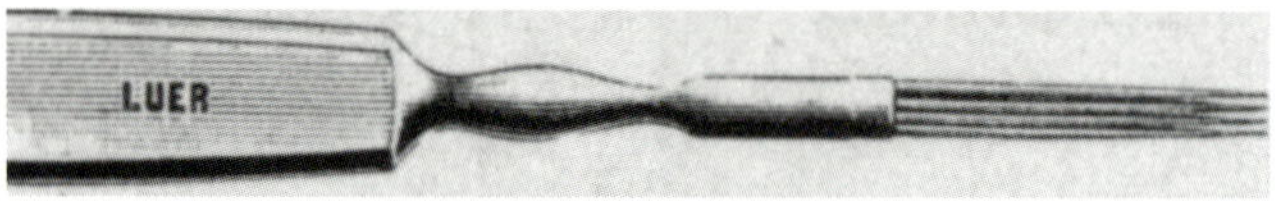

Fig. 1.4: Agnew's needle (Ziegler)

Ziegler's Period (1883–1973)

Born in Glenn Tannery, Luzerne, Pennsylvania, USA on November 1883, Dr Samuel Lewis Ziegler (Fig. 1.5) is considered the father of modern keratopigmentation. His research in corneal tattooing is revealed through this work titled "Multicolor Tattooing of the Cornea", published in 1922. Most of the aspects commented in this chapter, are known through his extensive knowledge on this matter.

He not only performed the corneal tattoo, but also recommended the type of pigments that should be used, commented his protocol and his technique, mentioned the instruments required to perform the surgical procedure, created a list of colors and their chemical composition and made a compilation of all the information, authors and their history, related to corneal tattooing available at that moment.

Dr Ziegler is going to be mentioned many times in this book because he had been the promoter of keratopigmentation in our times and his techniques remain valid after many years.

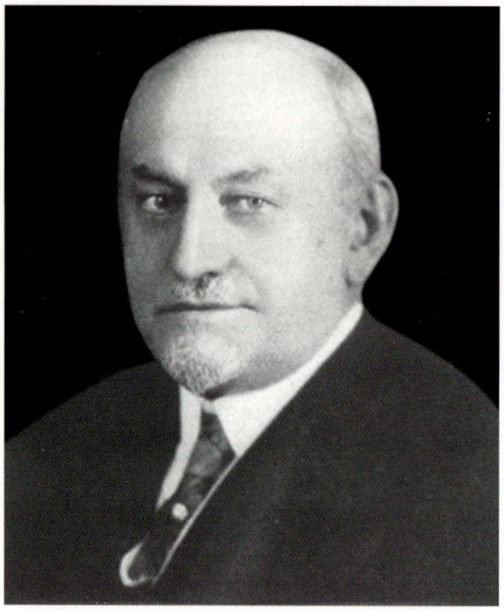

Fig. 1.5: Dr Samuel Lewis Ziegler

COLOR TATTOOING

It is interesting to note that Levis from Philadelphia, was the first American to advocate and practice tattooing with colors. Archer, at Utrecht, in 1874, made an exhaustive and valuable study of the various colored pigments, carrying his researches in three directions: (1) The fixity of colors; (2) modifications occurring in the corneal tissue, and (3) the disposition of dispersed pigment particles. He found gamboge so irritating that inflammation and exfoliation soon followed its use, thus throwing this pigment out of the corneal tissue. Ultramarine blue, terra Sienna, and India ink were better tolerated, but indigo and Prussian blue proved to be more irritating.[4]

No notable contributions on this subject were presented during the succeeding decade, but in 1887 Vacher,[18] of Orleans, contributed a paper of practical value, in which he emphasized the importance of using coloring-matter that was chemically pure, stable, and reduced to a very fine powder. He employed five pigments—calcium carbonate, carmin, Prussian blue, pale ochre, and India ink.[4]

During the next decade, Nieden[19] of Bochum, Cofler[20] of Trieste, Holth[21] of Christiania, and Chevallereau and Polack[22] of Paris, all contributed papers that greatly enhanced our practical knowledge of this interesting subject. Nieden, in 1901, devised a tattooing needle which was made on the principle of the fountain pen, suggested a trial of the Edison electric pen, and encouraged Merck to extract a brown pigment from the choroid of the ox, 26 eyes being required to produce 232 mgm of pigment.[19] This uveal pigment was difficult to produce, very expensive, and not especially advantageous. Like Archer, he condemns the use of gamboge. He further reports poor success from terra Sienna, sepia, burnt umber, and brown ochre, because of irritation and the extrusion of these pigments. As umber and ochre have both proved their worth in the hands of others, it is possible that his pigments were poorly prepared. He weakly favors ultramarine blue and Prussian blue.[4]

Cofler,[20] in 1902, procured Japanese colors from Tokyo in stick form, comprising yellow, blue, brown, and red. The cinnabar and cerulean blue—he found insoluble, harmless, and free from bacteria. He had great success from mixing cinnabar with India ink in securing all shades of brown, and by stippling his blue with radiations of black or brown he closely imitated the iris stroma.[4]

After trying Japanese stick colors, Holth abandoned them for finely ground French colors (1906), which he washed with water, alcohol, and ether in order to remove the oily and resinous impurities and thus secure a sterile, impalpable powder, free from irritating properties. He used lamp black, cinnabar, raw Sienna, burnt Sienna, raw umber, burnt umber, sepia, ultramarine blue, celestial blue (stannate of cobalt), powdered slate, calcium carbonate, gray earth, and China clay. He condemns green earth, ultramarine blue, Brunswick

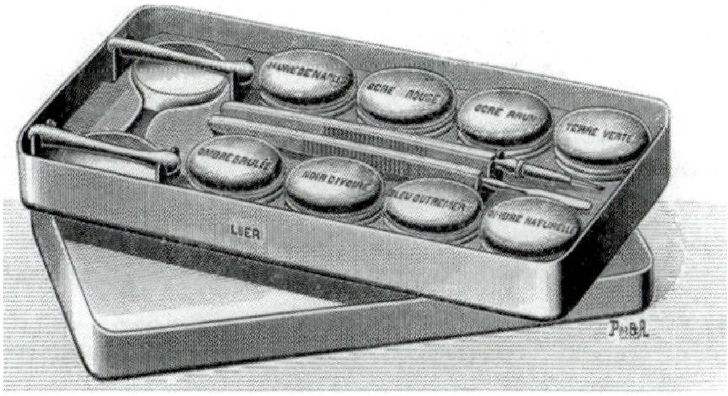

Fig. 1.6: Pigments palette (Ziegler)

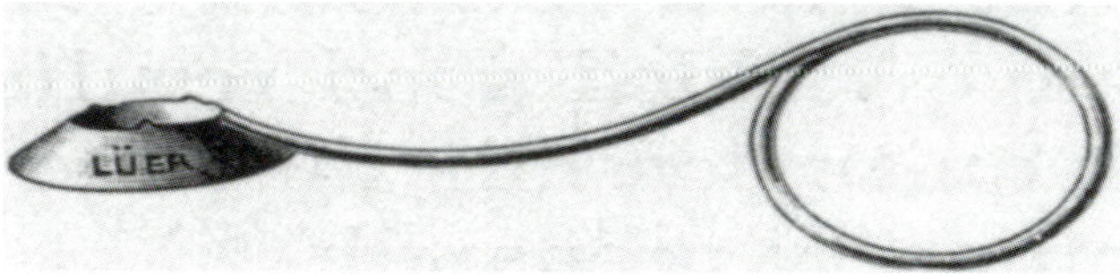

Fig. 1.7: Armaignae's pupillary ring (Ziegler)

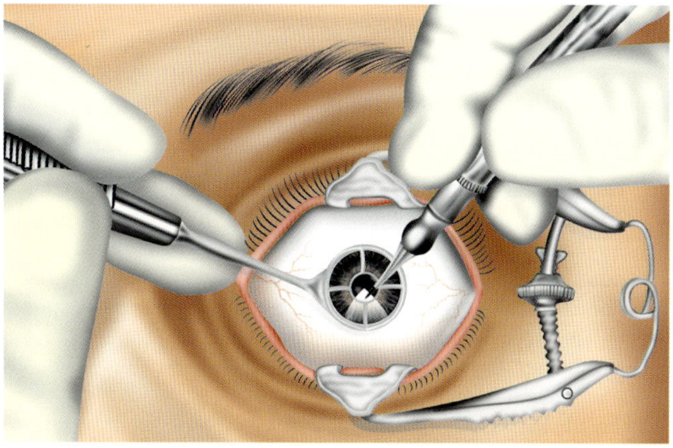

Fig. 1.8: Ziegler's fixation ring and Nieden's fountain pen (Ziegler 1922)

blue, mineral blue, Prussian blue, mountain blue, and yellow cadmium. As green earth and ultramarine blue have yielded good results in the hands of other surgeons, it is quite possible that the products available to him were not properly prepared.[4]

Palette of Colors

Chevallereau and Polack have worked out the best palette of colors (Figure 1.6), although their series comprises more shades of brown than were absolutely necessary. They suggest that this is an advantage, since few physicians are artists, but forget that the student of today must be quite familiar with microscopic stains and, therefore, well-versed in color nuances.[22]

The shades of blue are limited, but skillful mixing of the pigments on their palette will easily remedy this defect. They have tested many other pigments and abandoned them. Since their announcement in 1906, Ziegler tested all their colors and many more, and he was convinced that their palette can safely be adopted.[4]

Later studies were conducted by researchers as Nieden Bochum, Coffer of Trieste, Holth Christiania and Polack Paris, who greatly enriched the practical knowledge on this subject.[4,20]

TOOLS AND MATERIALS FORMERLY USED FOR KERATOPIGMENTATION

In 1896, authors like Czermak[23] used the von Hippel's trephine to delineate the pupil margin.[4]

Holth had been persistent and ingenious in the development of his instruments and techniques. Beginning in 1898, he started to use metal cylinders and tubular punches as corneal trephines in order more accurately to outline the margins of the pupil and the outer circle of the iris. He claims priority on this point over Armaignac,[24] who used for this purpose a large and a small funnel-shaped guide (Figure 1.7) provided with three spuds to fix in the cornea. He acknowledges Czermak's earlier use (1896) of von Hippel's trephine for the purpose of outlining the pupil.[23] He curetted the corneal epithelium from the proposed pupillary area before tattooing with pigment, which he mixed with a weak solution of gum Arabic as an excipient.[4]

Nieden, in 1901, devised a tattooing needle which was made on the principle of the fountain pen, and suggested a trial using this needle with Edison's electric pen (Figure 1.8). He found this electric tattooing needle faster than other traditional methods of tattoo.[4,19]

OTHER TECHNIQUES

Other physicians, such as Victor Morax, did not actually tattoo the cornea but still changed the external appearance of the cornea. His technique involved splitting the corneal tissue into two layers, introducing the coloring substance under the pedicle flap, and then applying a compressive dressing over the eye.[5]

It can be seen that along the history of keratopigmentation, various methods and pigments have been used. All these authors mentioned above have collaborated in the development of the procedure that has been forgotten for years, and that is taking great importance in today's ophthalmology.

REFERENCES

1. Holth S. Revival of Galen's corneal staining with copper sulfate and tannine should be abandoned. Am J Ophthalmol. 1931; 14:378-9.
2. Mannis MJ, Eghbali K, Schwab IR. Keratopigmentation: a review of corneal tattooing. Cornea. 1999;18: 633-7.
3. Van der Velden-Samdeerubun EM, Kok JH. Dermatography as a modern treatment for colouring leukoma corneae. Cornea. 1994;13:349-53.
4. Ziegler S. Multicolor tattooing of the cornea. Trans Am Ophthalmol Soc. 1922; 20:71-87.
5. Roy JN. Tattooing of the Cornea. The Canadian Medical Association Journal. 1938;436-8.
6. Kobayashi A, Sugiyama K. In vivo confocal microscopy in a patient with keratopigmentation (corneal tattooing). Cornea 2005;24:238-40.
7. De Weeker: Chirurg. Oculair., Paris, 1879, 181; Ocular Therapeut. trans. by Forbes, London, 1879, 147; Archiv. f. Augenheilk., ii, 1872, 84; Annal. d'Oeulist., August, 1897, 88 (As quoted by Ziegler S. Reference 4).
8. Pomier: Union Medicale, T. ix, 27, March, 1870, 363 (As quoted by Ziegler S. Reference 4).
9. Dunnage: Med. Times and Gaz., 1872, i, 294 (As quoted by Ziegler S. Reference 4).
10. Taylor: Brit. Med. Jour., 1872, 271; Amer. Jour. Med. Sci., 1872, 561 (As quoted by Ziegler S. Reference 4).
11. Woinow: Bericht. d. Gesel. Russ. Aerz., Moscow, 1872, No. 13 (As quoted by Ziegler S. Reference 4).
12. Hasner: Beitrag Z, Physiol U, Pathol D. Aug., 1873, 80 (As quoted by Ziegler S. Reference 4).
13. Archer: Arch F. Ophthal., xx, i, 1874, 225 (As quoted by Ziegler S. Reference 4).
14. Levis: Phila. Med. Times, Oct., 1872, 4 (As quoted by Ziegler S. Reference 4).
15. Williams: Boston Med. and Surg. Jour., July, 1873, 4 (As quoted by Ziegler S. Reference 4).
16. Thomson: Trans. Amer. Oph. Soc., 1873, 86 (As quoted by Ziegler S. Reference 4).
17. Mathewson: NY Med. Ree., 1874, 590 (As quoted by Ziegler S. Reference 4).
18. Vacher: Societ6 franqaise d'Ophtal., 1887, 248 (As quoted by Ziegler S. Reference 4).
19. Nieden: Bericht. Ophthal. Gesel., Heidelberg, 1901, 252 (As quoted by Ziegler S. Reference 4).
20. Cofler: Annali di Ottalmol., Pavia, 1902, fase. 3, 4, 5, 169 (As quoted by Ziegler S. Reference 4).
21. Holth: Soc. de medecin de Christiania, 1898, Fordhandlinger, 430; Annal. d'Oeulist., Nov., 1903, 333; Internat. Oph. Cong., Lucerne, 1904; B. 289; Soc. franq. d'Ophtal., 1906, 343 (As quoted by Ziegler S. Reference 4).
22. Chevallereau and Polack: Societe franqaise d'Ophtal., 1906, 331 (As quoted by Ziegler S. Reference 4).
23. Armaignae: Recueil d'Ophtal., August, 1903, 463 (As quoted by Ziegler S. Reference 4).
24. Czermak: Die Augen. Operat., 1896, 649 (As quoted by Ziegler S. Reference 4).

Pigments Selection

2

According to Ziegler, pigments should be chosen that are mineral in origin, indelible, easily sterilizable, non-irritating to the cornea, opaque to luminous light, and miscible in water but not soluble. When choosing colors for keratopigmentation, mineral colors are more permanent than vegetable colors when applied to human tissues, but it is obvious that irritating pigments, like the chromes, cadmium, cobalt, and gamboge, should not be employed.[1]

PIGMENTS TO AVOID

There are pigments that should not be used, such as chromes, cadmium, cobalt and gamboge. Chemical excipients, such as solutions of oxycyanid or bichlorid of mercury, should be omitted where there is danger of their forming troublesome chemical compounds when mixed with the pigments.[1]

STERILIZATION

Hamilton[2] has demonstrated the presence of a capsule bacillus in Chinese inks, and therefore sterilization is emphasized. This is difficult with the stick form, as it melts into great lumps in moist heat and cracks and hardens in dry heat so that it cannot be grated into a powder.[1]

The finely powdered French pigments can better stand sterihization in a dry sterihizer raised to 150°C, without undergoing change of color or consistency, and should not irritate the cornea when introduced.[1]

COLOR OF THE PIGMENT

Similarly, the pigments must be opaque enough to obscure a corneal scar or to intercept light rays in albinos in the presence of coloboma or keratoconus, and should not irritate the cornea when applied.[1]

As previously mentioned, the dye should match the iris color or be slightly darker, as it is possible that a pigment dispersion occurs following its injection into the corneal tissue —(a) by extrusion of the pigment due to the inflammation caused by chemical irritation; (b) by a slow migration of the pigment particles, and (c) by partial disolution.[(1)]

LOCALIZATION OF THE PIGMENT

According to Browicz,[3] Hirschberg[4] and Poncet,[5] the pigmentary deposits form irregular or fusiform clumps in the cells, vessels and interfibrillar spaces and lymphatic vessels, and typically penetrate deeper layers of the epithelium and the corneal stroma. Alt,[6] Parsons[7] and Terrien,[8] among others authors, confirmed these observations.

CHEMICAL COMPOSITION OF THE PIGMENTS

In order to make a graphic presentation of the palette of pigments, their chemical composition and the combinations required to yield the desired shade of iris color, Ziegler prepared the tables (Tables 2.1 and 2.2).[1]

Ziegler described that Naples Yellow is more useful than zinc white pigment to correct a corneal defect, because it can cover the error in a better way, by covering over or obscuring an irregular tattooing in darker color. He also noted that green earth is less stable than the other pigments, but can be very useful when mixed properly with most colors. When added to the brown tints, it often gives them a most natural appearance. Meanwhile red ochre, like cinnabar, can be mixed with ivory black to obtain any shade of brown.[(1)]

METALLIC AND NONMETALLIC PIGMENTS

Although it has been reported that metallic chemical tattoo is not as stable as the nonmetallic impregnation method, it has some important advantages: the technique is fast, simple, and provides better jet black color to recreate the pupil.[9-11]

In a metal ultrastructural corneal tattoo Olander et al. demonstrated the existence of extracellular and intracellular granules 10 years after the tattoo with platinum chloride.[10]

Sekundo observed that in all cases the granules were located in the keratocytes, in contrast to what happens in the metal tattoo where the granules were in the extracellular space.

Ultrastructural Study

Regarding skin tattoo, it has been observed that not only macrophages but also fibroblasts are capable of pigment endocytosis. Skin tattoos traditionally rely on nonmetallic

Table 2.1: Pigment composition[1]

Pigment (Spanish)	*Pigment (English)*	*Pigment (French)*	*Chemical composition*
Amarillo Nápoles	Naples yellow	Le Jaune de Naples	Calcined lead carbonate, biantimoniato potassium, ammonium chloride and dried alum
Verde tierra	Green earth	La Terre Verte	Copper carbonate hydrate with hydrated salts of aluminum, iron and manganese
Azul ultramarino	Ultramarine blue	Le Bleu d'Outremer	Sulfur, sodium and aluminum silicate
Marrón ocre Rojo ocre	Brown ochre Red ochre	L'Ocre Brun L'Ocre Rouge	Clay-containing iron and manganese oxides
Tierra de sombra natural	Raw umber	La Terre d'Ombre Naturelle	Clay-containing silicon, aluminum, iron and manganese oxide
Tierra de sombra tostada	Burnt umber	La Terre d'Ombre Brule'e	Scorched burnt umber, as described above.
Negro marfil	Ivory black	Le Noir d'Ivoire	Black calcined bone

Table 2.2: Iris color tones and required pigments[1]

Color tone	*Pigments required*
Yellow	Naples yellow
Light green or greenish blue	Green earth
Light blue	Ultramarine blue + Naples yellow
Dark blue	Ultramarine blue
Light brown or yellow	Brown ochre
Yellow brown	Brown ochre + green earth
Red brown	Red ochre
Brown	Raw umber
Greenish brown	Raw umber + green earth
Dark brown	Burnt umber
Very dark brown	Burnt umber or red ochre + Ivory black
Black (pupil)	Ivory black or Indian ink

colors[12-14] and the pattern and color of skin tattoos macroscopically remain unchanged throughout the life of the treated patient.

Lea and Pawlowski attributed these characteristics to the prominent connective tissue elements surrounding the fibroblasts containing the pigment particles.[13] However, even under proper fixation conditions, it has been described that the cornea tattooed with platinum (metallic tattoo) does not developed a membrane around the pigment particles.[10]

Apart from the location, another clear difference between the granules of metal and nonmetal tattoo was the ultrastructural appearance. Sekundo et al. reported intracellular dark granules (black) and light granules (gray) with sharp angled edges in all cases of nonmetallic tattoo. Instead, Olander et al. observed extracellular round black granules with partially indifferent edges in metallic tattoo. The absence of extracellular particles in Sekundo's cases suggested that endocytosis of organic substances is more permanent and stable than metal material endocytosis by human corneal fibroblasts.[1,10,15]

Although in Sekundo's research it is unclear whether these cells can migrate from the stroma as a result of a longstanding bullous keratopathy or can migrate from the corneal limbus as a result of a previous corneal disease, the interesting fact is that keratocytes may retain particles incorporated by endocytosis as they migrate through the corneal tissue.

Experimentally, this problem was addressed by Fujita et al. who showed that rabbits corneal fibroblasts can incorporate injected Indian ink particles by endocytosis within 3 to 4 days and keep them for at least 6 months. In Sekundo's study these results were confirmed in human corneas for a significantly longer period of time (up to 61 years). To explain this phenomenon, Fujita suggested that phagocytosis is a reaction of corneal fibroblasts, to protect the cornea from foreign materials injury or damage.[16]

Assuming that metallic pigments are more toxic than organic substances, it is expected an increased cellular degradation and subsequent more cellular debris are retained in the extracellular matrix of the cornea. Therefore, it is not surprising that the probability of extracellular granules is higher in metallic than in nonmetallic tattoos.[15]

In summary, the nonmetallic tattoo differs from metal tattoo, not only in the variable appearance of the particles, but also in the particles location, being exclusively intracellular even after many decades in nonmetallic cases. Keratocytes clean and control the extracellular matrix due to the ingestion and retention of the colored organic material (nonmetallic granules) over a long period of time.[15]

MICRONIZED MINERAL PIGMENTS

Micronized mineral pigments have an additional advantage over other natural pigments, because its particle size is reduced by processes of micronization. As small particles, 2.5 microns or smaller, the chance of developing a foreign body reaction against the pigment introduced into the corneal stroma, is much lower than with bigger particles.[17-20]

Another important advantage of micronized mineral pigments is the wide range of colors available. This is very convenient in keratopigmentation because the main goal is to accurately mimic the color of the patient's eye to get the best possible cosmetic result. The mixture of different pigments to achieve the desired color can make keratopigmentation a very laborious and time consuming process. However, micronized mineral pigments can be previously mixed and prepared and then properly sterilized, reducing the operating time.[17-20]

REFERENCES

1. Ziegler S. Multicolor tattooing of the cornea. Trans Am Ophthalmol Soc.1922;20: 71-87.
2. Hamilton: Centralbl. F. Bakt. U. Parasit., 1898. iv, ii, 6 (As quoted by Ziegler S; Reference 1).
3. Browiez: Arch f. Ophthal, 1877, iii, 212 (As quoted by Ziegler S; Reference 1).
4. Hirschberg: Arch f. Ophthal, 1882, 269 (As quoted by Ziegler S; Reference 1).
5. Poncet: Gaz. des Hop., No. 28,1876,210. (As quoted by Ziegler S; Reference 1).
6. Alt: Amer. Jour. Ophthal., April, 1884, 8 (As quoted by Ziegler S; Reference 1).
7. Parsons: Pathol. of the Eye, 1904, i, 253 (As quoted by Ziegler S; Reference 1).
8. Terrien: Chirurg. de l'Oeil, 1902, 45: 1921, 51 (As quoted by Ziegler S; Reference 1).
9. Duke-Elder S, Leigh AG (1965). System of ophthalmology. In Disease of the outer eye, part 2. St Louis, CV Mosby.
10. Olander K, Kanai A, Kaufman HE An analytical electron microscopic study of a corneal tattoo. Ann Ophthalmol. 1983;15:1046-9.
11. Anastas CN, McGhee CN, Webber SK, Bryce IG. Corneal tattooing revisited: excimer laser in the treatment of unsightly leucomata. Aust N Z J Ophthalmol. 1995;23:227-30.
12. Christensen HE, Schmidt H. The ultrastructure of tattoo marks. Acta Pathol Microbiol Scand A. 1972;80: 573-6.
13. Lea PJ, Pawlowski A. Human tattoo. Electron microscopic assessment of epidermis, epidermal-dermal junction, and dermis. Int J Dermatol. 1987;26:453-8.
14. Fujita H, Nishii Y, Yamashita K, Kawamata S, Yoshikawa K. The uptake and long-term storage of India ink particles and latex beads by fibroblasts in the dermis and subcutis of mice, with special regard to the non-inflammatory defense reaction by fibroblasts. Arch Histol Cytol. 1988;51:285-94.
15. Sekundo W, Seifert P, Seitz B, Loeffler KU. Long-term ultrastructural changes in human corneas after tattooing with non-metallic substances. Br J Ophthalmol. 1999;83: 219-24.
16. Fujita H, Ueda A, Nishida T, Otori T. Uptake of india ink particles and latex beads by corneal fibroblasts. Cell Tissue Res. 1987;250:251-5.
17. Alió JL, Rodríguez AE, Toffaha BT, et al. Femtosecond-assisted keratopigmentation for functional and cosmetic restoration in essential iris atrophy. J Cataract Refract Surg. 2011;37:1744-7.
18. Alió JL, Rodríguez AE, Toffaha BT, et al. Keratopigmentation (corneal tattooing) for the management of visual disabilities of the eye related to iris defects. Br J Ophthalmol. 2011; 95:1397-1401.
19. Alió JL, Rodríguez AE, Toffaha BT, et al. Femtosecond-assisted keratopigmentation double tunnel technique in the management of a case of Urrets-Zavalia Syndrome. Cornea. 2012; 31:1071-74.
20. Sirerol B, Walewska-Szafran A, Alió JL, et al. Tolerance and biocompatibility of micronized black pigment for keratopigmentation simulated pupil reconstruction. Cornea. 2011;30: 344 50.

Corneal Tolerance and Biocompatibility to Micronized Mineral Pigments

3

Several studies have demonstrated the biocompatibility and corneal tolerance of micronized inorganic pigments for keratopigmentation. Those experiments and studies are going to be discussed in this chapter.

FIRST EXPERIMENTAL STUDY USING MICRONIZED MINERAL PIGMENTS

In the Figures 3.1A to D, histopathological findings of the first keratopigmentation experiment using micronized mineral pigments are illustrated. The aim of this study was to determine the tolerance and toxicity of micronized mineral pigments, using a black color obtained from iron oxide, and brown Leghorn hens as the *in vivo* experimental model. No signs of corneal toxicity were found in this experiment, which suggests that this type of pigment is a valid alternative for corneal tattooing.[1]

Hematoxylin-eosin staining was applied to analyze the histological sections using the standard protocol of this staining, and histology was performed using the Nikon Eclipse E400 microscope.

The results after a 3 months follow-up are described below:

- The corneal epithelium was intact, no ulcers, erosions or edema was observed. No hyperplasia or atrophy were found, keeping the normal thickness of the epithelium

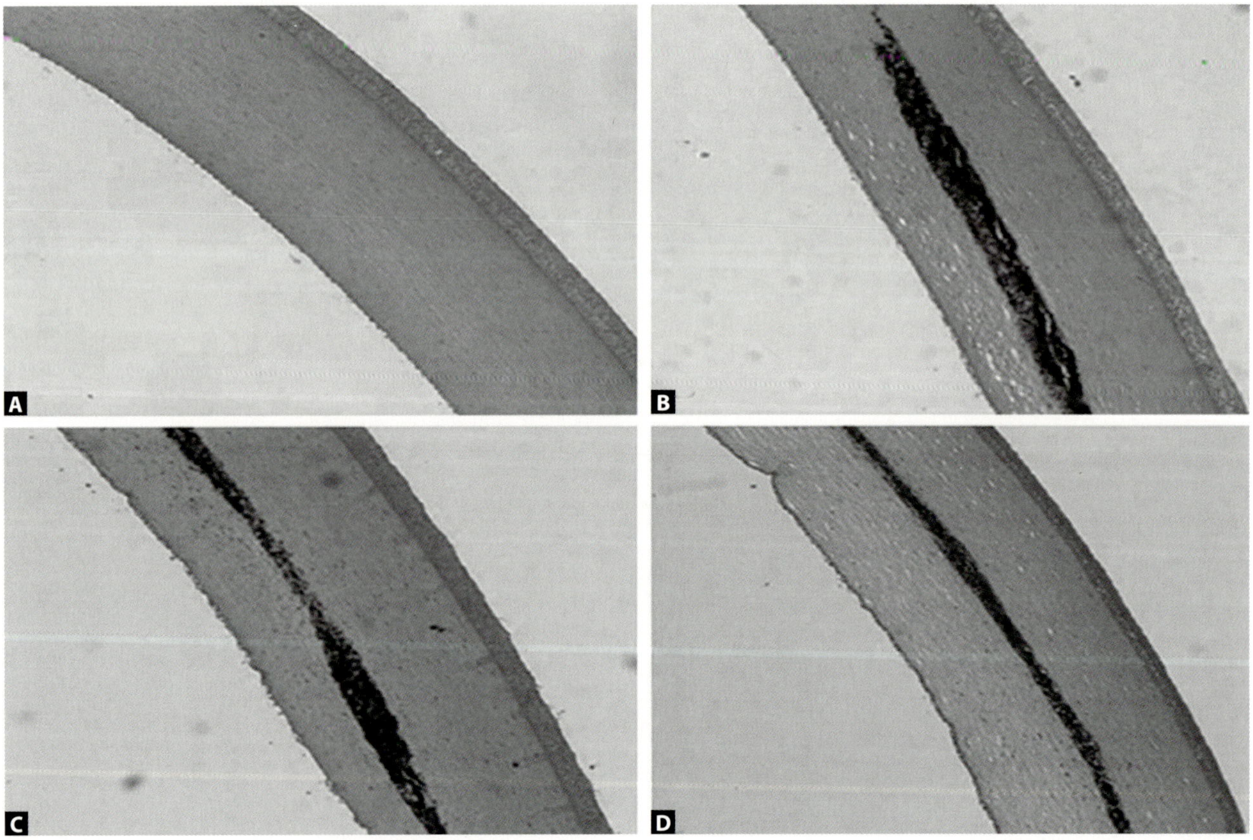

Figs 3.1A to D: Histopathological results. (A) Control eye; (B) Pigmented eye with no signs of inflammation or neovascularization after 1 month; (C) One of the cases with minimal inflammation; (D) Absence of inflammatory cells or neovascularization 3 months after surge[1]

(3–5 cells). Bowman's membrane was not examined because rabbits do not have this structure despite the great similarity with the human cornea (Figures 3.2 to 3.4).

- Keratocytes around the pigment were activated, they were larger and many keratocytes adopted a starry appearance. The cytoplasm was eosinophilic. The cell nucleus was discreetly bigger but with increased cromasia without visible or very small nucleolus. The existence of small pigmented fine granules were found inside the cytoplasm of many corneal keratocytes that were nearby the pigmented area (Figure 3.5).
- The corneal stroma in both, pigmented eyes and controls, showed no signs of stromal scarring or fibrosis. Collagen fibers maintained their undulating shape and not exaggerated adhesion between these fibers were found. The predominant type I collagen was demonstrated by immunohistochemical staining, follow-up by type III. The extracellular stromal matrix was intact, and in the middle portion of the corneal stroma was evident a linear presence of pigment in all tattooed eyes. The cohesiveness of the pigment was demonstrated, although in some areas, dense pigmented clusters were found, not affecting

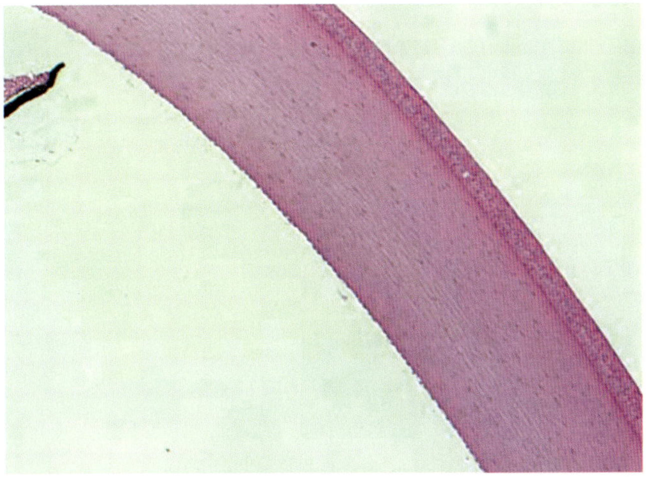

Fig. 3.2: Control. No inflammatory cells or neovascularization changes are observed in the stroma

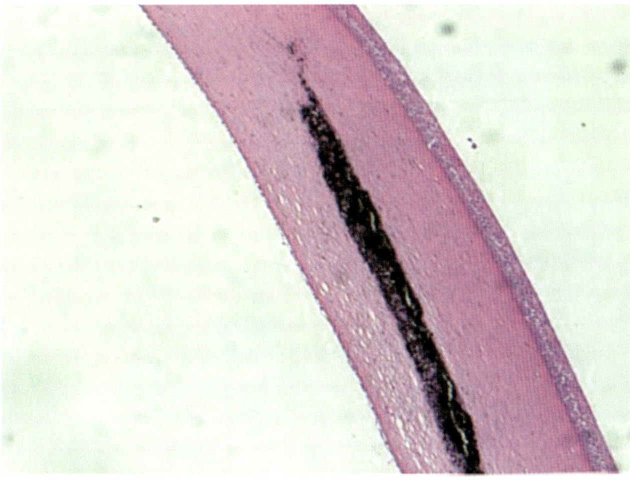

Fig. 3.4: Retained pigment 3 months after keratopigmentation. No inflammation or neovascularization associated

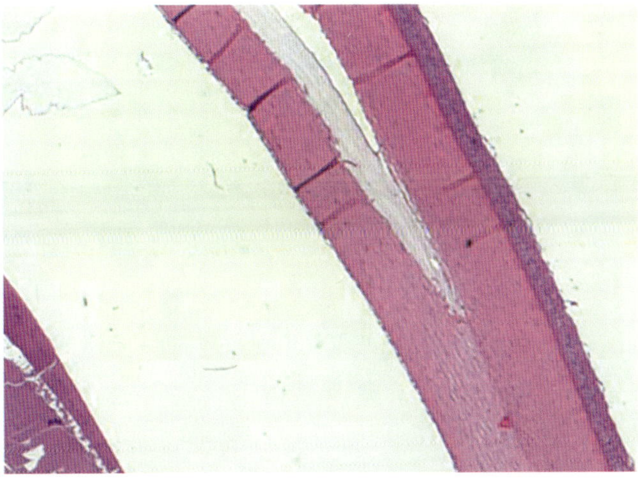

Fig. 3.3: No inflammation was observed. The epithelium and endothelium are unaffected

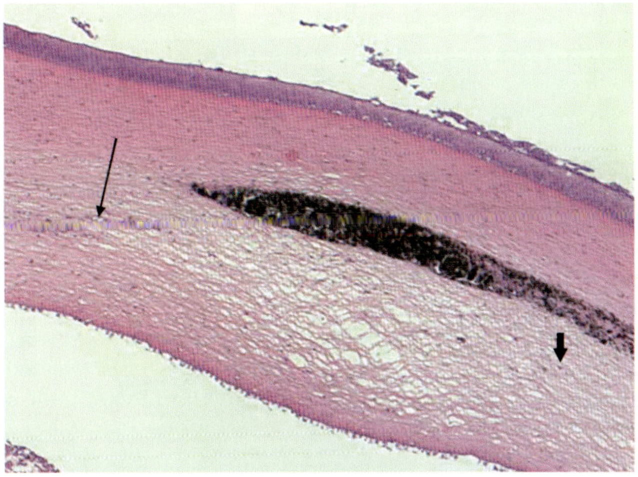

Fig. 3.5: Mild lymphocytic infiltrate present in the stroma (long arrow). Activated keratocytes with larger nuclei (short arrow)

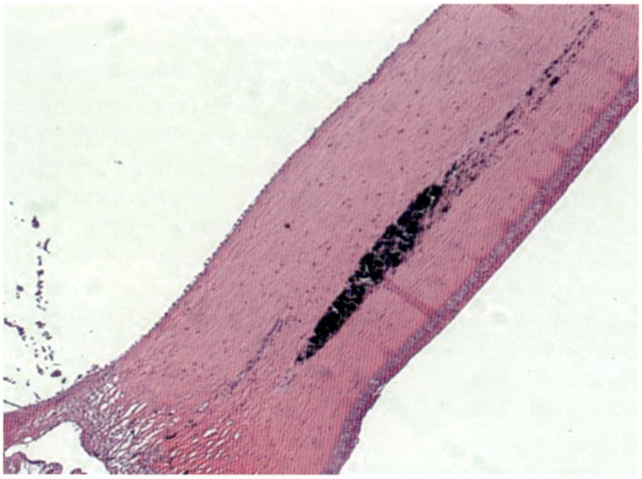

Fig. 3.6: The pigment remains 3 months after surgery, and in some areas dense clusters dominate and in others areas the pigment is thinner and less abundant. However, no pigment dispersion is identified

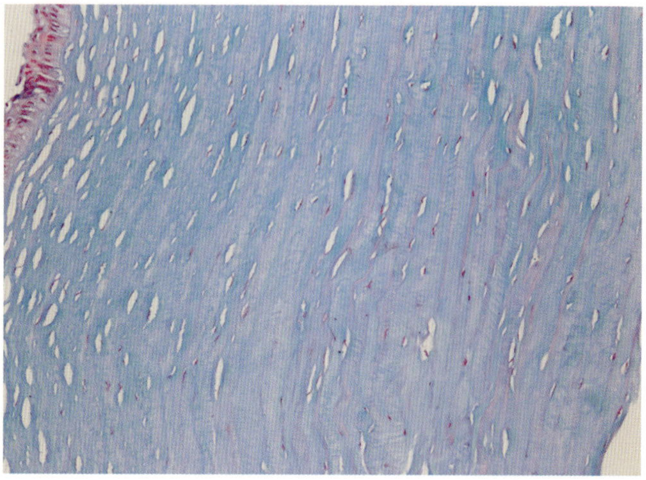

Fig. 3.8: Alcian blue staining. Stromal matrix remains unchanged

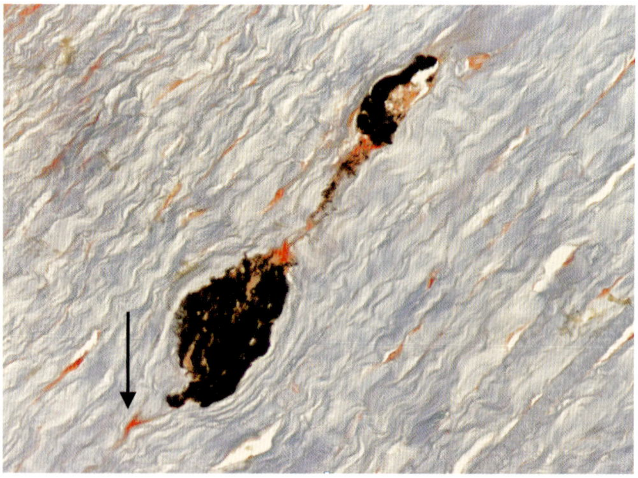

Fig. 3.7: Masson trichrome staining. The pigment remains within the stroma, without dispersion but in clusters of variable size. Activated keratocytes (arrow) and some neuronal cells are recognized around the pigmented area

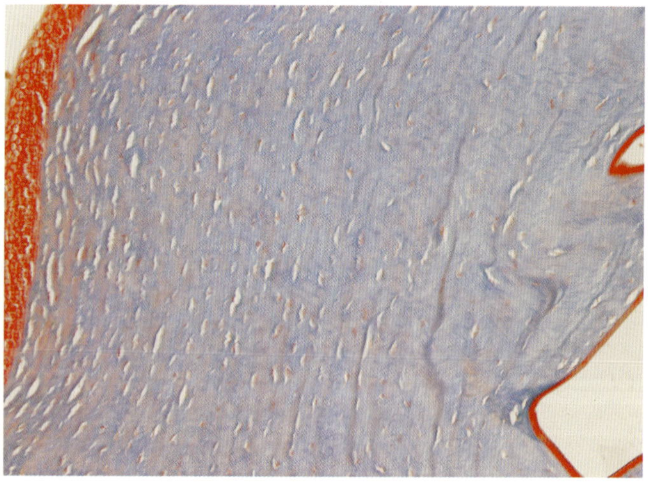

Fig. 3.9: Masson trichrome stain. No abnormalities are observed in the stromal collagen

the cosmetic appearance. The edges of the pigmented areas were clear without dispersion (Figures 3.6 to 3.11).

- The peripheral corneal nerves were in perfect condition, maintaining corneal sensitivity and achieving a quicker recovery after the surgery. The pockets eyes (treated but not pigmented) also maintain the biomechanical properties of the peripheral cornea which provides greater stability.
- No histological abnormalities were found in endothelial layers of all animals, tattooed and controls. No changes were identified in Decement's membrane in any eye examined.

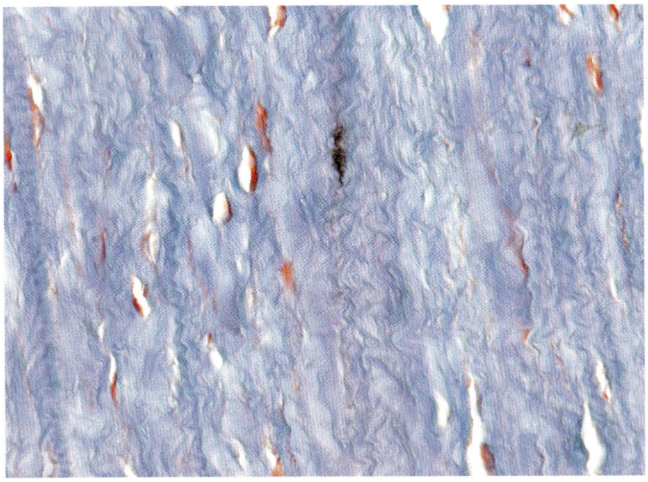

Fig. 3.10: Masson trichrome stain. Note the wavy arrangement of collagen fibers. Activated keratinocytes are identified

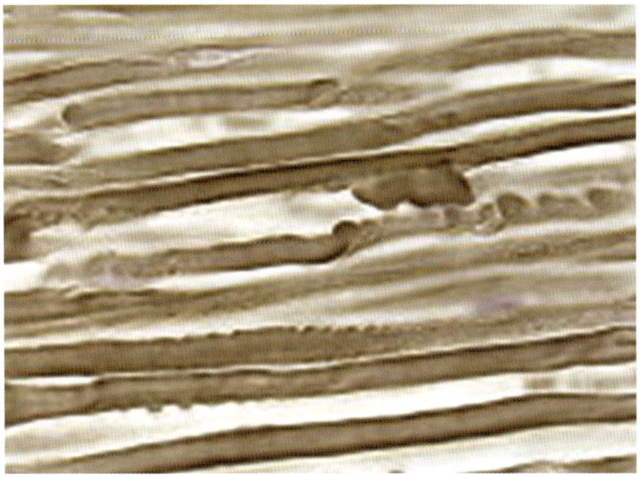

Fig. 3.11: Immunohistochemical staining with anticollagen I, predominant in the corneal stroma

FIRST CLINICAL STUDY USING MINERAL PIGMENTS

The aim of this study was to investigate keratopigmentation with micronized mineral pigments as a surgical alternative to improve cosmetic appearance in severely impaired eyes.

Forty eyes underwent keratopigmentation alternatively to invasive cosmetic reconstructive surgery. Corneal staining with mineral micronized pigments was performed using an intralamellar or superficial technique.

One year postoperatively, all but two patients (95%) were satisfied. Pigmented eyes were improving patient's appearance. Eight cases needed a second keratopigmentation. Two patients with preoperative corneal edema did not obtain an adequate cosmetic appearance due to progressive pigment clearance observed from 6 months postoperatively. Three eyes with traumatic aniridia observed good cosmetic outcome and a significant reduction in glare.

In 95% of cases of keratopigmentation, a brownish-black color was used and a bluish-green color for 5% of the cases. Pupil diameters were different, 4 mm being the most frequent (Figures 12A to I). In 10 cases of keratopigmentation by ICS, it was performed in two consecutive stages (retattooing) to adjust the cosmetic results to the needs of the case and the patient's expectations.

Pre- and postoperatory pictures of patients from this study are shown, where the biocompatibility and stability of these pigments are demonstrated.

Figures 3.13A and B show pre- and postoperative appearances of selected patients.

Figures 3.14A and B show pre- and 1-year postoperative images of a 65-year-old male patient affected by multiple retinal detachments resulting in complete blindness corneal leucoma and strabismus. Severe restrictions to ocular motility prevented an adequate alienation of the axial axis. For partial iris reconstruction, three different pigments were used to mimic the appearance of the LE.

Figure 3.15A shows a 55-year-old patient with total aniridia and aphakia due to ocular trauma before anterior segment reconstruction including a sulcus-sutured intraocular lens. To more accurately match the bluish color of the LE, initially, the pigmentation for iris reconstruction was performed using only blue pigment (Figure 3.15B) and completed with a secondary pigmentation of the LE (Figure 3.15 C).

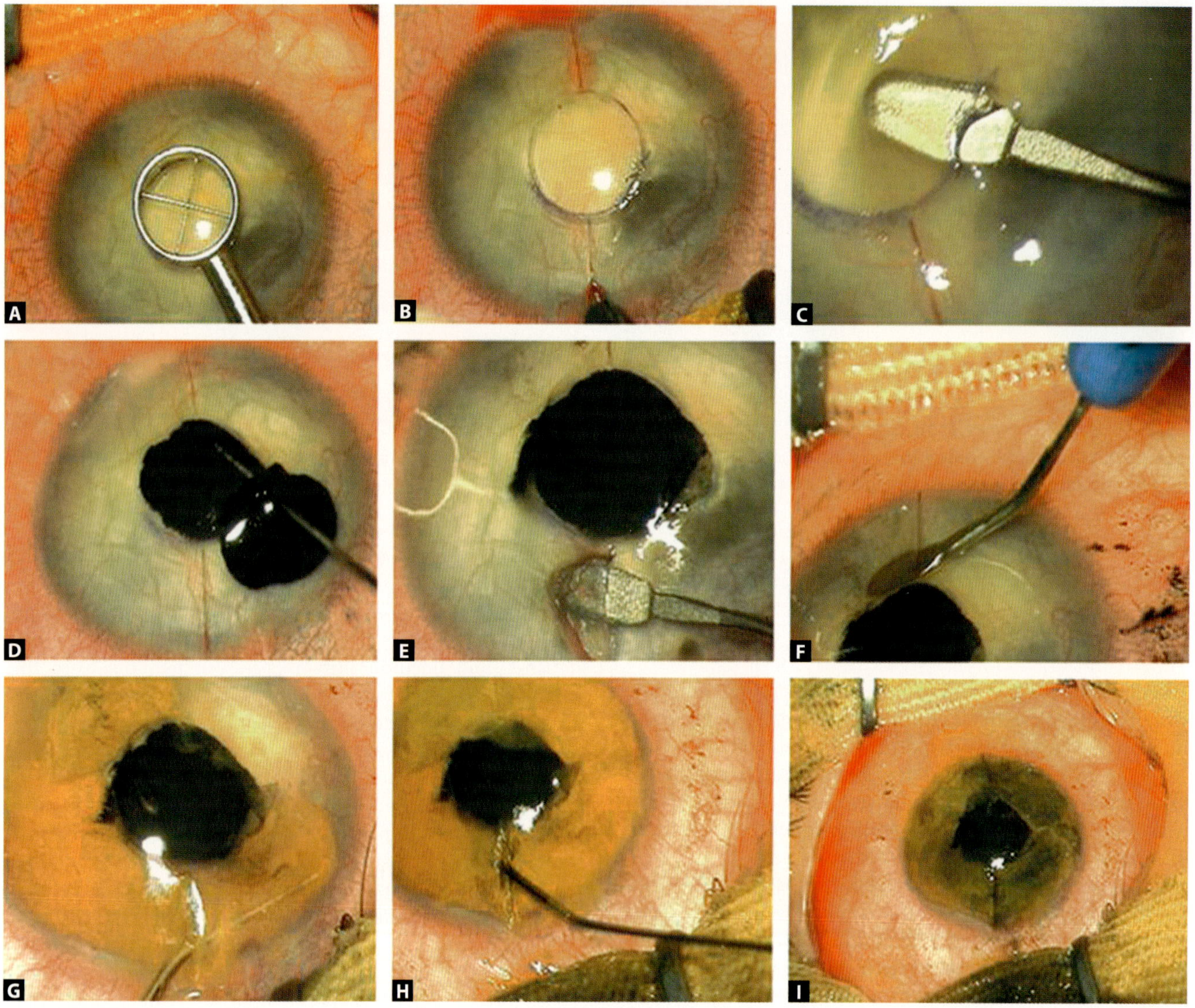

Figs 3.12A to I: Intralamellar corneal staining (ICS). (A) Pupil diameter of 4 mm previously estimated following the low mesopic pupil and marked with an RK optic marker; (B) 3–4 incisions with a prephased diamond ring of 1 mm; (C) Cornea dissected intralamellary with a microcrescent knife (Sharpoint); (D) Pupil stained with the adequate dark color (0.1 cm^3) with a 30-gauge cannula; (E) Dissection of peripheral cornea top side; (F) Dissection of peripheral cornea bottom side; (G) Coloring peripheral cornea in an irregular format to recreate better the iris crests; (H) Mixing black and yellow-brown colors to give the right color for the fellow eye; (I) Final result of the corneal tattooing

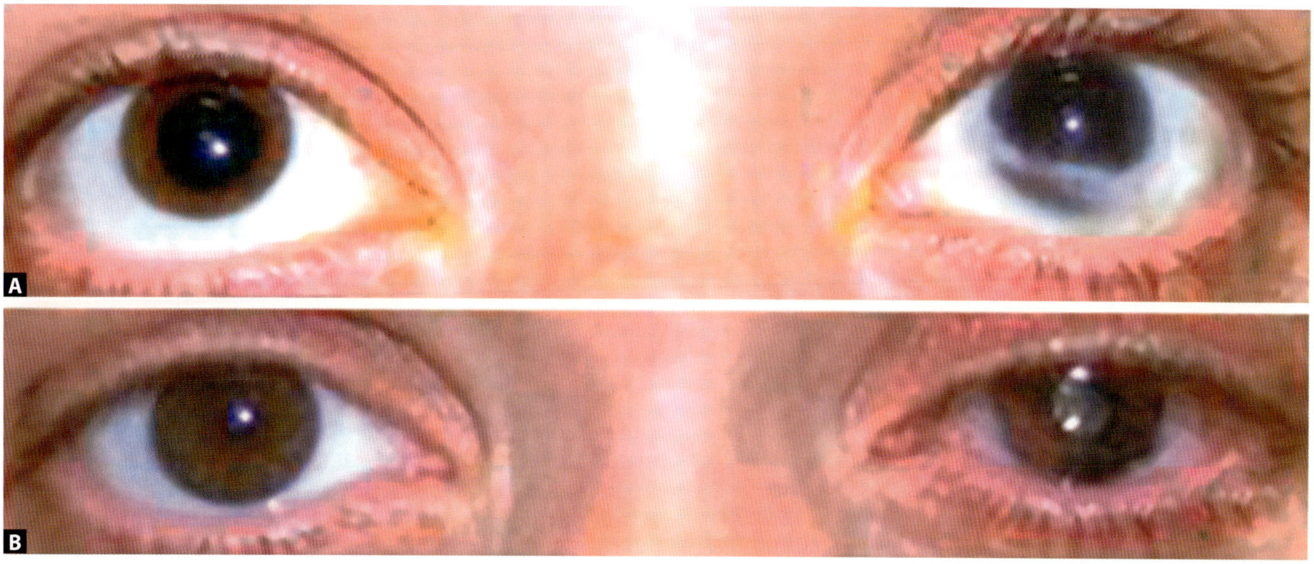

Figs 3.13A and B: (A) Preoperative appearance of the left eye (LE); (B) Results 1 year after iris appearance reconstruction and pupil simulation

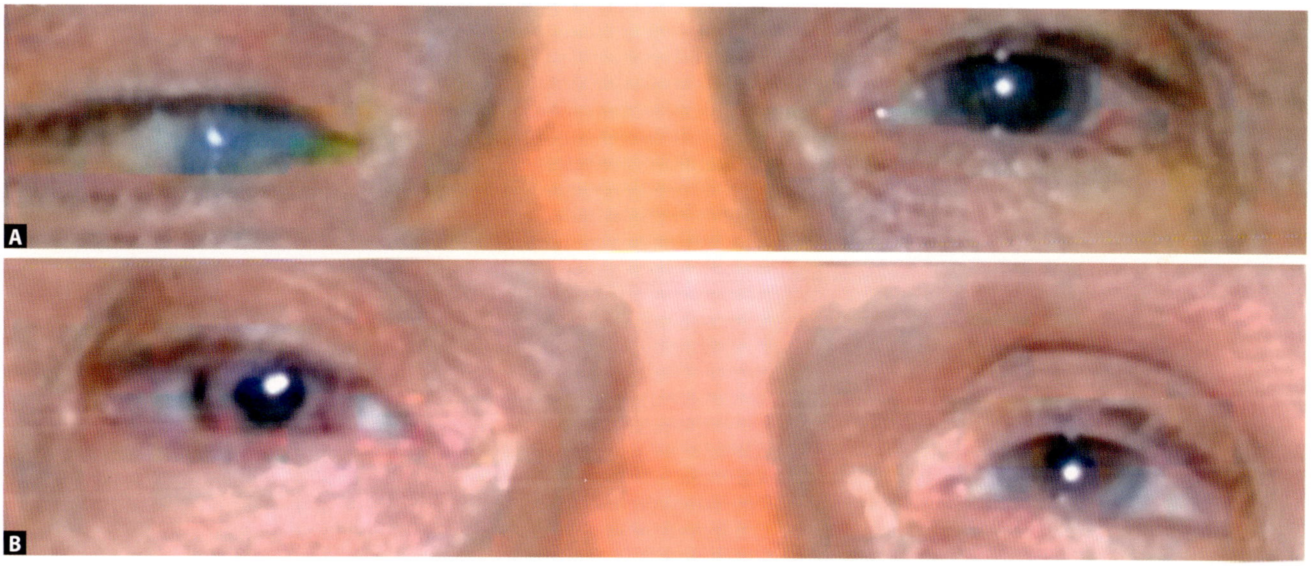

Figs 3.14A and B: (A) Preoperative aspect of a patient with partial iris atrophy; (B) Appearance of the patient 1 year after sectoral iris simulation

A 44-year-old female patient with a history of childhood ocular trauma leading to partial iris atrophy (Figure 3.16A underwent corneal KTP for sectoral iris simulation. Figure 3.16B shows the appearance of the patient 1 year after surgery.

There were no cases of inflammatory reactions or side effects associated with keratopigmentation procedures such as pain, foreign-body reaction, corneal de-epithelization or color loss throughout this study, which demonstrate the good corneal tolerance and biocompatibility of these pigments for their use in human corneas[2] (Figure 3.17).

In summary, the use of micronized mineral pigments for corneal tattooing, could be considered as an alternative for

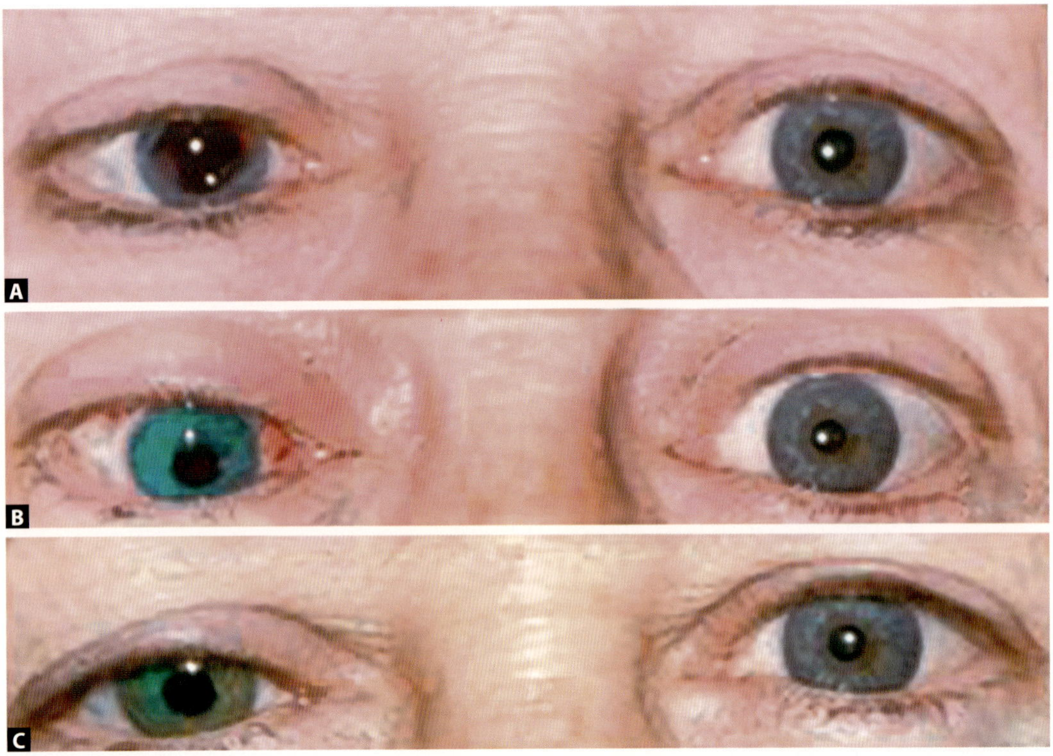

Figs 3.15A to C: Pre- and postoperative appearances of selected patients. (A) Preoperative appearance before anterior segment reconstruction including a sulcus-sutured intraocular lens; (B) First pigmentation using only blue pigment; (C) Second pigmentation to better match the appearance of the LE

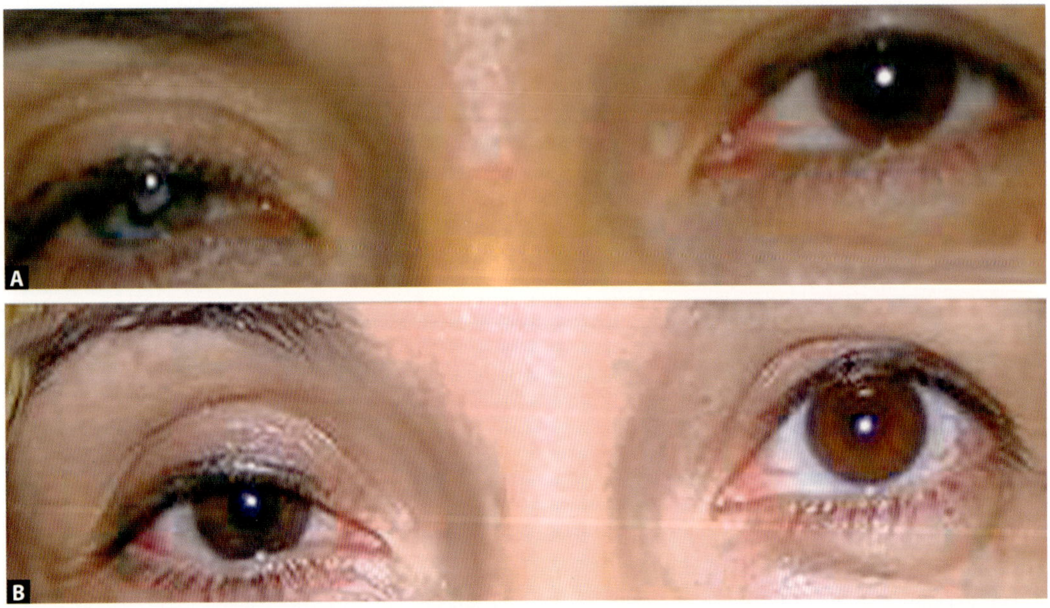

Figs 3.16A and B: Pre- and postoperative appearances of selected patients. (A) Preoperative aspect of patient with corneal leucoma and strabismus; (B) Results 1 year after strabismus surgery and partial iris reconstruction and color simulation in LE

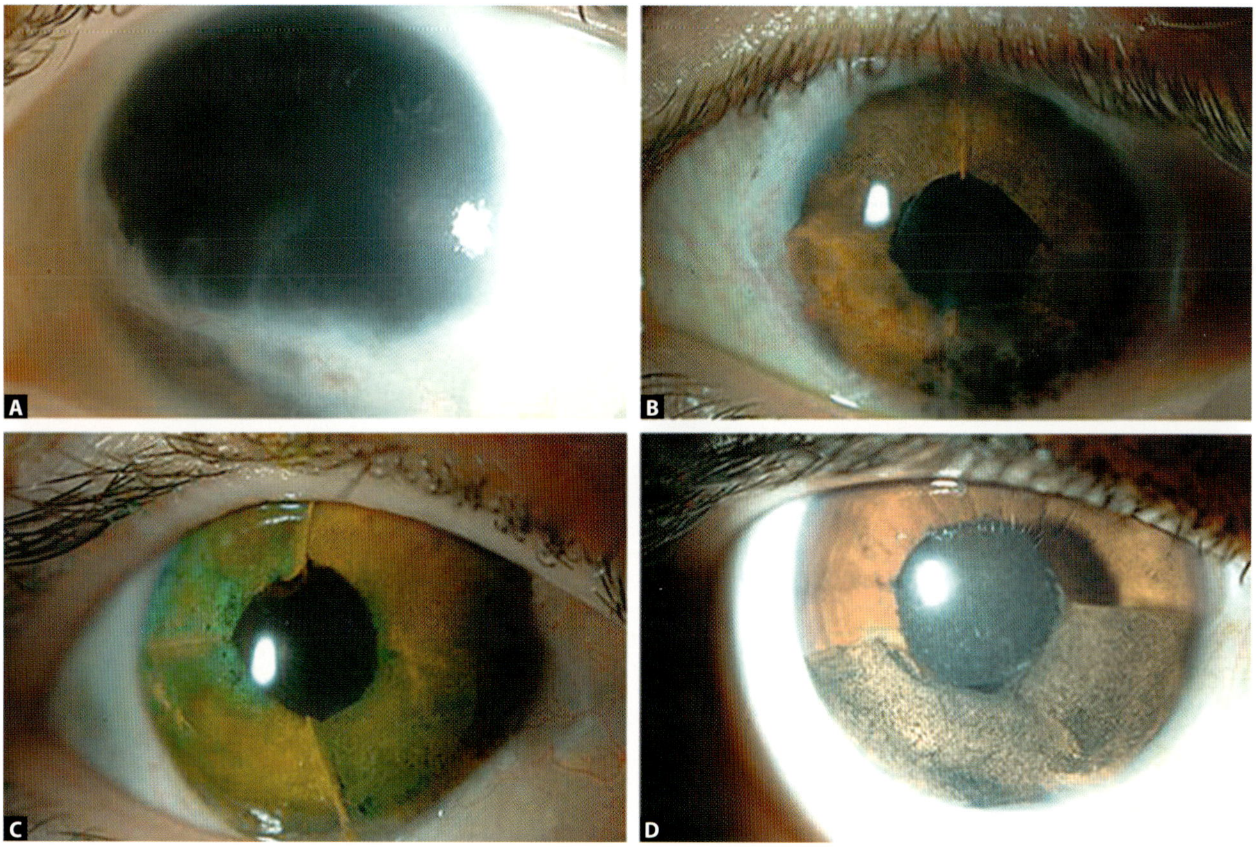

Figs 3.17A to D: Pre- and postoperative slit-lamp examination of selected patients. (A) Aspect of LE of the patient under a slit-lamp before keratopigmentation; (B) Slit-lamp image of the cosmetic result achieved in LE of the patient 1 year after corneal pigmentation; (C) Detail of the sectoral iris simulation of the patient as seen with slit-lamp; (D) Slit-lamp detail of the sectoral iris simulation of the patient

patients in whom evisceration, enucleation, prosthesis and orbital implants would otherwise be used to improve their cosmetic appearance. Corneal tattooing can be a procedure for long-term or permanent correction of cosmetic eye deformities in patients who have cosmetically disabling corneal scars.[2]

We can conclude that keratopigmentation achieves stable and satisfactory cosmetic results, with high patient satisfaction, to treat corneal scars and aniridias.

According to these results, keratopigmentation is a safe surgical procedure that is easy to learn and perform, does not require expensive materials and avoids more extensive and invasive reconstructive ocular procedures. Further investigations are necessary for a better understanding of the long-term biological effects in keratopigmented corneas.

OTHER EXPERIMENTS USING MICRONIZED MINERAL PIGMENTS IN RABBITS

The aim of the study was to determine the tolerance and biocompatibility of micronized mineral pigments for corneal cosmetic pigmentation in an experimental model.[3]

Corneal intralamellar keratopigmentation was performed in 28 New Zealand white rabbits using micronized mineral pigments. Prophylactic actions using intraoperative antibiotic prophylaxis and gamma radiation of the pigment mixtures were performed to avoid infection. Animals were examined regularly by slit-lamp to detect any sign of inflammation, pigment diffusion, color changes or neovascularization. Histopathological examination was performed to determine the level of pigment diffusion, the level of inflammation and the presence of neovascularization.[3]

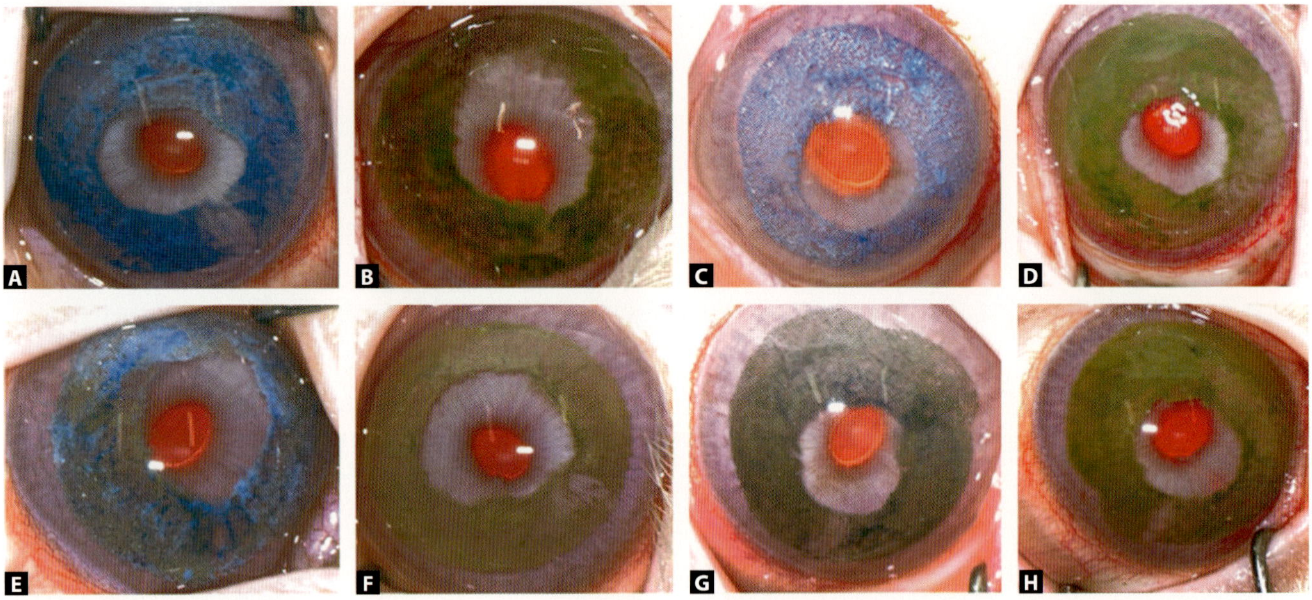

Figs 3.18A to H: Two months after the surgery. (A and C) blue pigment, (B and D) green pigment, (E and G) blue mixed with brown, (F and H) green mixed with brown[3]

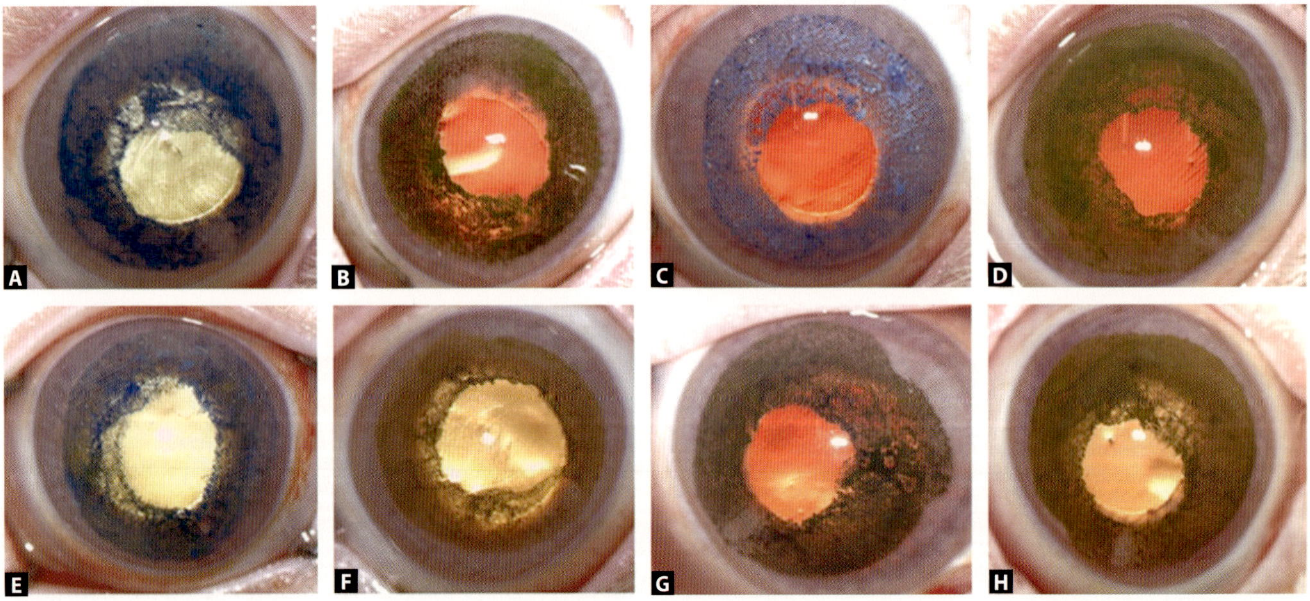

Figs 3.19: Three months after the surgery. (A and C) blue pigment, (B and D) green pigment, (E and G) blue mixed with brown, (F and H) green mixed with brown[3]

No pigment diffusion or changes in color, inflammation or neovascularization were detected in the eyes treated (Figures 3.18 and 3.19). Histopathological examination corroborated clinical results regarding inflammation. Pigmented corneas showed a good cosmetic appearance without signs of ocular toxicity.[3]

CONCLUSION

After all these studies we have concluded that micronized mineral pigments could be a valid alternative treatment for cosmetic keratopigmentation. Intralamellar keratopigmentacion technique presented good cosmetic appearance without adverse effects in the eyes treated.[1-3]

REFERENCES

1. Sirerol B, Walewska-Szafran A, Alió JL, et al. Tolerance and biocompatibility of micronized black pigment for keratopigmentation simulated pupil reconstruction. Cornea. 2011;30:344-50.
2. Alió JL, Sirerol B, Walewska-Szafran A, Miranda M. Corneal tattooing (keratopigmentation) to restore cosmetic appearance in severely impaired eyes with new mineral micronized pigments. Br J Ophthalmol. 2010;94:245-9.
3. Amesty MA, Alio JL, Rodriguez A. Corneal tolerance to micronized mineral pigments for keratopigmentation. Br J Ophthalmol. 2014;98:1756-60.

Instruments Required for Keratopigmentation

4

For any operation, including corneal tattooing, the appropriate instruments must be available. If instruments are not available, or are blunt, or do not function properly, it may be necessary to delay or postpone surgery. Using such instruments in an operation can result in a poor outcome, or even pose a risk to surgeons and their assistants. The impact is therefore considerable.[1]

Making sure surgical instruments are in good working order requires the following:

- Purchasing high-quality instruments, as these are likely to be more robust and will last longer. The companies supplying them are also more likely to offer service warranties.[1]
- Cleaning the instruments carefully after each operation, checking them to make sure they are still in good working order, packing them carefully, and sterilizing them using appropriate methods.[1]
- Checking that everyone working in the operating theater and sterilization areas knows how to handle instruments carefully. If sterilization is centralized, those used to handling the large, robust instruments used in general surgery, orthopedics, or obstetrics will have to be trained in handling ophthalmic instruments, which are small and delicate with fine points or very short blades.[1]

INSTRUMENTS USED FOR KERATOPIGMENTATION

Ancient Needles Used for Tattooing

There were several instruments used for corneal tattooing, for example, Wecker's tattoo grooved needle, or the needles designed by Agnew or Taylor.[2]

Wecker abandoned his single-grooved needle (Figure 4.1) for Taylor's bundle of needles (Figure 4.2) with two, five or eight needles together, which since then were called Wecker's needles. Meanwhile, Ziegler preferred to use only two needles. On the other end of the handle was placed Wecker's metal spatulla, which is useful both in mixing the color paste and in applying it to the cornea. Agnew preferred four long needles set tandem (Figure 4.3).[3,4]

Tyson[5] has improved on this technic by using shorter needles set in a solid matrix, so as to avoid perforation of the cornea. Thomson utilized for this purpose the "Gillott's Crow-Quill Lithographic Pen." He turned it upside down, so as to hold the ink in reserve for the complete tattooing, like a fountain pen, and mixed his pigment with glycerin. Borsch,[6] who was formerly Wecker's chief of clinic, rightly states that only a single needle should be used to perform the most delicate work, such as optical tattooing for diffuse nebulse, outlining the iris circle, or making separated pricks for the iris stroma.[3]

Other Historical Instruments

Electric Tattooing Needle

Ziegler designed an electric tattooing needle, which has been made from a dental mallet, and therefore, has sufficient force to drive the pigment through the corneal epithelium. The Edison Electric Pen, or Neostyle, utilized to perforate a sheet of paper to be used as a die for mimeographing, was no longer on the market by that time, but the few examples that Ziegler, examined have demonstrated their adaptability for the purpose of electric tattooing.[3]

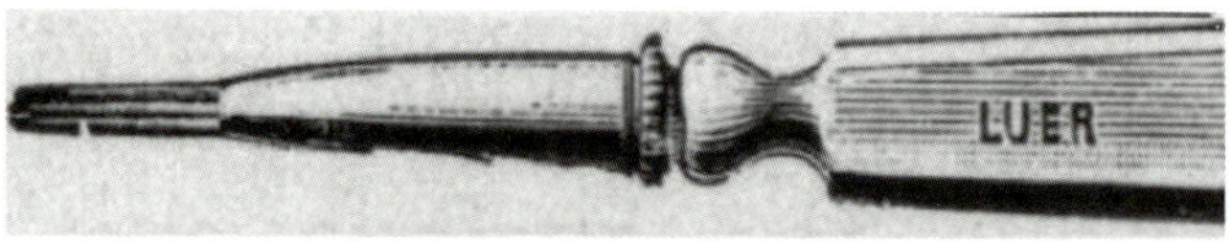

Fig. 4.2: Taylor's bundle of needles

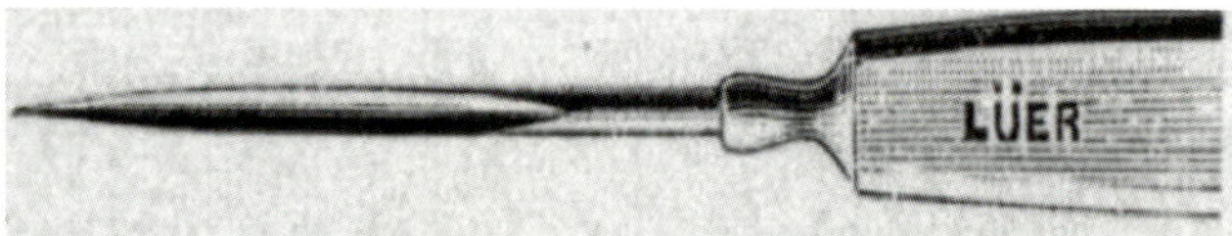

Fig. 4.1: Wecker's single-grooved needle

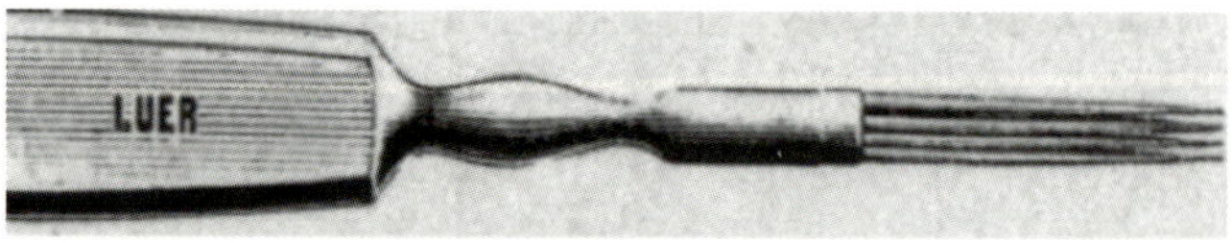

Fig. 4.3: Agnew's needle set

Toothed Curets

The toothed curets of Skeel or Ziegler were used to carry out the technic of Czermak[7] or Holth,[8] both of whom removed the surface epithelium from the pupillary area. Oblique scarification or cross-hatching with a knife accomplished a similar purpose. Frohlich sliced off the superficial corneal layer with a keratome or cataract knife, but Holth claimed that the color of the exposed cicatricial tissue modified the pupillary black to a bluish shade.[8,9]

Ziegler's Limbal Fixation Ring

Fixation forceps cannot be used, since the grasp of the teeth would be immediately filled with pigment. Smooth-bladed epilation forceps may be utilized to grasp the superior rectus and thus steady the eye. But Ziegler preferred to use his limbal fixation ring of 11 mm (Figure 4.4), which was divided into quadrants attached to a pupillary ring of 3.5 mm. Its edges were sharp enough to keep the globe from rotating, and at the same time cut into the cornea like a trephine, and so outline both the pupil and the peripheral iris circle. It was possible to confine the pigment to a single quadrant and thus work expeditiously and efficiently. In a large surface to be tattooed, it will be wiser to limit our tinting to only one quadrant at each seance.[3]

Corneal and Pupillary Trephines

If a corneal trephine is preferred, the mechanical one of von Hippel or Mackay can be used, but the hand trephine of Ziegler or Elliot is quite sufficient.

The pupillary trephine can be introduced through Ziegler's fixation ring if desired. The double trephine of Barck can also be used to outline the pupillary and iris circle. Either of these methods will yield an accurately centered pupil, which is so necessary.[3]

INSTRUMENTS CURRENTLY USED FOR CORNEAL TATTOOING

Intralamellar Corneal Staining (ICS)

Some of the instruments that are going to be mentioned are shown in Figure 4.5. The center of the cornea should be marked with a calliper and the pupil size diameter determined by an RK optic zone marker of 3, 3.5, 4 or 4.5 mm (Katena, New York, USA). Free hand incisions could be performed using a diamond blade or another corneal blade from the limbus to the border of the marked pupil to match the low mesopic pupil diameter of the healthy eye, estimated with a Holladay gauge or an infrared pupillometer of 4 mm (Procyon, Bausch & Lomb Surgical, Rochester, New York, USA).[10-13]

From radial incisions, the cornea is dissected intralamellarly and circularly with a microcrescent knife (Sharpoint, Surgical Specialties Corporation, Reading, PA; USA). Three or four incisions are usually necessary and the dissection is made until the dissector reached the nearest incision on both sides. Finally, the whole cornea is dissected from the periphery to the corneal pupil. The adequate color is injected through the tunnel created using a 30 gauge cannula on a 1 ml syringe. For keratopigmentation itself no stitches are required.[10-13]

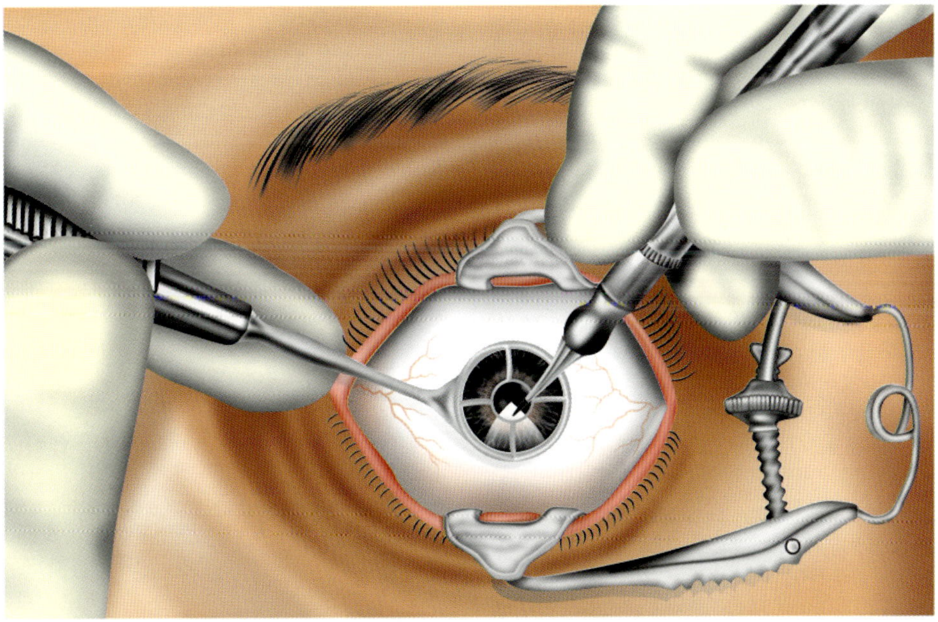

Fig. 4.4: Ziegler's fixation ring and Nieden's pen[3]

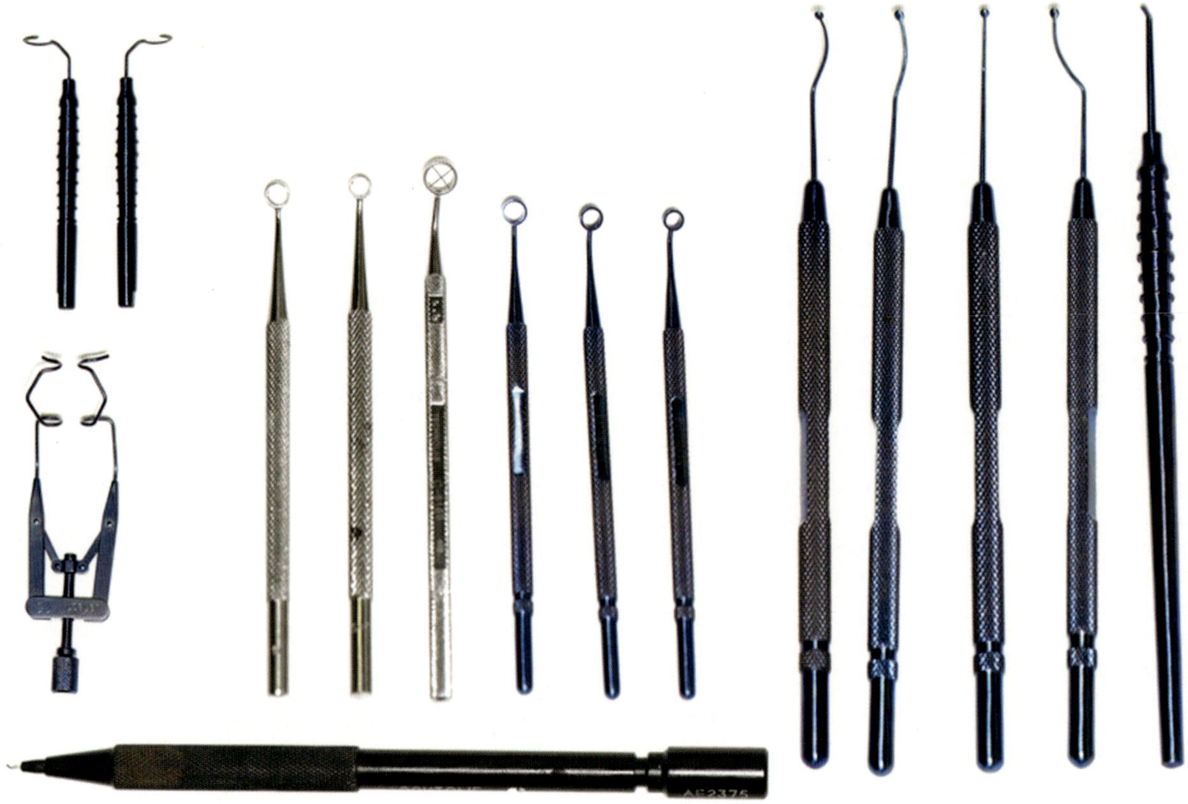

Fig. 4.5: Instruments used for corneal tattooing

To create the intralamellar tunnel, a pigtail or helical dissector (pigtail or spiral corneal dissector CPK, Epsilon, Irvine CA, USA) can also be used because it facilitates the creation of the tunnel requiring just one radial incision and avoiding unnecessary extra incisions. This instrument dissects intrastromally and circumferentially along the route of the pupil margin 180° clockwise and 180° counterclockwise, leaving the pupillary area intact.

The instruments seen in Figure 4.5 are the most commonly used for intralamellar keratopigmentation. In this picture, we can observe some of them: titanium corneal markers (Ø 3.0 mm, Ø 3.5 mm, Ø 4.0 mm), titanium helicoidal tunnel corneal dissector right and titanium helicoidal tunnel corneal dissector left, some titanium pupil creator corneal dissectors (straight, right and left), a titanium flat corneal dissector (90°), a titanium speculum, another three steel pupil markers and one 400 µ sapphire blade.

Superficial Corneal Staining (SCS)

For this type of keratopigmentation, the instruments required to measure the pupil size are mentioned previously. Then, a drop of the adequate stain is placed on the corneal surface, and then micropunctures are performed down to the superficial layers of the stroma using a 30-gauge needle. The maneuver is repeated, until the adequate amount of pigment is introduced into the superficial cornea to achieve an acceptable cosmetic appearance.[10-13]

Femtosecond-assisted Keratopigmentation (FAK)

Before the surgery, pachymetry and tomography are measured in different areas of the cornea by means of the time-domain Visante optical coherence tomography system (Carl Zeiss Meditec AG) to decide the appropriate lamellar depth for the femtosecond tunnels. Two types of surgeries can be performed, creating just one stromal tunnel or two stromal tunnels. A double layer technique with two stromal tunnels mimics the anatomy of the iris, where the light-colored pigment is applied to the superficial layer and the dark-colored pigment is applied to the deepest layer.[10-13]

Afterward, the white-to-white horizontal and vertical diameters are measured using callipers to determine the diameter of the lamellar dissection. Two intrastromal tunnels can be created using the 60-kHz femtosecond laser (IntraLase AMO, Irvine, CA). The deepest tunnel could be performed first at a 400 microns depth from the surface with an inner diameter of 6 mm and an outer diameter of 9.5 mm. The energy should be set at 2 mJ, with a vertical incision at 6 o' clock. A second superficial tunnel could be performed at 200 microns depth, with an inner diameter of 6 mm and an outer diameter of 9.5 mm. The energy should be set at 2 mJ with a vertical incision at 12 o' clock (Figure 4.6).[10-13]

A lamellar dissector (KTP corneal dissector, Epsilon; Irvine, CA) is required to open the intralamellar femtosecond tunnels from each one of the incisions. Then, the pigments are injected using a 30-gauge cannula into the deeper and superficial tunnels through the superior and inferior incisions (Figures 4.7 and 4.8).

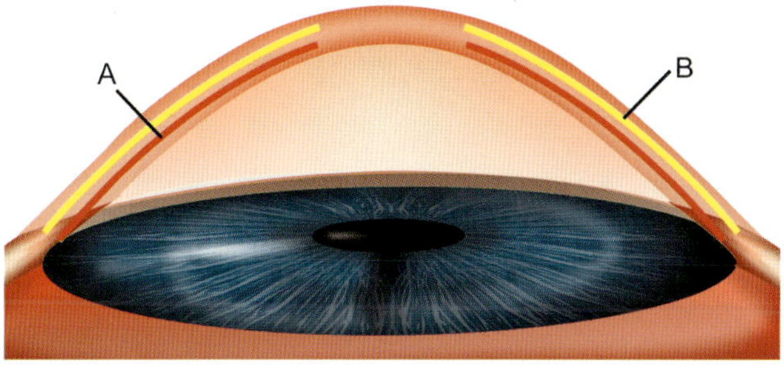

Fig. 4.6: A, The deep darker layer to absorb the light and prevent it from entering the eye and hence eliminating visual function symptoms. B, Superficial light-colored layer that matches the color of the contralateral eye and hence improving the cosmetic appearance of the patient

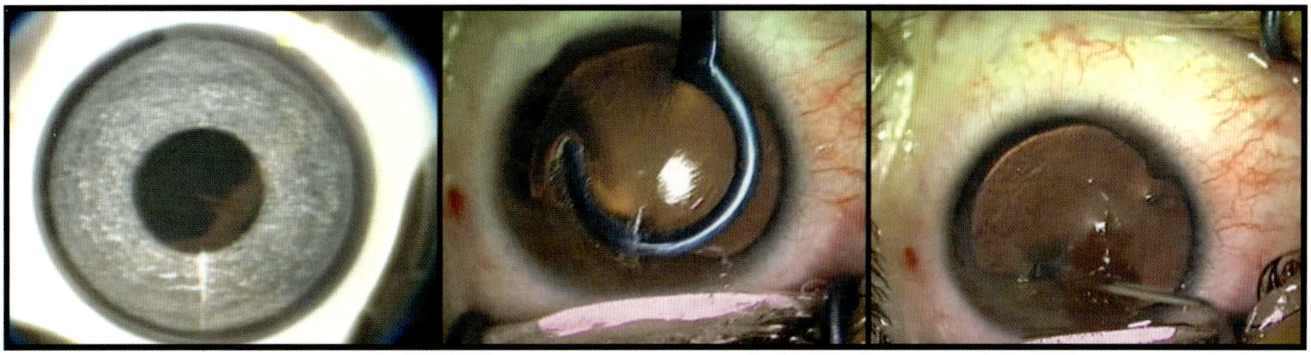

Fig. 4.7: Photographs using Intralase for femtosecond-assisted keratopigmentation (FAK)

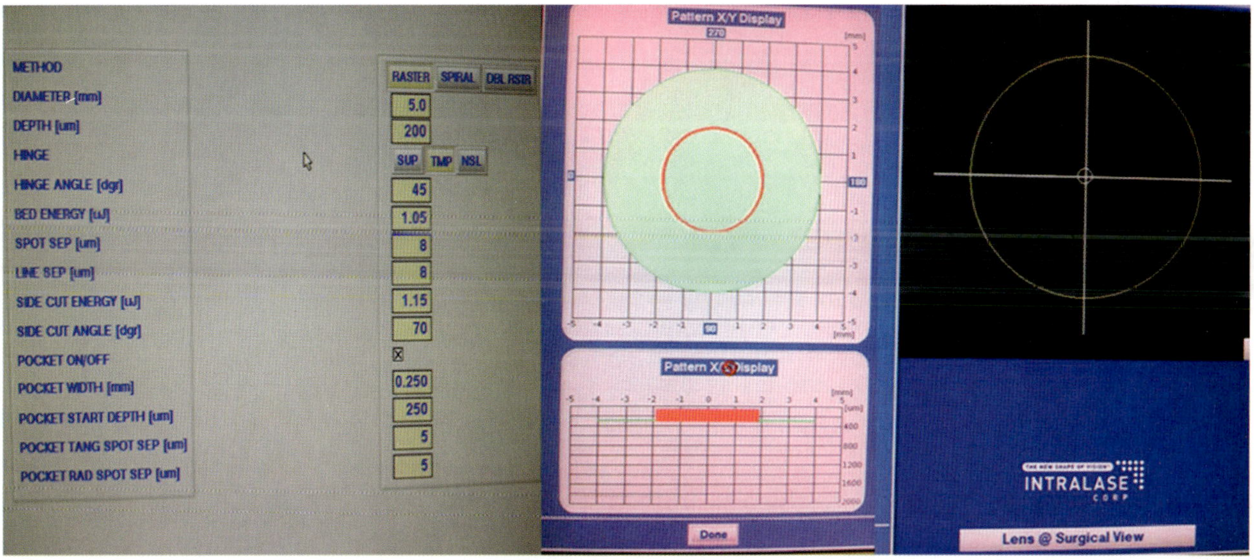

Fig. 4.8: Intralase for FAK

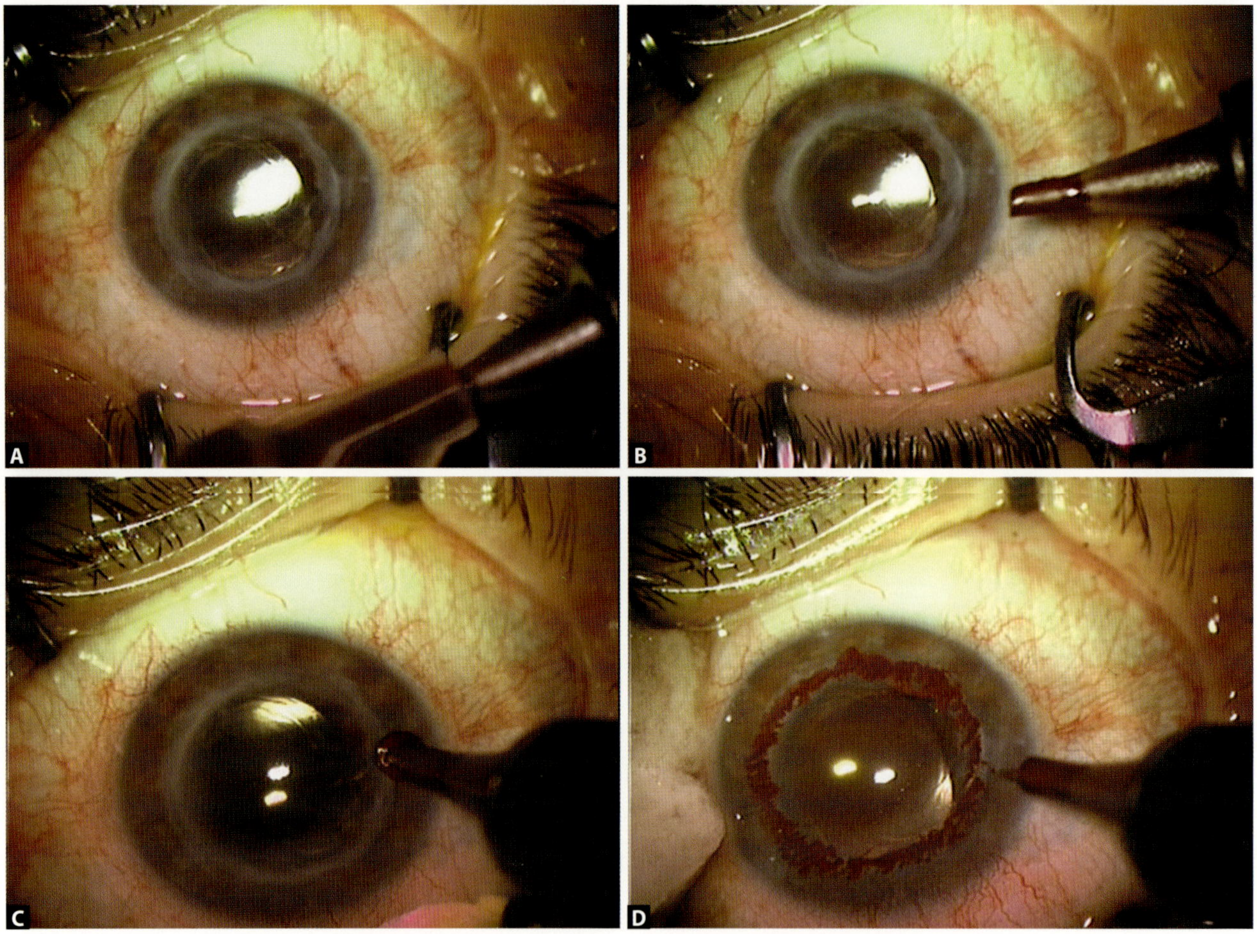

Figs 4.9A to D: Superficial automated keratopigmentation

Superficial Automated Keratopigmentation (SAK)

After FAK, the peripheral cornea could be treated in some areas with superficial automated keratopigmentation, to create an optimal cosmetic result (Figs 4.9A to D). The superficial automated keratopigmentation procedure is performed using a prototype of a punctural device (Vissum Eye MP System, Madrid, Spain; Apl. No.2.949.539). Automatic micropunctures are performed, puncturing the superficial layers of the stroma to an approximate depth of 120 microns from the corneal surface. The penetration depth of the needles is controlled by the length of the longitudinal axial vibration of the tip.[10-13]

If we compare the instruments used in the past for corneal tattooing and the instruments currently used, we can see the great improvement in the surgical technique since we have much more reliable advanced instruments that allow us to achieve better and more consistent keratopigmentation results.

REFERENCES

1. Patel D, Hoare P. Instruments for cataract surgery. Community Eye Health. 2011;24(76):26-9.
2. Taylor: Brit. Med. Jour., 1872, 271; Amer. Jour. Med. Sci., 1872, 561. (As quoted by Ziegler S. Reference 3)
3. Ziegler S. Multicolor Tattooing of the Cornea. Trans Am Ophthalmol Soc. 1922;20:71-87.
4. De Weeker: Chirurg. Oculair., Paris, 1879, 181; Ocular Therapeut. trans. by Forbes, London, 1879, 147; Archiv. f. Augenheilk., ii, 1872, 84; Annal. d'Oeulist., August, 1897, 88. (As quoted by Ziegler S. Reference 3).
5. Tyson N.Y. Med Rec, June 1894, 709. Wood's System of Ophthal. Operations, 1911:11,1002. (As quoted by Ziegler S. Reference 3).
6. Borsch: Ophthal. Rec., 1902, 476. (As quoted by Ziegler S. Reference 3).
7. Czermak: Die Augen. Operat., 1896, 649. (As quoted by Ziegler S. Reference 3).
8. Holth S. Revival of Galen's corneal staining with coppersulfate and tannine should be abandoned. Am J Ophthalmol. 1931;14: 378-9.

9. Frohlich: Klin. Monats. f. Augenheilk., 1897, 301. (As quoted by Ziegler S. Reference 3)
10. Alió JL, Rodríguez AE, Toffaha BT, et al. Femtosecond-assisted keratopigmentation for functional and cosmetic restoration in essential iris atrophy. J Cataract Refract Surg. 2011;37:1744-7.
11. Alió JL, Rodríguez AE, Toffaha BT, et al. Keratopigmentation (corneal tattooing) for the management of visual disabilities of the eye related to iris defects. Br J Ophthalmol. 2011;95:1397-401.
12. Alió JL, Rodríguez AE, Toffaha BT, et al. Femtosecond-assisted keratopigmentation double tunnel technique in the management of a case of Urrets-Zavalia syndrome. Cornea. 2012;31:1071-74.
13. Alió JL, Sirerol B, Walewska-Szafran A, Miranda M. Corneal tattooing (keratopigmentation) to restore cosmetic appearance in severely impaired eyes with new mineral micronized pigments. Br J Ophthalmol. 2010;94:245-9.

Ancient and Current Protocol for Surgical Keratopigmentation

5

The practice of corneal tattooing or keratopigmentation is by no means a new surgical technique. In fact, it was practiced in a very rudimentary way in ancient times and it was sporadically used to treat corneal opacities.[1,2]

Ziegler is considered the father of modern keratopigmentation and his contribution gave us the foundations to develop the current keratopigmentation protocols.

In this chapter, Ziegler's surgical protocol is going to be discussed and compare to the modern available protocols.

ANCIENT ZIEGLER'S SURGICAL PROTOCOL

It is important to have a protocol for keratopigmentation and follow certain steps to achieve good results. The steps for corneal tattooing are as follows:

Anesthesia

In the past, the anesthesia was achieved using hyoscine hypodermic injections and injections of morphine or novocaine.[3]

Asepsis

Ziegler recommended to maintain asepsis by irrigation, as it was done in the past, for other eye operations, using a sterile solution of boric acid.[3]

Color Pigments Selection

It is important to match as much as possible the color of the patient's healthy eye, so that should be studied in detail. The size of the pupil, the size and color of the circle of the iris, iris types of radiation, and the exact color of the iris stroma.[3]

In the past, the colors were mixed dry and they were preserved, in case it was necessary to use them for the other eye, to ensure that the colors were the same. The pupil size should also match and produce the same response to exposure to daylight than the healthy eye, and the pupil size should never exceed 3 to 4 mm; otherwise, it would seem that the eye with corneal tattoo is staring. The ivory black ends up being a "dead" black, while the Indian ink is slightly transparent, which could provide a more natural sheen to the surface. Ziegler used to prepare Indian ink in sterile syringes that a Parisian chemist named Guillaumin prepared for him.[3]

Inks Sterilization

Ziegler preferred using French powdered pigments and sterilization was performed using purifying resin, then rinsed with alcohol, ether and water to remove other impurities. The remaining powder was treated with ether, which produced fine powder grains separating the coarse grains of the fine grains. These fine grains were then decanted and dried over a sand bath, which left an impalpable powder. After all this work, the dust is sterilized and then mixed with sterile water. The sterilization was done using a dry steam sterilizer at 150°C. To mix the pigments, a porcelain dish and a small glass mortar was used. The flexible Wecker's metal spatula was often replaced by that glass mortar (Figure 5.1).[3]

In the case of Indian ink, Wecker and Ziegler used this ink as brick or rod (Figure 5.2). This brick was "sliced" with a sharp knife or "scratched" with a steel grater. Subsequently, it was sterilized and dried in an electrical sterilizer to a temperature of 1500°C, and then mixed into a slurry with sterile water on a porcelain plate with a metal spatula, or it was also mixed to make a paste and then sterilized in a steam sterilizer.[3]

It is possible to add a drop of glycerin to this paste. Occasionally, Ziegler preferred to soften the color moistening the end of its color swab in sterile water. The polychromatic pigments are generally used in a slimmer solution or layer than black, since the iris stroma does not need the opacity of the pupil area.[3]

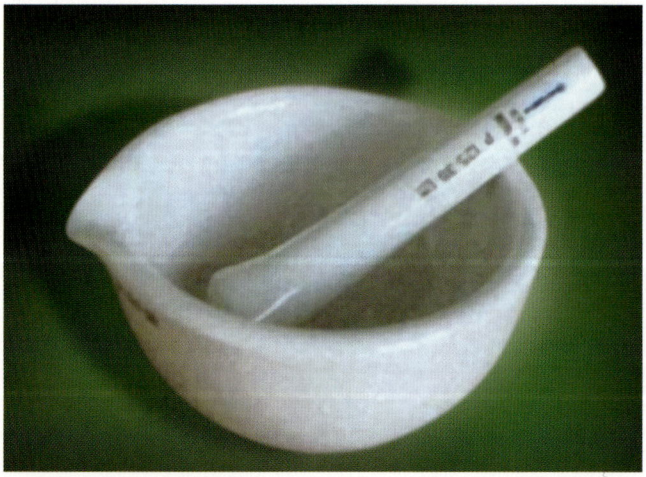

Fig. 5.1: Porcelain mortar

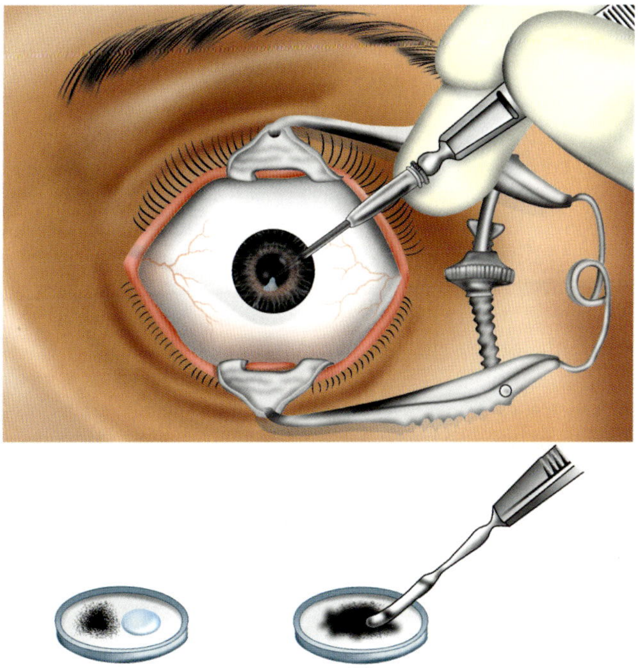

Fig. 5.2: Tattooing pupil. De Wecker's method using India ink (sliced or grated) with drop of water. Then mixing ink with spatula

ZIEGLER'S OPERATIVE TECHNIQUE

First Stage

Brilliant illumination is always necessary. Ziegler's speculum was used because it holds the eyelids away from the globe. Pressing the limbal fixation ring (Figure 5.3) against the cornea with the left hand, the trephine is lightly applied through the central ring to outline the pupillary area, after which the epithelial surface may be scarified or curetted. If preferred, the margin of the pupil can be outlined with the tattooing needle alone (Figure 5.3A).[3]

Second Stage

(a) Either the electric needle or the fountain pen (both of which carry their own ink) were used rapidly to cover the pupillary area; or (b) the pigment paste (black) was spread over the pupillary area by the metal spatula and the tattooing needle rapidly pricked through the paste into the leukomatous cornea, first vertically and then obliquely.[3]

When the corneal surface appears to be thoroughly covered and impregnated, it should be irrigated to see whether more pigment is needed. If some untinted spaces remain, the pigment paste should be rubbed in with the metal spatula, the needle-pricks repeated, and the surface irrigated as before.[3]

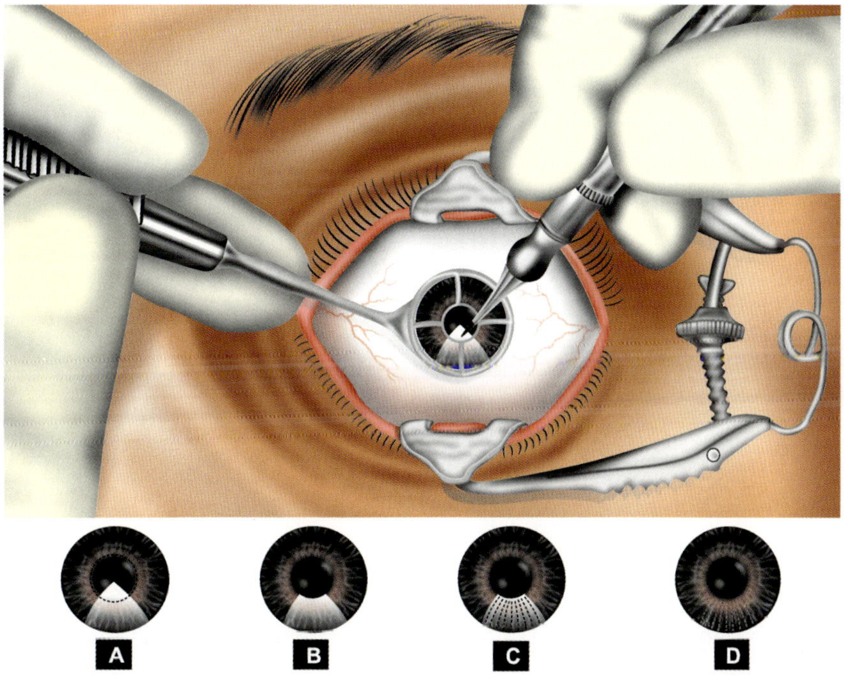

Figs 5.3A to D: Ziegler's fixation ring and Nieden's fountain pen. From left to right: (A) Margin of pupil outlined in black; (B) Iris circle in black. Pupil finished; (C) Iris radiations in black; (D) Iris stroma in color (Ziegler 1922)

If, when finished, the pupillary margin looks irregular, or a spur of pigment juts out, it should be covered or obscured by tinting the spur with Naples yellow. In optical tattooing, the single needle should always be held vertically, as oblique pricking may raise the epithelium. A moistened pledget of cotton should be placed at the inner canthus, to catch the tears or wipe off any displaced pigment.[3]

Third Stage

The peripheral iris circle (Figure 5.3B) was similarly treated with the proper shade of color, preferably black or brown; but a darker shade of the iris pigment may be indicated, since the appearance of the other eye should be closely imitated.[3]

Fourth Stage

The iris radiations (Figure 5.3C) were lightly stippled in with black, after which the proper shade of iris pigment was spread over the quadrant and tattooed (Figure 5.3D). This was allowed to dry or was fanned or the hot-air Phon turned on it for a minute or two. A transparent epicornea of celluloid, glass, or oiled silk (Figure 5.4) was laid over the tattooed surface, the eye was closed, and the dressing retained for twenty-four hours.[3]

After treatment Eserin or pilocarpine was instilled where a glaucomatous tendency is manifested or suspected. Ice pads should be promptly used in case of pain or inflammation. If a second tattooing is necessary, an interval of two weeks should be allowed to elapse.[3]

OTHER ASPECTS TO CONSIDER BEFORE CORNEAL TATTOOING

Good judgment will indicate that every contraindication shall be eliminated before tattooing is attempted.[3]

If there is chronic conjunctivitis, active treatment should be instituted. If the tear-duct is at fault, rapid dilatation should be performed at least two weeks in advance of tattooing. In adherent leukoma, synechiotomy or iridectomy should be performed. If the cornea is vascular, the leash of blood-vessels should be obliterated by touching them with the galvanocautery point and waiting until thorough cicatrization has taken place. Application of a pencil of carbon dioxide snow for two seconds will have a similar effect. Sometimes adrenalin is sufficient to accomplish temporarily this purpose, while the needle punctures and introduction of pigments tend to obliterate the vessels. As calcareous deposits are very disturbing, the curette and cautery should be resorted to. If the staphyloma is amenable to operation, it should be excised by keratectomy and the corneal wound allowed to harden for at least six months and possibly a year. The suggestion of Pontius to use adrenalin (1:1000) freely in order to strengthen and regenerate the weakened cornea has proved valuable in Ziegler's hands.[4] This is especially applicable in cases of acute staphyloma and keratoconus. In a phthisis bulbi that is quiet De Wecker's suggestion to cause "compensating exophthalmos" by dividing all the recti muscles sometime prior to the tattooing is worthy of consideration. Where the conjunctiva has contracted onto the cornea it is possible so to blanch it by adrenalin as to be able to outline the peripheral iris circle on the ischemic conjunctiva and thus more clearly imitate the normal eye.[3]

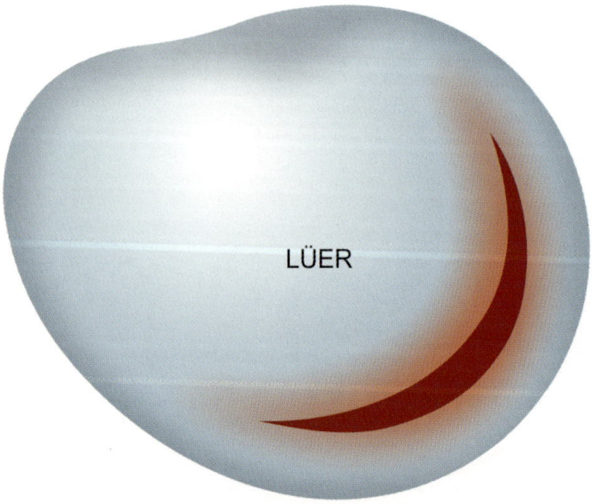

Fig. 5.4: Celluloid epicorneal dressing[3]

CURRENT TECHNIQUE AND PROTOCOL FOR INTRALAMELLAR OR INTRASTROMAL KERATOPIGMENTATION[5-10]

The procedure involve the following steps:

Anesthesia

Topical anesthesia is required to perform this type of surgery. Oxybuprocaine/tetracaine could be used for this purpose. It can also be performed under general, retrobulbar or peribulbar anesthesia.

If the procedure is performed in an animal model, systemic anethesia is also required, using an intramuscular injection of ketamine 40 mg/kg and xylazine 10 mg/kg.

Surgical Technique

Aseptic and antiseptic actions are performed using iodine solutions as in any invasive procedure.

Pupil is Marked

The center of the cornea is marked and a calliper is used to designed and delineated the pupillary margin. A RK optical zone marker of 5 mm can be used (Katena, New York, EEUU).

Incisions

One free hand radial incision to midstromal depth is performed with a 45° knife from the limbus to the border of

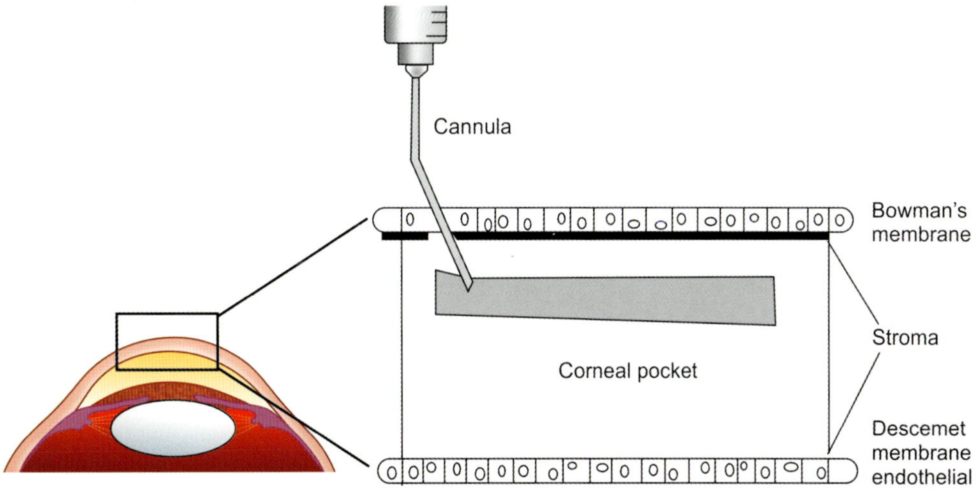

Fig. 5.5: Intrastromal keratopigmentation technique

the marked pupil at 12 O'clock (Sharpoint, Surgical Specialties Corporation, Reading, Pennsylvania, USA).

Intrastromal Tunnel

From the radial incision, the cornea is dissected intralamellarly in the same plane with a microcrescent knife (Sharpoint, Surgical Specialties Corporation, Reading, Pennsylvania; USA) and then with a helical dissector (pigtail or spiral corneal dissector CPK, Epsilon, Irvine California, USA) 180° clockwise and 180° counterclockwise intrastromally and circumferentially along the route of the pupil margin (leaving the pupillary area intact).

Pigment Injection

The desired color is injected inside the intrastromal tunnel with a 30-gauge irrigation cannula (Figure 5.5). Two or more different colors can be used to create a more natural iris color. Sometimes it is necessary to irrigate or wash out the tunnel with saline to remove some pigment if the color appears to be very dark compare to the other eye. No corneal sutures are required with this technique.

Antibiotics Prophylaxis

Antibiotic prophylaxis is topically applied. Ciprofloxacin hydrochloride 3 mg/mL and chloramphenicol ointment can be used postoperatively. Cyclopentolate hydrochloride 10 mg/mL could be also applied topically twice a day for a few days.

Additional prophylactic actions can be taken to avoid infection using intraoperative antibiotic and gamma radiation of the mixtures as preoperative sterilization of the pigments.

Postoperative Protocol

The postoperative treatment using antibiotics-antiinflammatory drops and analgesia is crucial to achieve good results and prevent infections, as in any invasive surgical technique. Slit-lamp examination is recommended 1 day, 4 days and 1 week after the surgery to detect possible complications.

REFERENCES

1. Holth S. Revival of Galen's corneal staining with coppersulfate and tannine should be abandoned. Am J Ophthalmol.1931;14: 378-9.
2. Mannis MJ, Eghbali K, Schwab IR. Keratopigmentation: a review of corneal tattooing. Cornea.1999;18: 633-7.
3. Ziegler S. Multicolor Tattooing of the Cornea. Trans Am Ophthalmol Soc. 1922;20:71-87.
4. Pontius. Treatment of Acute Staphyloma of the Cornea, N. Y. Med. Jour., September, 1912, 637 (As quoted by Ziegler S. Reference 3).
5. Alió JL, Rodríguez AE, Toffaha BT, et al. Femtosecond-assisted keratopigmentation for functional and cosmetic restoration in essential iris atrophy. J Cataract Refract Surg. 2011;37:1744-7.
6. Alió JL, Rodríguez AE, Toffaha BT, et al. Keratopigmentation (corneal tattooing) for the management of visual disabilities of the eye related to iris defects. Br J Ophthalmol. 2011;95:1397-1401.
7. Alió JL, Rodríguez AE, Toffaha BT, et al. Femtosecond-assisted keratopigmentation Double Tunnel Technique in the Management of a case of Urrets-Zavalia Syndrome. Cornea. 2012;31:1071-4.
8. Alió JL, Sirerol B, Walewska-Szafran A, Miranda M. Corneal tattooing (keratopigmentation) to restore cosmetic appearance in severely impaired eyes with new mineral micronized pigments. Br J Ophthalmol. 2010;94:245-9.
9. Sirerol B, Walewska-Szafran A, Alió JL, et al. "Tolerance and Biocompatibility of Micronized Black Pigment for Keratopigmentation Simulated Pupil Reconstruction. Cornea. 2011;30: 344-50.
10. Amesty MA, Alio JL, Rodriguez A. Corneal Tolerance to Micronized Mineral Pigments for Keratopigmentation. Br J Ophthalmol. 2014;98:1756-60.

6 Keratopigmentation Techniques

Different methods have been suggested to perform corneal tattoo. The instruments most commonly used were described in previous chapters (Figure 6.1).

There are mainly two different types of keratopigmentation techniques currently in use.

1. Superficial keratopigmentation (superficial corneal staining)
   - Superficial corneal staining (SCS)
   - Superficial automated keratopigmentation (SAK)
2. Intrastromal keratopigmentation (Intralamellar/intrastromal corneal staining)
   - Manual intrastromal keratopigmentation (MIK)
   - Femtosecond-assisted keratopigmentation (FAK).

The selection of a correct technique depends on the objective of the corneal pigmentation, that could be a cosmetic purpose or a therapeutic tattoo.

The selected technique could also depends on the location of the corneal scar. In general intrastromal keratopigmentation is recommended but some corneal scars might not be amenable using this technique and might require more superficial methods.

For a better understanding of this topic, it is reasonable to comprehend the methods used in the past.

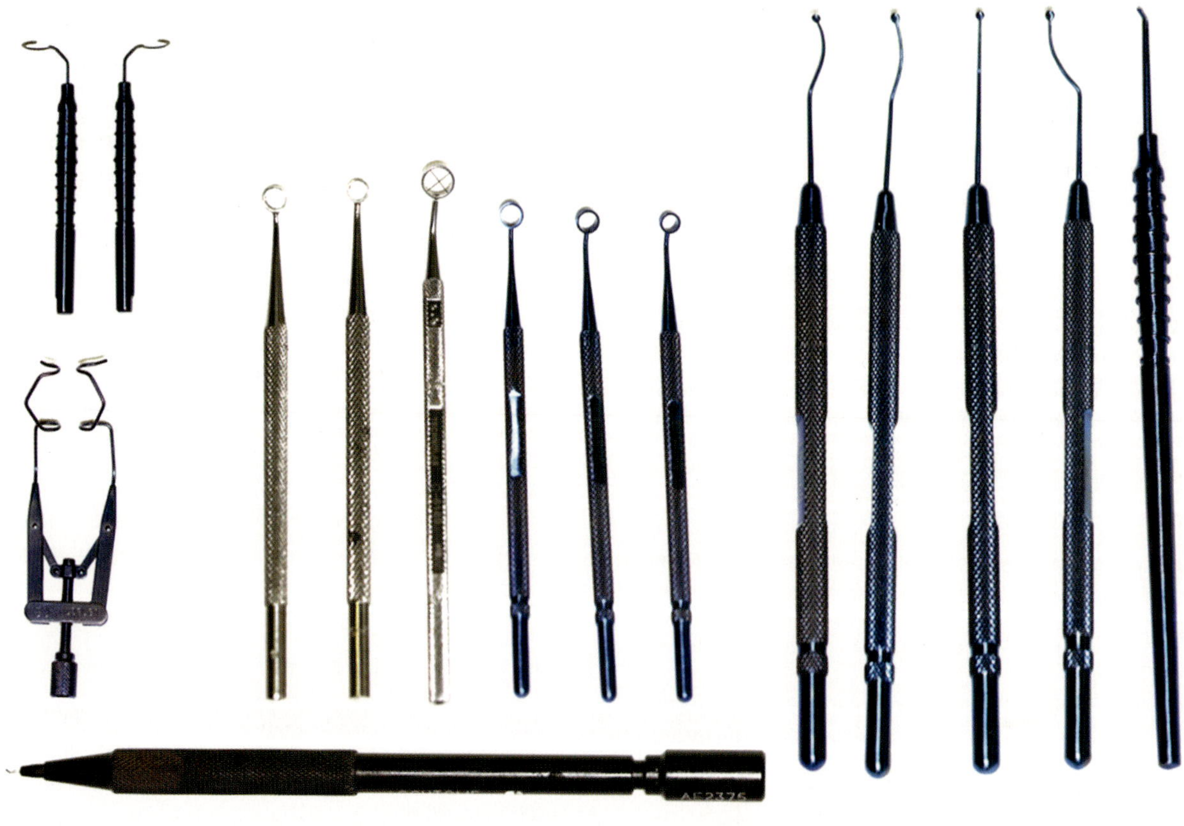

Fig. 6.1: Instruments used for corneal tattooing

SUPERFICIAL KERATOPIGMENTATION TECHNIQUES

Unlike the methods currently used, formerly completely different methods for superficial corneal tattooing were known.

Keratopigmentation could be achieved either by creating the precipitation of the pigment in the corneal tissue by a chemical reaction with a solution of metals, such as gold chloride,[1,2] silver nitrate,[2-4] or platinum chloride,[1,2,4] or alternatively, injecting directly[5,6] an insoluble pigment such as indian ink,[1] iron oxide[1,7] or titanium dioxide[8,9] into the corneal stroma.[10] In many cases the prior techniques were not satisfactory due to fading, discoloration and anterior segment inflammation.[11]

The first of them was based on a chemical reaction, and that is why it was called chemical staining. It was mainly used in the West countries due to the pioneering work of Knapp, Kerautbauer, Bietty and other collaborators.[12] Another method was performed using carbon impregnation. The chemical tattoo was easier and faster than the carbon impregnation method, but faded faster than nonmetallic techniques.[13]

Different instruments have been used to introduce the pigments into the cornea, including a simple needle,[1,14] a bundles of fine needles,[15] or more complex devices like dermograph also used for dermatological treatments and dermopigmentation (Figure 6.2).[16]

For this type of keratopigmentation the instruments required to measure the pupil size are the previously seen in Figure 6.1. A drop of the adequate stain is placed on the corneal surface, and then micropunctures are performed down to the superficial layers of the stroma using one of the needles previously mentioned. The maneuver is repeated, until the adequate amount of pigment is introduced into the superficial cornea to achieve an acceptable cosmetic appearance.[17-20]

Another type of superficial corneal tattooing is the automated keratopigmentation procedure, which is performed using a prototype of a punctural device (Vissum Eye MP System, Madrid, Spain; Apl. No. 2.949.539). Automatic micropunctures are performed, puncturing the superficial layers of the stroma to an approximate depth of 120 microns from the corneal surface. The penetration depth of the needles is controlled by the length of the longitudinal axial vibration of the tip.[17-20]

The inconvenience with this type of superficial procedure is that the corneal epithelium is affected and it could cause more discomfort and pain postoperatively. However it is important to consider this technique specially in cases where the scar is located in the anterior stroma.

INTRASTROMAL KERATOPIGMENTATION TECHNIQUES

Newer approaches have recently been described using the lamellar corneal structure anatomical advantage, suggesting the possibility that it may get a more accurate distribution and uniform reproducible pigmentation.[5-6,17-21]

Manual Intrastromal Keratopigmentation

In 1984, Panda et al.[5] described a keratopigmentation series of cases in which they compared the intralamellar tunnel technique with the superficial pigmentation technique. The intralamellar procedures were associated with less inflammation and significantly less fading than the superficial techniques.

In 1998, Beekhuis et al.[21] described the lamellar stromal keratography to treat the uncomfortable photophobia in patients with aniridia. The pigments were also injected intrastromally after a lamellar dissection of the stroma.

Burris et al.[6] investigated the intrastromal lamellar technique as a possible treatment modality to correct iris defects, for optical and cosmetic benefits. They used samples from an eye bank to develop their investigation.

A few years later Alió et al.[20] conducted a study comparing the superficial corneal staining technique and the intrastromal corneal staining, using micronized mineral pigment, in severely impaired eyes. The idea emerged to avoid invasive cosmetic reconstructive surgery like enucleation and

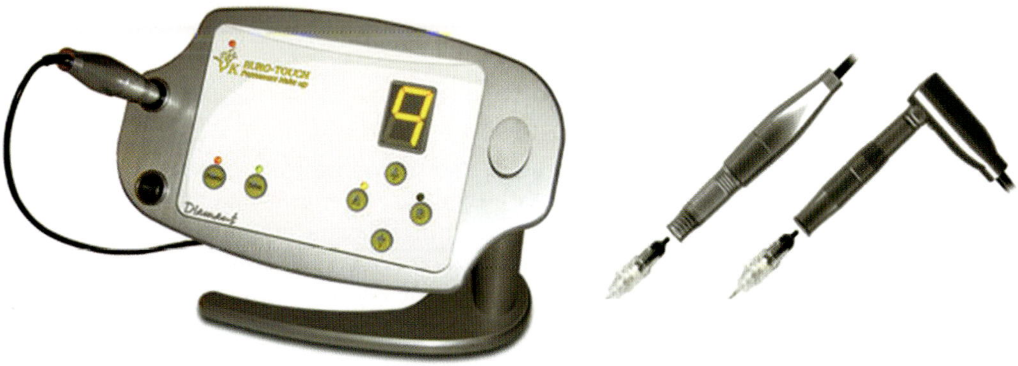

Fig. 6.2: Dermograph for micropigmentation

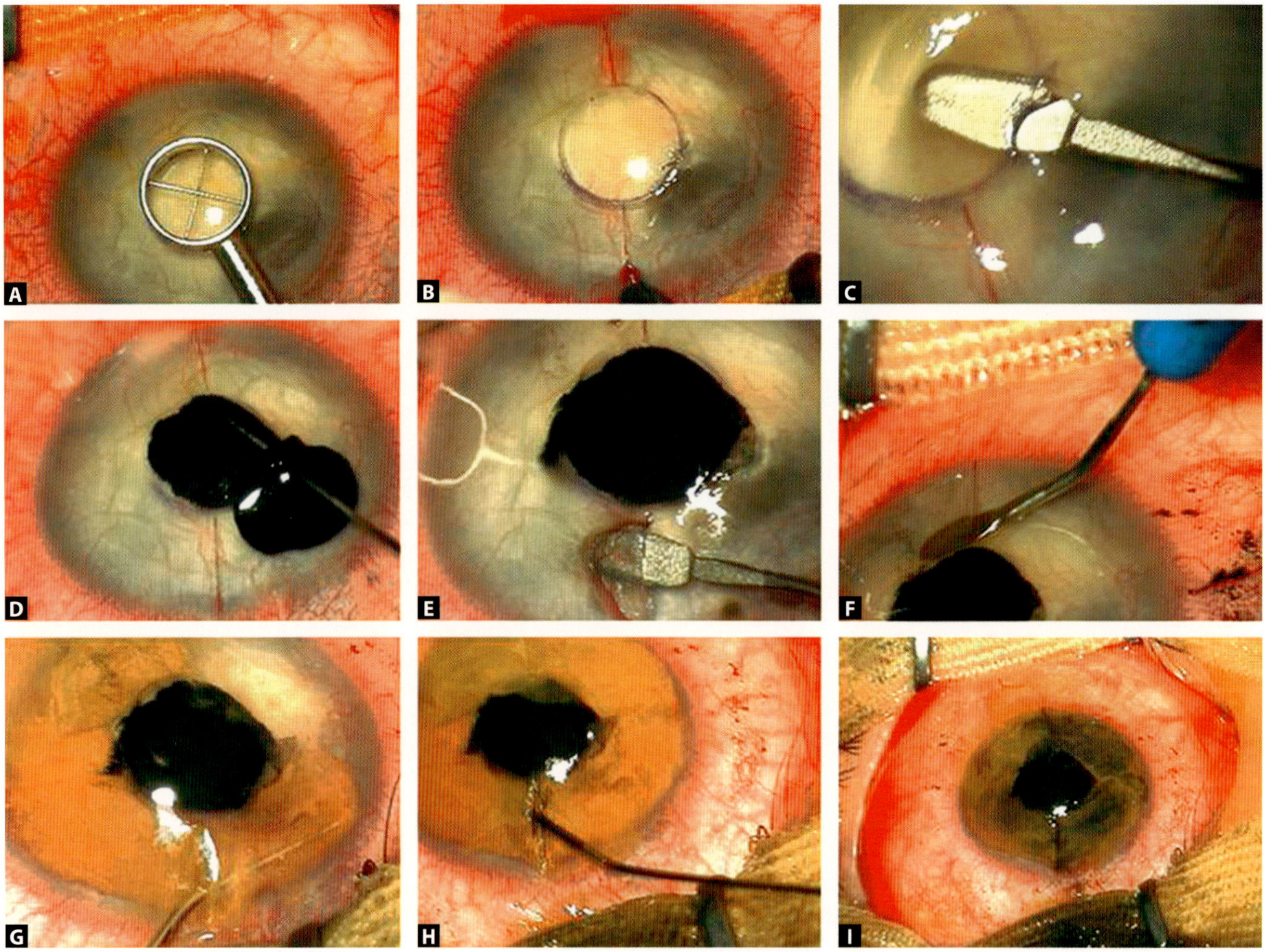

Figs 6.3A to I: Intralamellar corneal staining technique[20]: (A) Pupil diameter is marked (in this case 4 mm); (B) 3 or 4 radial incisions are performed using a 1 mm diamond blade previously calibrated; (C) Corneal intrastromal dissection in the pupil area using a microcrescent blade (Sharpoint; Surgical Specialties Corporation, Readying, Pennsylvania); (D) Intralamellar staining in the pupil area with black using a 30G cannula; (E and F) Peripheral corneal intrastromal dissection through the radial incisions previously performed; (G) Intralamellar peripheral corneal staining using brown pigments to mimic the iris color; (H) This pigment is then mixed with a darker pigment to simulate a normal iris color and to match the color of the other eye; (I) Outcomes after the intrastromal staining technique[20]

evisceration procedures in those eyes. The study concluded that intrastromal staining resulted more beneficial than superficial staining, providing a more homogeneous appearance of the pigmented area, the surgical procedure was faster, the patients also showed a faster and less symptomatic recovery postoperatively. An additional advantage is that the corneal surface remains unchanged and the epithelium is not affected, and the pigments are not in contact with the tear film which reduces the risk of fading (Figures 6.3A to I).[20]

Another way to dissect the intralamellar tunnel is through just one radial incision using a pigtail corneal dissector, also called Helicoidal Tunnel Corneal Dissector, 180° clockwise and 180° counterclockwise along the pupil margin. This instrument is shown in Figure 6.1.[17-20,22]

Finally, the adequate color is injected through the tunnel using a 30 gauge cannula on a 1 mL syringe. For keratopigmentation itself no stitches are required.[17-20,22]

Femtosecond-assisted Intrastromal Keratopigmentation

Femtosecond-assisted keratopigmentacion is a new technique. One or two intrastromal tunnels can be created and the pigments are injected inside those tunnels. When two tunnels are performed, there is a different purpose for each one. The deep tunnel has a functional purpose, which consists in blocking the light using a dark color that should be injected into this tunnel, while the superficial tunnel is

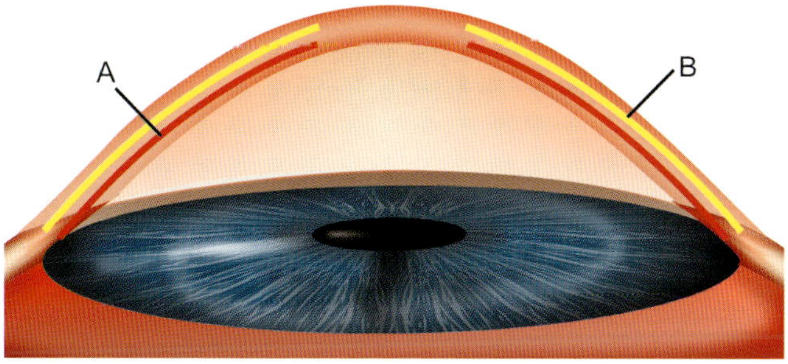

Figs 6.4A and B: (A) Darker and deep, light absorbing layer, (B) Surperficial layer, light-colored to match the color of the other eye[19]

for cosmetic purposes, to mimic the color of the other eye (Figure 6.4A).[17-19]

Before the surgery, pachymetry and tomography are measured in different areas of the cornea by means of the time-domain Visante optical coherence tomography system (Carl Zeiss Meditec AG) to decide the appropriate stromal depth for the femtosecond tunnels.

Two types of surgeries can be performed, creating just one intrastromal tunnel or two stromal tunnels using the 60 kHz femtosecond laser (for example, the IntraLase AMO, Irvine, CA).

Afterward, the white-to-white horizontal and vertical diameters are measured using calipers to determine the diameter of the lamellar dissection. The deepest tunnel could be performed first at a 400 microns depth from the surface with an inner diameter of 6 mm and an outer diameter of 9.5 mm. The energy should be set at 2 mJ, with a vertical incision at 6 o'clock. A second superficial tunnel could be performed at 200 microns depth, with an inner diameter of 6 mm and an outer diameter of 9.5 mm. The energy was set at 2 mJ with a vertical incision at 12 o'clock (Figure 6.4B).[17-20]

A lamellar dissector (KTP corneal dissector, Epsilon; Irvine, CA) is required to open the intralamellar femtosecond tunnels from each one of the incisions (at 12 o'clock and at 6 o'clock). Then the pigments are injected using a 30-gauge cannula into the deeper and superficial tunnels through the superior and inferior incisions.

A double layer technique with two intrastromal tunnels mimics the anatomy of the iris, where the light-colored pigment is applied to the superficial layer and the dark-colored pigment is applied to the deepest layer.[17-20]

REFERENCES

1. Ziegler S. Multicolor tattooing of the cornea. Trans Am Ophthalmol Soc. 1922;20:71-87.
2. Clark EH. Tattooing of corneal scars with insoluble pigments. Plast Reconstr Surg. 1946;2:44-59.
3. Gifford S, Steinberg A. Gold and silver impregnation of cornea for cosmetic purposes. Am J Ophthalmol. 1927;10:240-7.
4. Pischel DK. Tattooing of the cornea with gold and platinum chloride. Arch Ophthalmol. 1930;3:176-81.
5. Panda A, Mohan M, Chawdhary S. Corneal tattooing—experiences with lamellar pocket procedure. Indian J Ophthalmol. 1984;32:408-11.
6. Burris TE, Holmes-Higgin DK, Silvestrini TA. Lamellar intrastromal corneal tattoo for treating iris defects (artificial iris). Cornea. 1998;17: 169-73.
7. Van der Velden-Samdeerubun EM, Kok JH. Dermatography as a modern treatment for colouring leukoma corneae. Cornea. 1994;13:349-53.
8. Reed JW. Corneal tattooing to reduce glare in cases of traumatic iris loss. Cornea. 1994;13: 401-5.
9. Reed JW, Beran RF. Elimination of monocular diplopia by corneal tattooing. Ophthalmic Surg. 1988;19:437-9.
10. Muller H, Van der Velden/Samderubun EM. Tattooing in maxillo-facial surgery. J Craniomaxillofac Surg. 1988;16:382-4.
11. Wiegmann E. Is tattooing according to knapp entirely without danger? Am J Ophthalmol. 1929;12:431.
12. Duke-Elder S, Leigh AG. System of ophthalmology. In Disease of the outer eye, part 2. St Louis, CV Mosby. 1965.
13. Olander K, Kanai A, Kaufman HE. An analytical electron microscopic study of a corneal tattoo. Ann Ophthalmol. 1983:15:1046-9.
14. Von Wecker L. Tatouage de la cornee. Union Med. 27:41 (As quoted by Ziegler S. Reference 1).
15. Taylor CB. On the Modern Art of Tinting Opacities of the Cornea. Br Med J 1872:2;271 (As quoted by Ziegler S. Reference 1).
16. Wessels IF, Wessels GF. Mechanized keratomicropigmentation: corneal tattooing with the blepharopigmentor. Ophthalmic Surg Lasers. 1996;27:25-28.
17. Alió JL, Rodríguez AE, Toffaha BT et al. Femtosecond-assisted keratopigmentation for functional and cosmetic restoration in essential iris atrophy. J Cataract Refract Surg. 2011;37:1744-7.
18. Alió JL, Rodríguez AE, Toffaha BT et al. Keratopigmentation (corneal tattooing) for the management of visual disabilities of the eye related to iris defects. Br J Ophthalmol. 2011;95:1397-1401.
19. Alió JL, Rodríguez AE, Toffaha BT et al. Femtosecond-assisted keratopigmentation Double Tunnel Technique in the Management of a case of Urrets-Zavalia Syndrome. Cornea. 2012;31:1071-74.
20. Alió JL, Sirerol B, Walewska-Szafran A, Miranda M. Corneal tattooing (keratopigmentation) to restore cosmetic appearance in severely impaired eyes with new mineral micronized pigments. Br J Ophthalmol. 2010;94:245-9.
21. Beekhuis WH, Drost BH, Van der Velden/Samderubun EM. A new treatment for photophobia in posttraumatic aniridia: a case report. Cornea. 1998;17:338-41.
22. Amesty MA, Alio JL, Rodriguez A. Corneal tolerance to micronized mineral pigments for keratopigmentation. Br J Ophthalmol. 2014;98:1756-60.

Indications and Contraindications

7

It is very important to consider which cases are amenable for corneal tattooing and the selection of the technique according to each case. The main goal of corneal tattooing is one of the following: cosmetic purpose, therapeutic purpose or both.[1.]

COSMETIC KERATOPIGMENTATION

Among the indications for cosmetic purposes are:

- Corneal scar without anterior synechiae
- Corneal scar + synechiae, only if the iris is not exposed
- Cicatricial keratitis
- Vascularized scars, only in cases that are controlled with adrenaline
- Phthisis bulbi
- To cover leukocoria secondary to cataract, if cataract surgery, it is not recommended.

Tenotomy of recti muscles is also combined with corneal tattooing to treat the enophthalmos in cases of phthisis bulbi, to induce an exophthalmos and achieve better results.[2]

THERAPEUTIC KERATOPIGMENTATION

Since 1872, Wecker emphasized the importance to perform corneal tattoo for optical purposes. Corneal opacities are optically translucent and this characteristic can produce blurriness. To resolve this problem, Wecker conducted an experiment in which he created a pinhole pupil slightly downward and inward, and he covered the rest of the central cornea with an opaque black pigment, achieving excellent results.[1,2]

In 1907, Mayeda[3] made some photographic experiments in Nagoya-Japan, using an opaque black color and a Zeiss lens (15 mm of aperture). First, he smeared the lens with a paste, and then he covered the dough with a black opaque pigment, demonstrating that:

- If there was a translucent paste in the lower half of the lens = the image was blurred.
- If same translucent dough was covered with a black opaque pigment = the image was clear.

Thus, Mayeda determined that the opaque black pigment returned definition back to normal in each case. After his study, he also treated 30 unique cases of corneal opacities and concluded that the vision improved in all cases, 2 to 10 times, than before tattooing the corneal opacity.[3]

These studies have proven beneficial results after corneal tattooing for optical reasons. Therefore, it is important to describe the indications for this type of keratopigmentation.

Among the indications for optical or functional purposes are:

- Albinism
- Aniridia
- Coloboma
- Iridodialysis
- keratoconus
- Diffuse corneal opacity and related glare
- Essential iris atrophy[4]
- Urrets-Zavalia syndrome[5]

CONTRAINDICATIONS TO CORNEAL TATTOO

Contraindications for corneal tattoo, either for optical purposes or for cosmetic purposes are the following:

- Corneal scar + anterior synechiae if the iris is exposed
- Iridocyclitis
- Staphyloma
- Glaucoma
- Some cases of irritation or anterior segment inflammation
- Band keratopathy or any calcareous deposit
- Nasolacrimal obstruction and chronic infections (dacryocystitis)
- Ocular surface chronic inflammation
- Severe-moderate dry eyes.

RECENT INDICATIONS FOR CORNEAL PIGMENTATION: SOME EXAMPLES

Due to the satisfactory progress of penetrating keratoplasty and deep anterior lamellar keratoplasty, the list of indications for corneal pigmentation has been reduced significantly.[6]

Another reason that reduces the number of indications are the recent advances in reconstructive surgery of the ocular surface, increasing the popularity of colored contact lenses. These cosmetic contact lenses, enucleation and evisceration associated with external orbital prosthesis or lamellar epithesis are the methods most commonly used to improve the esthetic appearance in cosmetically unacceptable eyes.[7-9]

However, contact lenses can cause inflammation, infection or pain,[1] and keratoplasties can develop infection and graft failure, plus it is ethically unacceptable to perform keratoplasties for purely cosmetic purposes. That is why corneal tattooing or keratopigmentation is useful in selected cases, especially for patients complaining of visual impairment secondary to light scattering. In these cases, it is considered an excellent alternative or the only way to improve visual acuity.[4-6,10]

It is important to consider the presence or absence of pain in these patients. If ocular pain is present, corneal pigmentation is not recommended and other procedures like evisceration-enucleation should be considered.

KERATOPIGMENTATION FOR FUNCTIONAL OR OPTIC REASONS: OUR EXPERIENCE

Essential iris atrophy is a unilateral progressive disease, more frequent in women of 20–50 years of age. It is characterized by iris atrophy with corectopia and polycoria and sometimes with increased intraocular pressures. The endothelium is abnormal and shows guttata like changes with a low cell density count. In advanced late cases, the cornea may show signs of decompensation with corneal edema and require corneal graft surgery.[4] Treatment options for this condition are limited; they include cosmetic contact lenses, iris suturing, or implantation of an artificial iris. In Figures 7.1A to D, we present a case where all these options were of limited value.[4]

Although cosmetic contact lenses were a good option decreasing the photophobia at the beginning, it could not resolve the problem of monocular diplopia when the atrophy progressed and the inner edge of the iris was centered in the visual axis (Figure 7.1C). Iris repair by suturing was impossible because the iris was significantly atrophied and very irregular; surgery in this abnormal anatomical pattern was extremely difficult. An artificial iris was also a nonviable option because of the corneal endothelial dysfunction.[4]

Furthermore, both iris repair and artificial iris have risks for intraoperative complications, and it must be remembered that the preoperative visual acuity of the patient was 20/25.[4]

Femtosecond laser technology allows the surgeon to perform intralamellar dissections for tattooing different types of corneal areas using the options provided by the software associated with the femtosecond laser, as illustrated by this case. The technique for corneal tunnel creation is more precise and safe and easier to perform (Figure 7.2.), with minimal postoperative reaction and faster recovery time, than

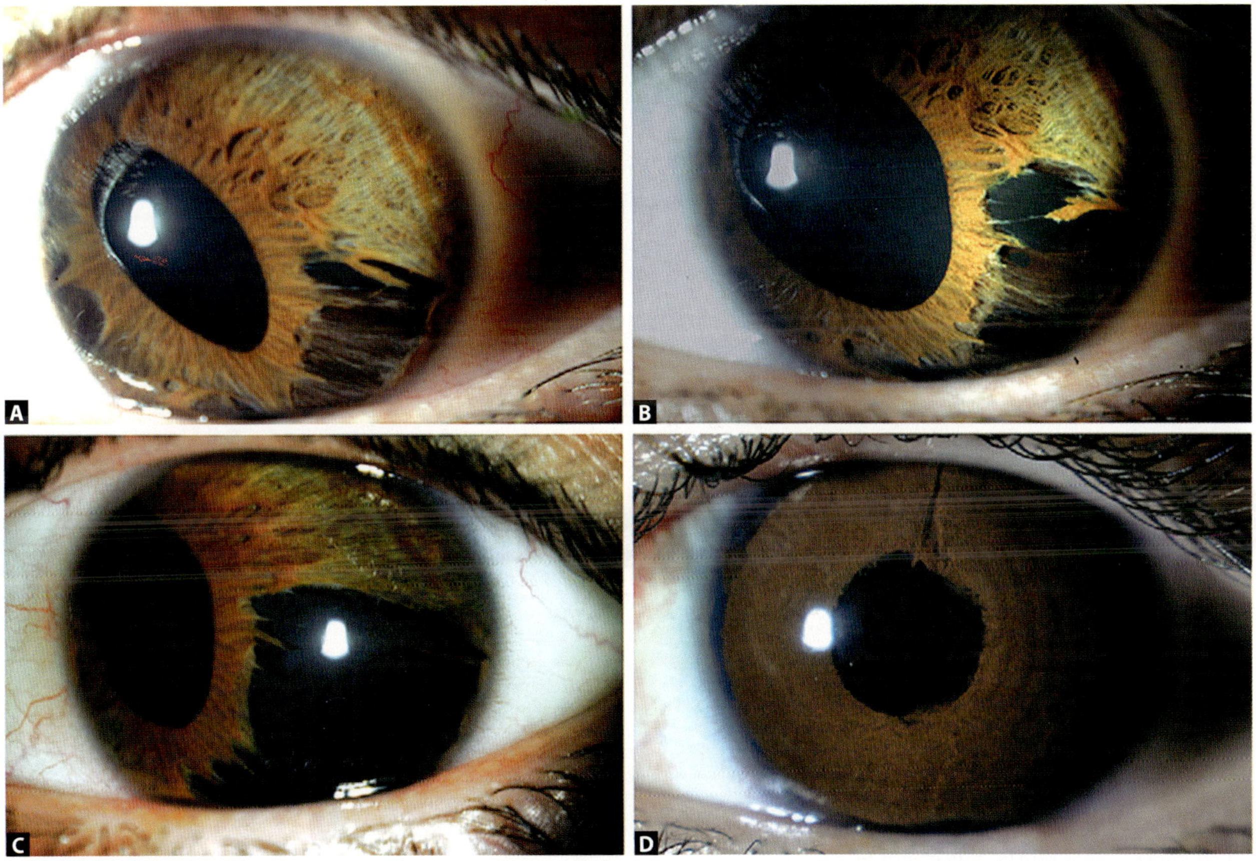

Figs 7.1A to D: Frontal image obtained with a slit-lamp biomicroscope of the essential iris atrophy; (A) First visit (oval pupil and atrophic iris holes); (B) Second visit, 3 months later (larger irregular pupil and more atrophic areas); (C) Third visit, 3 months later (typical polycoria and corectopia); (D) Postoperative visit, 3 days after femtosecond-assisted KTP[4]

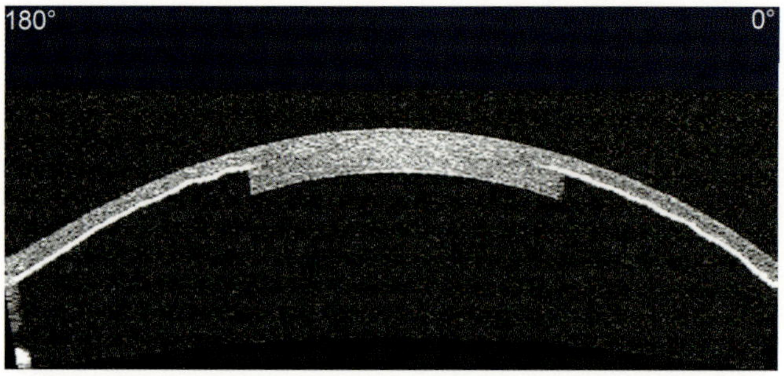

Fig. 7.2: Optical coherence tomography high-resolution corneal image of the eye having femtosecond-assisted KTP. A regular, uniform layer of pigment was localized in the anterior stroma

other keratopigmentation (KTP) techniques such as manual intralamellar staining and superficial corneal staining.[11] Furthermore, manual dissection was necessary in this case because of the limitation of the software to create a wide peripheral corneal tunnel by the femtosecond laser. This case of essential iris atrophy is an example of the applicability of keratopigmentation to the restoration of functional problems created by iris defects. In our case, the femtosecond-assisted keratopigmentation was very effective and could solve the patient's symptoms and provide an excellent cosmetic result.

In Figures 7.3 to 7.5, we can appreciate more examples of keratopigmentation for functional reasons. The use of micronized mineral pigments with an adequate toxicology study,[11-13] is an essential step in the modern development of keratopigmentation. Our experience using this pigment has demonstrated it to be safe during a 5-year follow-up. Future studies of the stability of this pigment are necessary to determine its half-life in the corneal stroma.

Keratopigmentation is minimally invasive and results demonstrated a significant decrease in the subjective glare and photophobia, and even in monocular diplopia in all our treated cases. The cosmetic outcome was also very favorable. These techniques may allow the surgeon to correct the visual disabilities associated with iris defects in a new, more accessible way, thus avoiding more aggressive intraocular procedures.[4-5,12,13]

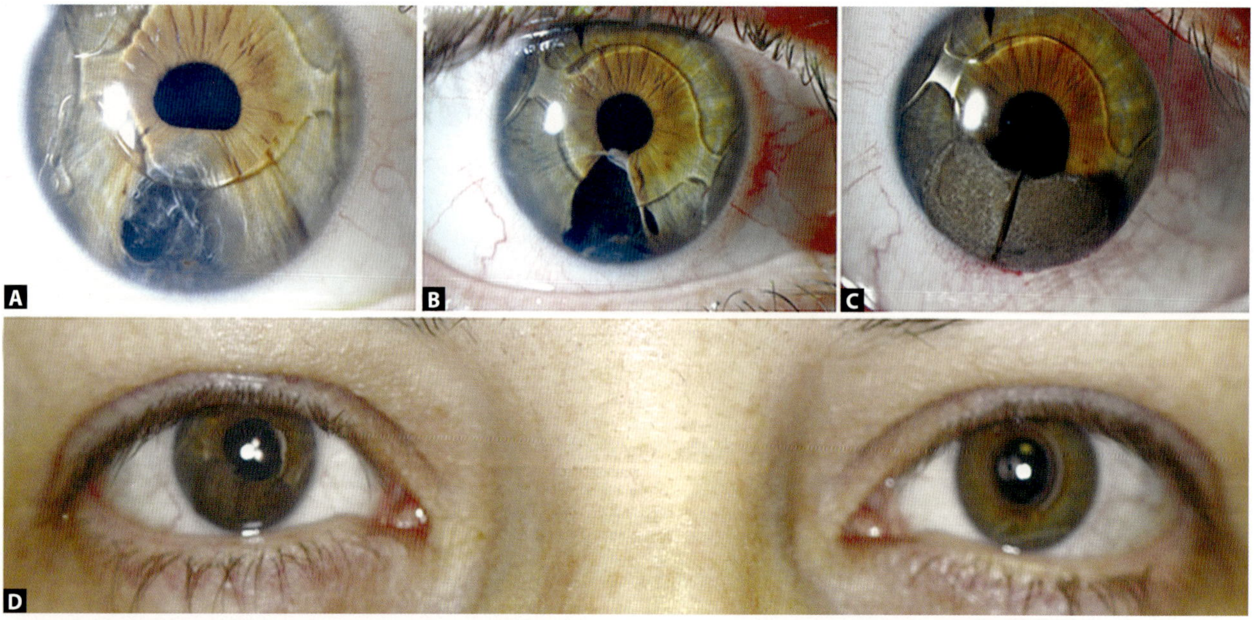

Figs 7.3A to D: Patient's iris defect secondary to epithelial iris cyst in her right eye. (A) Aspect of the eye after two unsuccessful attempts of intracyst mitomycin injection; (B) Aspect of the eye after sectorial iridectomy and iris suturing of the peripheral pupil edges. The patient complained of polyopia and incapacitating glare; (C and D) Postoperative aspect of the patient after manual intralamellar keratopigmentation[10]

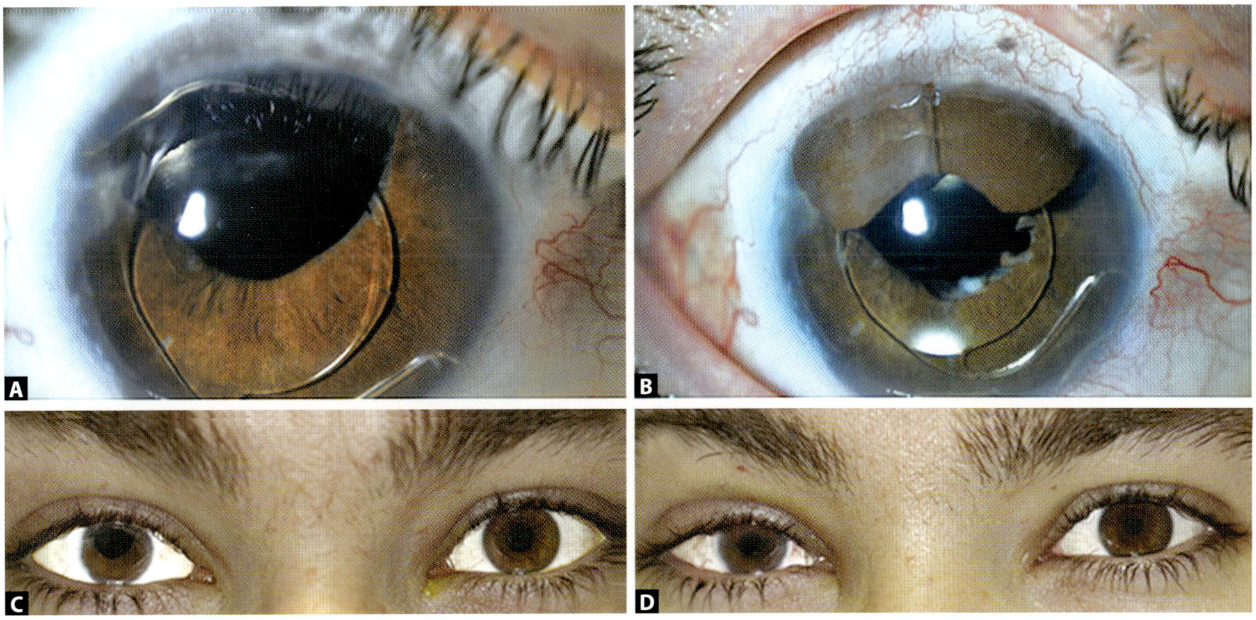

Figs 7.4A to D: (A to C) Preoperative aspect of the patient complaining of debilitating glare owing to traumatic coloboma; (B to D) Postoperative appearance after restoration of the iris defect with manual intralamellar keratopigmentation. A significant decrease in glare was reported by the patient[10]

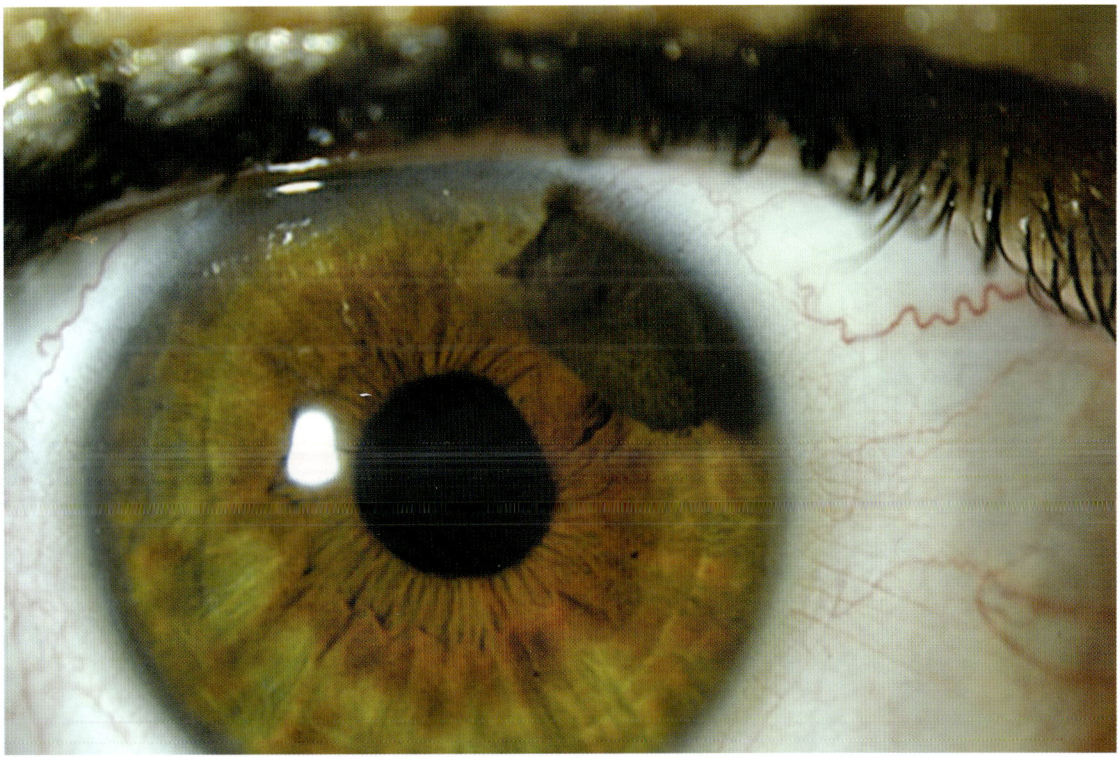

Fig. 7.5: Postoperative slit-lamp examination of a patient suffering from monocular diplopia at night following the implantation of a posterior chamber phakic intraocular lens owing to an inadequately performed peripheral iridotomy. A manual intralamellar keratopigmentation procedure was indicated at the area of the iridectomy. Total disappearance of the symptoms was achieved[10]

REFERENCES

1. Ziegler S. Multicolor Tattooing of the Cornea. Trans Am Ophthalmol Soc. 1922;20:71-87.
2. Von Wecker L (1870). Tatouage de la cornee. Union Med 27: 41 (As quoted by Ziegler S. Reference 1).
3. Mayeda (1908) Beitrag. Z. Augenheilk., 233 (As quoted by Ziegler S. Reference 1).
4. Alió JL, Rodríguez AE, Toffaha BT, et al. Femtosecond-assisted keratopigmentation for functional and cosmetic restoration in essential iris atrophy. J Cataract Refract Surg. 2011;37:1744-7.
5. Alió JL, Rodríguez AE, Toffaha BT, et al. Femtosecond-assisted keratopigmentation Double Tunnel Technique in the Management of a case of Urrets-Zavalia Syndrome. Cornea. 2012;31:1071-4.
6. Sekundo W, Seifert P, Seitz B, Loeffler KU. Long-term ultrastructural changes in human corneas after tattooing with non-metallic substances. Br J Ophthalmol. 1999;83:219-24.
7. Hallock GG. Cosmetic trauma surgery. Plast Reconstr Surg. 1995;95:380-1.
8. Hoeyberghs JL. Fortnightly review: cosmetic surgery. BMJ. 1999;318:512-6.
9. Kuzan WM Jr. Plastic surgery. J Am Coll Surg. 1999;188:171-7.
10. Alió JL, Rodríguez AE, Toffaha BT, et al. Keratopigmentation (corneal tattooing) for the management of visual disabilities of the eye related to iris defects. Br J Ophthalmol. 2011;95:1397-401.
11. Alió JL, Sirerol B, Walewska-Szafran A, Miranda M. Corneal tattooing (keratopigmentation) to restore cosmetic appearance in severely impaired eyes with new mineral micronized pigments. Br J Ophthalmol. 2010;94:245-9.
12. Sirerol B, Walewska-Szafran A, Alió JL, et al. Tolerance and Biocompatibility of Micronized Black Pigment for Keratopigmentation Simulated Pupil Reconstruction. Cornea. 2011;30:344-50.
13. Amesty MA, Alio JL, Rodriguez A. Corneal Tolerance to Micronized Mineral Pigments for Keratopigmentation. Br J Ophthalmol. 2014;98:1756-60.

Histopathology

8

Histological examination is crucial to determine the tolerance and biocompatibility of the pigments used for keratopigmentation. Some authors have investigated about this important topic and the results they have achieved in their studies is going to be commented in this chapter.

HISTOPATHOLOGICAL RESULTS

Sekundo et al. performed corneal tattooing in human corneas and the histopathological examination revealed pigmented granules inside the keratocytes when the pigment used was a nonmetallic dye, unlike what occurred in patients treated with metallic pigments.[1] They concluded that keratocytes can actively ingest and retain particles of nonmetallic dyes in their cell membranes for a very long period of time (Figures 8.1 and 8.2).

It is possible to distinguish in Figure 8.1, a higher concentration of pigment particles in the middle stromal layers of the cornea (hematoxylin and eosin staining, 40x from the original).[1]

It is also evident in Figure 8.2, a subepithelial keratocyte with pigment particles agglomerations. The adjacent extracellular matrix does not show any foreign material or pigment.[1]

Fujita et al. experimentally demonstrated that rabbit corneal fibroblasts can ingest by endocytosis injected ink particles in a period of 3 to 4 days and then stored those particles for at least 6 months.[2]

Takahashi et al. also examined corneas from three Japanese patients who underwent keratopigmentation 12, 20 and 34 years earlier. They described Indian ink particles both intracellularly and extracellularly in these three patients.[3]

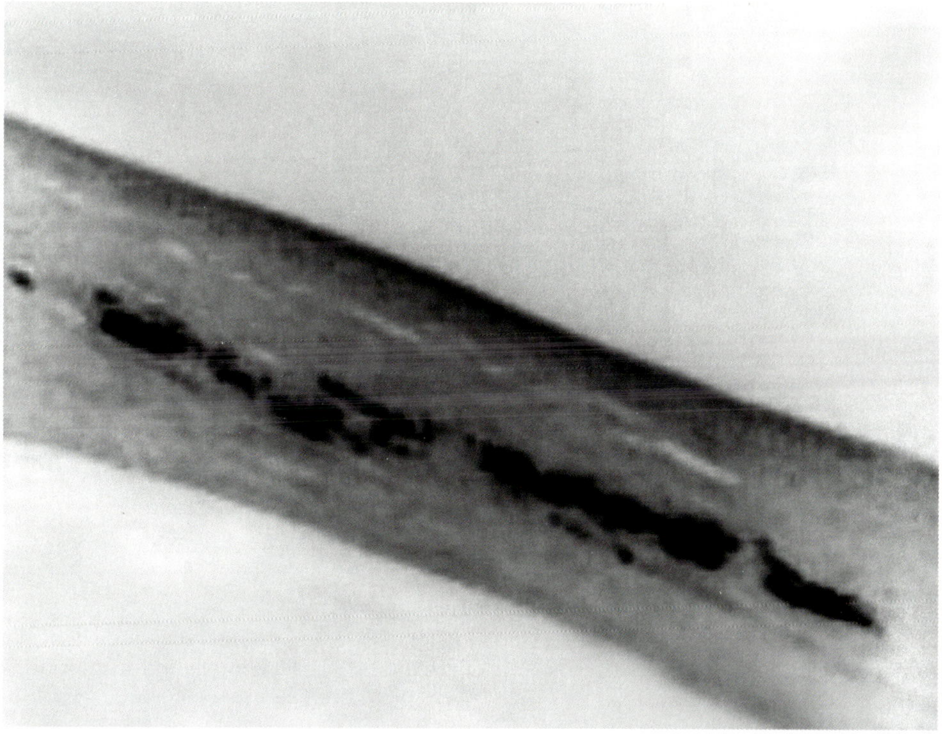

Fig. 8.1: Midstromal tattoo pigment particles hematoxylin and eosin staining

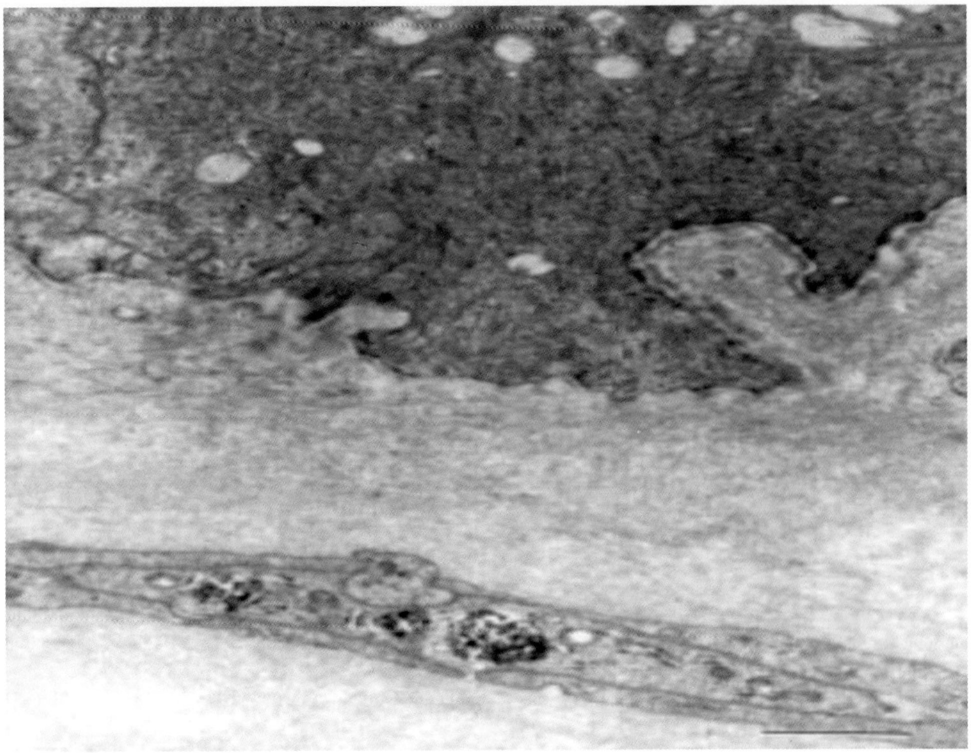

Fig. 8.2: Subepithelial keratocyte with pigment particles agglomerations

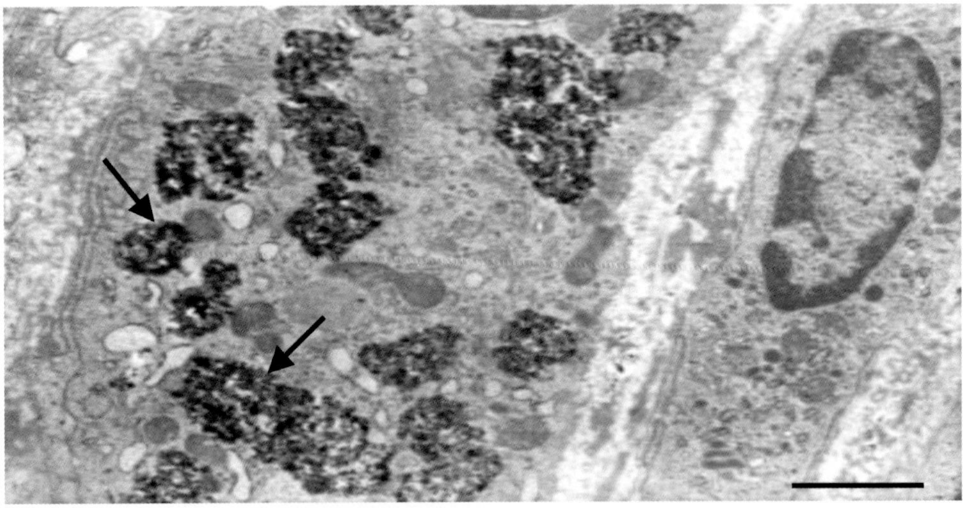

Fig. 8.3: Keratocyte with several intracellular tattoo particles

These different conclusions in the previous mentioned studies suggest that the ink that was used in Japan could have had different ingredients to those used in the western countries.

To conclude, ultrastructural studies comparing metalic tattoo with nonmetallic tattoo demonstrated intracellular granules inside the keratocytes in the nonmetallic one (Figure 8.3), and intracellular and extracellular granules after the metalic tattoo with platinum chloride.[1,4]

The absence of extracellular particles in nonmetallic tattoo suggests that endocytosis of organic substances by the human cornea fibroblasts is more permanent and stable than

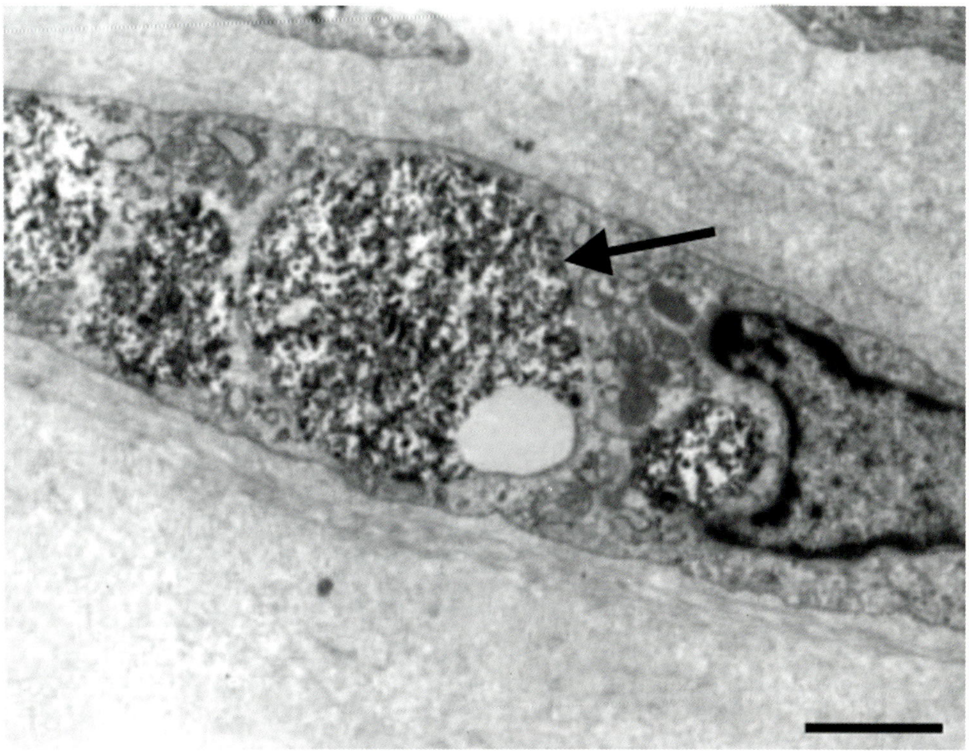

Fig. 8.4: Middle stromal keratocyte with pigment granules of different electronic densities

endocytosis of metalic dyes which easily are found located extracellularly. Thus, there are differences between human corneas and other species with respect to the intracellular or extracellular location of the pigments and their chemical nature, either metallic or nonmetallic. Figure 8.4 shows a middle stromal keratocyte with pigment granules of different electronic densities. These granules clusters are surrounded by a membrane (arrow).[1]

Fujita et al.[2] suggested that phagocytosis by fibroblasts is the consequence of the corneal reaction to protect themself from injuries and damages due to nontoxic foreign materials. Assuming that metal salts are more toxic than organic substances, is reasonable to expect higher quantity of cellular debris in the extracellular matrix of the cornea in metallic tattoos. This characteristic could also induce a low-grade inflammation, with subsequent softening and melting in the corneal stroma.[5]

Hematoxylin-eosin Staining

In our studies, microscopic examination using hematoxylin-eosin staining, revealed that stromal pigmentation is observed as blackish bands, parallel to the corneal surface, of variable length and thickness, which appears to be located between the stromal collagen lamellae (Figures 5 and 6).[7,8]

Sometimes pigment granules are also observed inside of stromal cells, which can be located at different distances from the pigmented area.[8,9]

Because of the strong black discoloration of the pigments seen microscopically, it is not possible to secure the intra- or extracellular location, but in our opinion, it is mainly located extracellularly between the collagen fibers, and promptly inside of a cell (fibroblasts or stromal keratocytes), which sometimes have an increased size.[7]

All pigments showed the same blackish color microscopically, regardless of the color that was used for intrastromal micropigmentation. Only in samples pigmented with blue or bluish brown, small precipitates with blackish blue could be observed (Figure 8.6). No inflammatory cells were observed after stromal keratopigmentation in our studies.[7]

Masson's Trichrome Staining

Regarding the organization of the collagen fibers, no changes were seen in their lamellar arrangement using the Masson's trichrome staining (Figure 8.7A).[6,8]

However lamellar collagen pattern could be altered in some areas as we can appreciate in Figure 8.7B (arrow).[7]

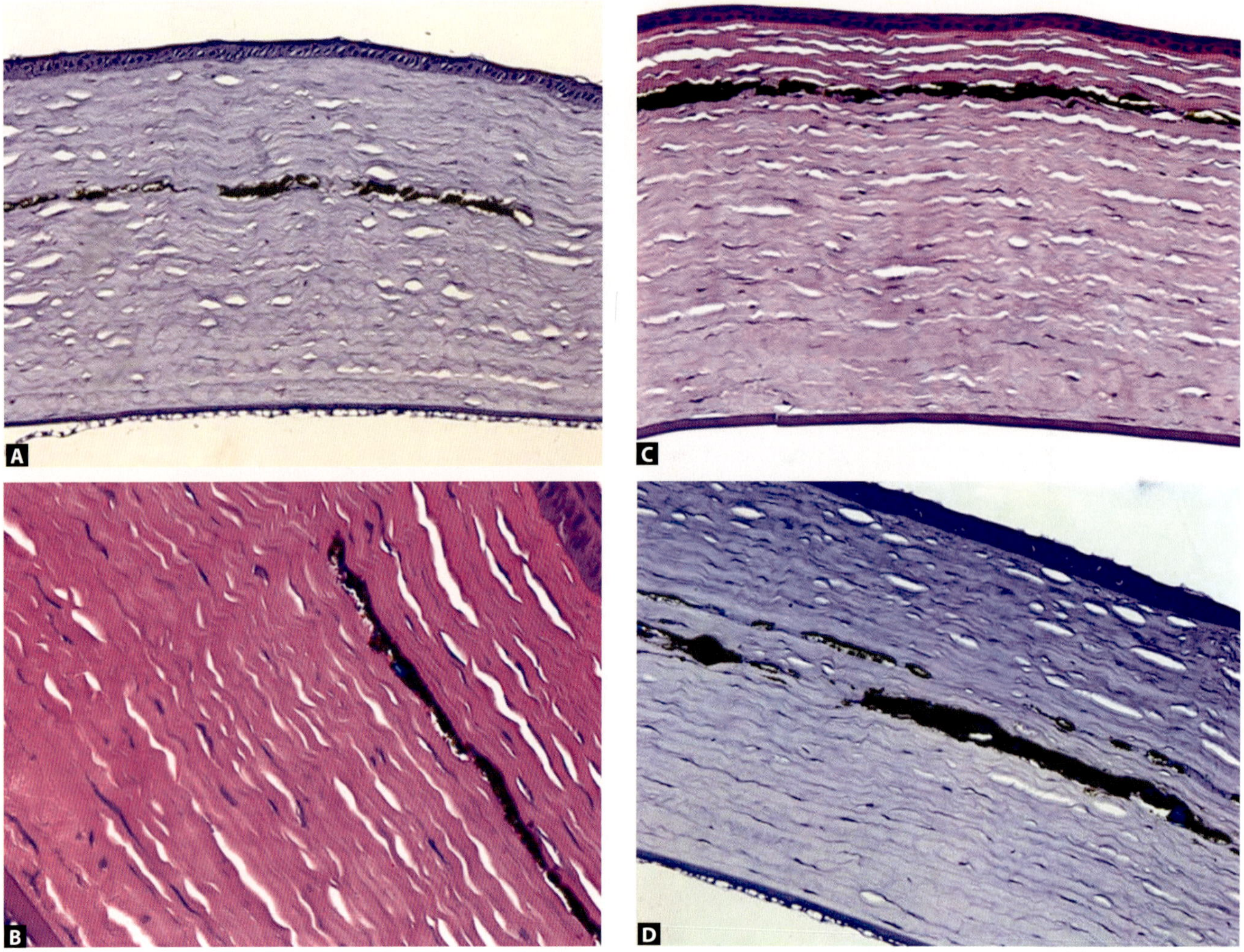

Figs 8.5A to D: Hematoxylin-eosin staining[6]

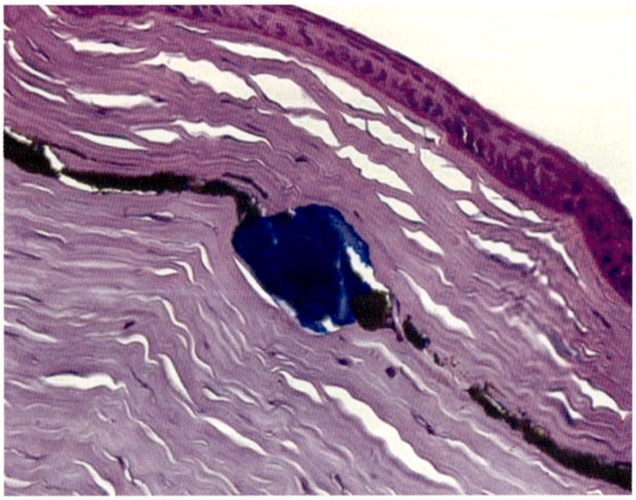

Fig. 8.6: Hematoxylin-eosin staining, in a sample pigmented with blue[6]

These specific changes in the collagen lamellar arrangement are commonly seen near the pigmented area. It is common to observe several "swirls" in the samples, which may have irregular lines and pigmentation spots inside (Figure 8.7B).[7]

MORPHOMETRIC ANALYSIS

Morphometric analysis could be performed to determine the exact location of the pigment expressed as a percentage, both relative to the entire thickness of the cornea, as compared to stromal thickness. In our experience, the image analysis program *Image ProPlus 7.0 from Media Cybernetics* could be used for this purpose.[7]

A representative picture of the measures of the pigment depth is presented in Figure 8.8.[7]

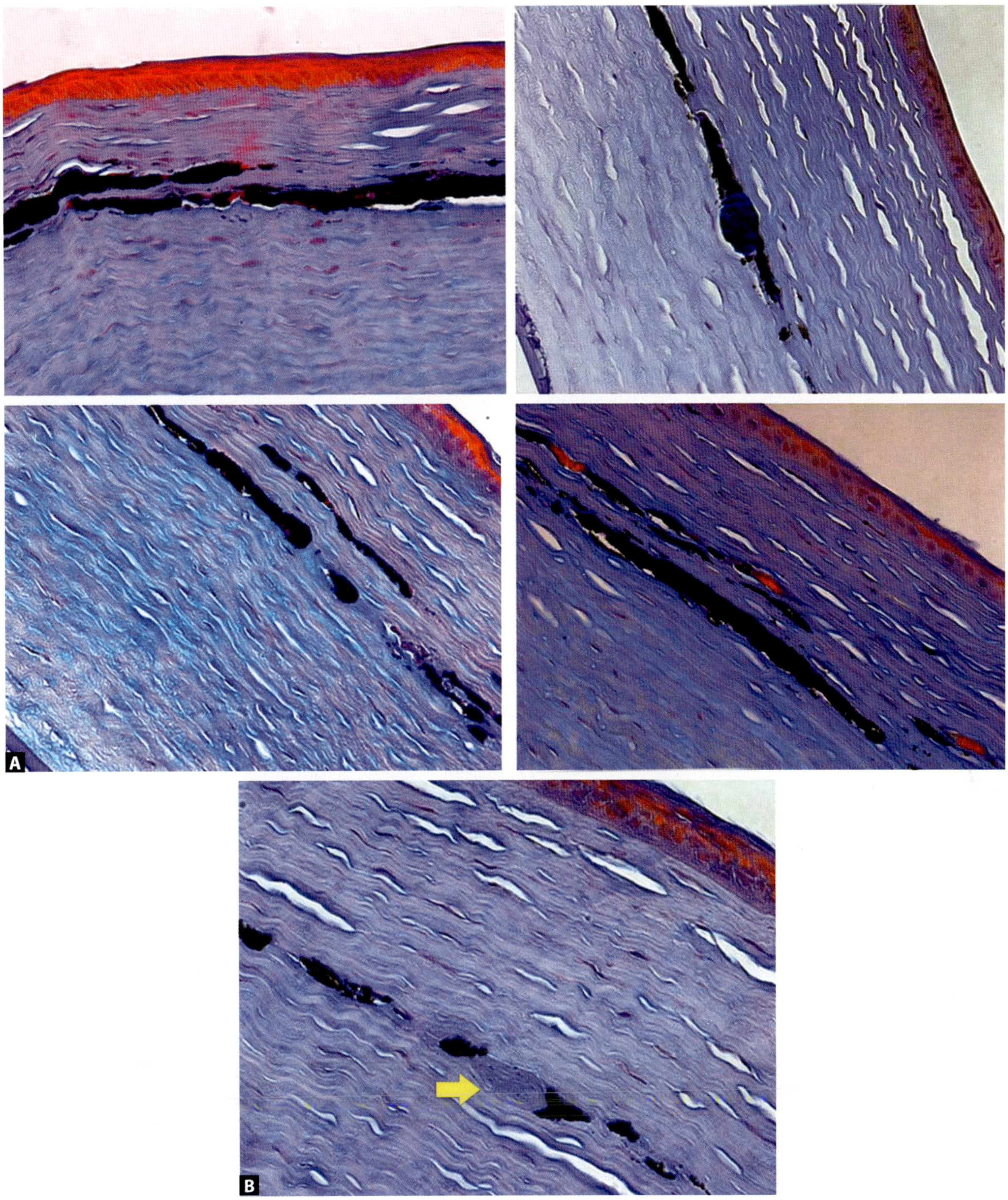

Figs 8.7A and B: Masson's trichrome staining[6]

LEUKOCYTE COMMON ANTIGEN IMMUNOSTAINING

Protein tyrosine phosphatase receptor type C also known as PTPRC is an enzyme that, in humans, is encoded by the *PTPRC* gene. PTPRC is also known as CD45 antigen (CD stands for cluster of differentiation), which was originally called leukocyte common antigen.[10]

LCA is a type I transmembrane protein that is in various forms present on all differentiated hematopoietic cells except erythrocytes and plasma cells that assists in the activation of those cells (a form of co-stimulation). It is expressed in lymphomas, B-cell chronic lymphocytic leukemia, hairy cell leukemia, and acute nonlymphocytic leukemia. A monoclonal antibody to CD45 is used in routine

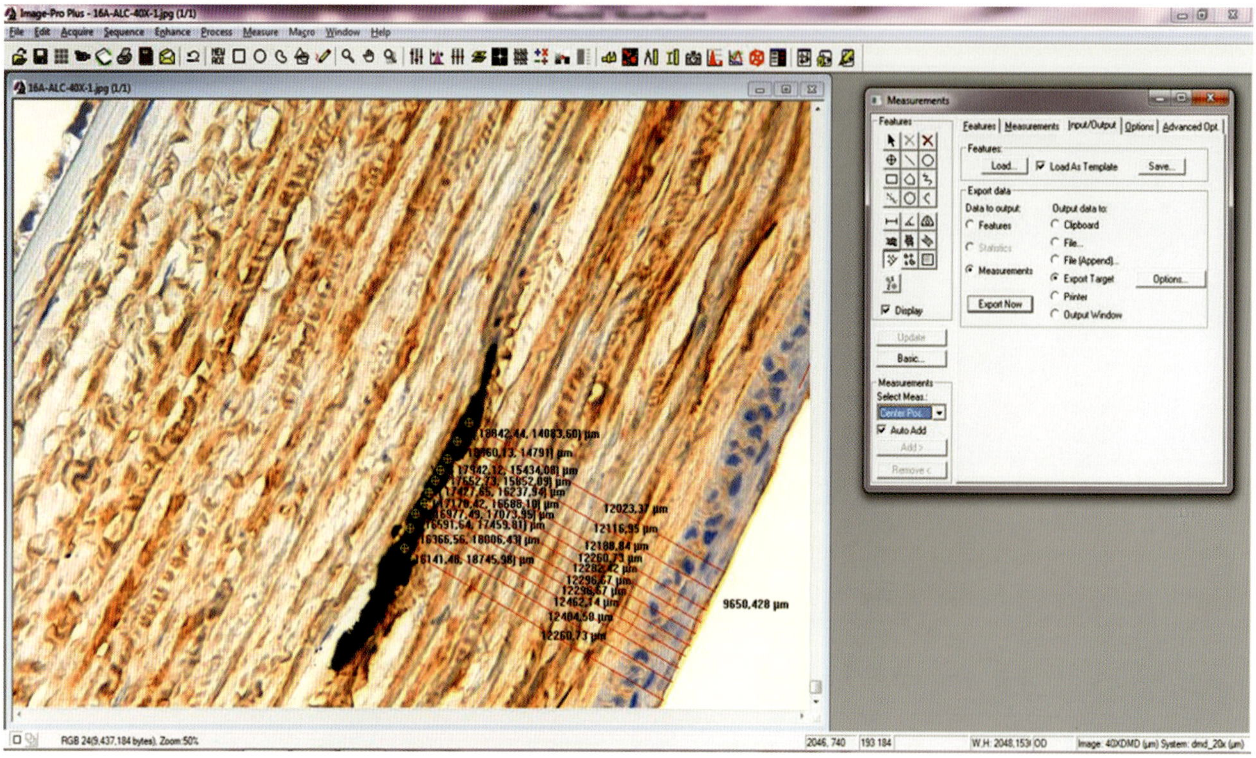

Fig. 8.8: Image analysis program Image ProPlus 7.0 [7]

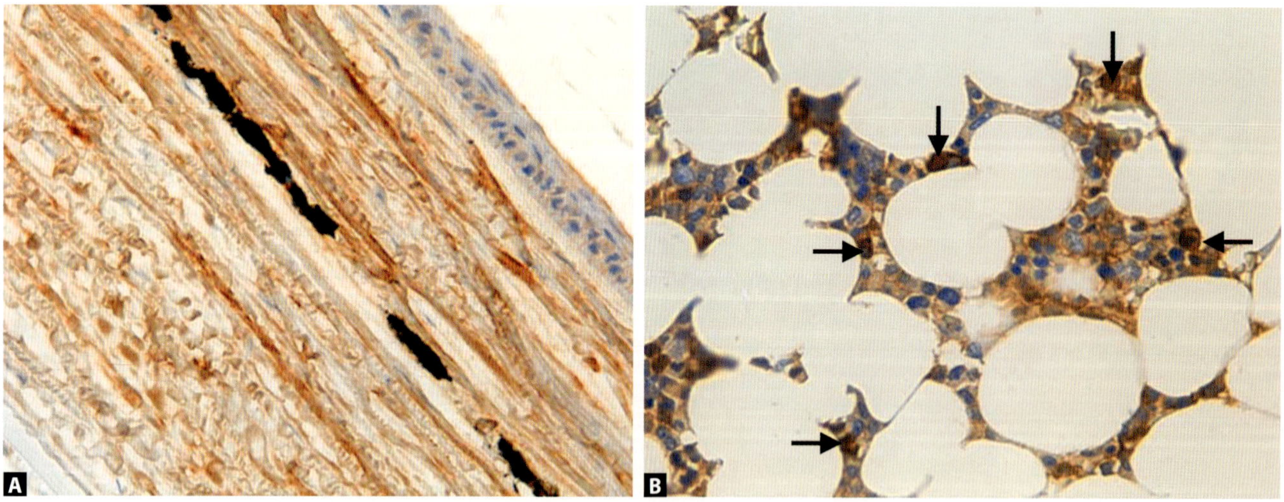

Fig. 8.9: Leukocyte common antigen immunostaining. (A) Nonspecific immunostaining is observed in this rabbit cornea; (B) Cells showing immunoreaction in same rabbit bone marrow (arrows)[7]

immunohistochemistry to differentiate between histological sections from lymphomas and carcinomas.[11]

To assess the presence of inflammation, a leukocyte common antigen (LCA) immunostaining, monoclonal antibody antimouse, can be performed, using standard techniques. The rabbit bone marrow could be used to compare as a positive control (Figure 8.9).[7]

This type of immunostaining reveals the presence of leukocytes in the treated cornea. It is possible to appreciate in Figure 8.9 that the staining is negative, concluding that the pigments did not arouse any inflammatory reaction in this preparation (Figure 8.9A), while in the positive control used (rabbit bone marrow) immunoreactive cells were detected (Figure 8.9B).[7]

To determine the presence or absence of inflammation is crucial to prove the tolerance and biocompatibility of the cornea for keratopigmentation using these mineral pigments. There is sufficient evidence that confirms that this micronized mineral pigments are safe to use in human cornea, and many more experiments would be needed to explore different colours and types of dyes before they can be used in patients.

REFERENCES

1. Sekundo W, Seifert P, Seitz B, Loeffler KU. Long-term ultrastructural changes in human corneas after tattooing with non-metallic substances. Br J Ophthalmol. 1999;83: 219-24.
2. Fujita H, Ueda A, Nishida T, Otori T. Uptake of India ink particles and latex beads by corneal fibroblasts. Cell Tissue Res. 1987;250:251-5.
3. Takahashi J, Sakimoto T, Kitano S. The phagocytosis in the stroma of tattooed cornea. Atarashii Ganka. 1990;7:725-28.
4. Olander K, Kanai A, Kaufman HE. An analytical electron microscopic study of a corneal tattoo. Ann Ophthalmol. 1983;15: 1046-49.
5. Lea PJ, Pawlowski A. Human tattoo. Electron microscopic assessment of epidermis, epidermal-dermal junction, and dermis. Int J Dermatol. 1987;26:453-8.
6. Amesty MA, Alio JL, Rodriguez A. Corneal tolerance to micronized mineral pigments for keratopigmentation. Br J Ophthalmol. 2014;98:1756-60
7. Amesty MA (2014) Tolerancia y Biocompatibilidad corneal tras Queratopigmentación con pigmentos minerales micronizados. Directores: Jorge L. Alió, José L Encinas. Tesis Doctoral. Departamento de Cirugía. Universidad Autónoma de Madrid.
8. Rey S (2013). "Queratopigmentación: Histopatología, toxicidad, reactividad biológica. Estudio Experimental." Director: Jorge L. Alió. Tesis Doctoral. Departamento de Patología y Cirugía. Universidad Miguel Hernández, Elche-Alicante.
9. Sirerol B, Walewska-Szafran A, Alió JL, et al. Tolerance and biocompatibility of micronized black pigment for keratopigmentation simulated pupil reconstruction. Cornea. 2011;30:344-50.
10. Kaplan R, Morse B, Huebner K, et al. Cloning of three human tyrosine phosphatases reveals a multigene family of receptor-linked protein-tyrosine-phosphatases expressed in brain. Proc. Natl. Acad. Sci. USA. 1990;87:7000–4.
11. Leong, Anthony S-Y, Cooper, Kumarason; Leong, F Joel W-M. Manual of Diagnostic Cytology (2 edn). Greenwich Medical Media, Ltd. pp. 2003;121-124. ISBN 1-84110-100-1.

Section 2

Experimental Atlas of Keratopigmentation

Editors: Jorge L Alió, Alejandra Rodríguez

Experimental Atlas of Keratopigmentation

9

SURGICAL INSTRUMENTS FOR KERATOPIGMENTATION

In this section, we present the surgical instruments specially designed for keratopigmentation (Figures 9.1 to 9.3).

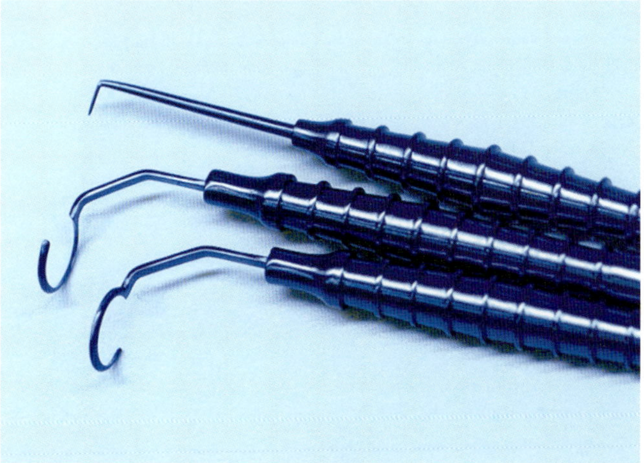

Fig. 9.1: Helicoidal corneal dissector (Epsilon, USA) used for iris simulation

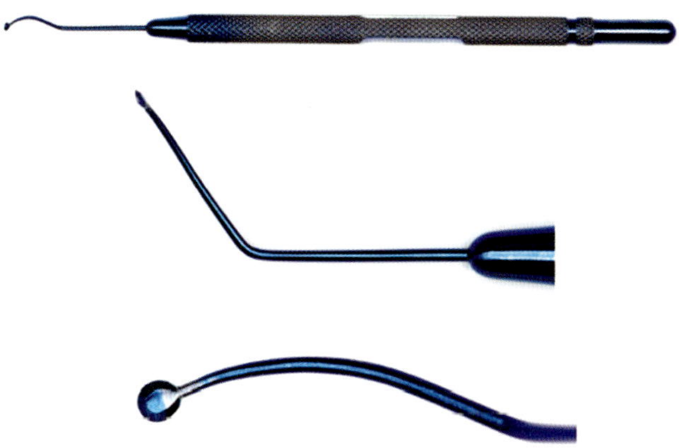

Fig. 9.2: Curve pupil corneal dissector (Epsilon, USA) used for pupil simulation

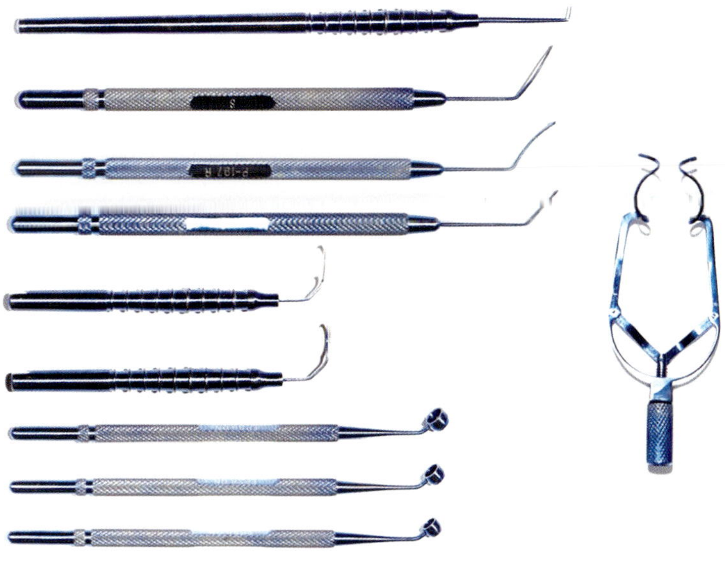

Fig. 9.3: Instruments tray used for keratopigmentation, including helicoidal corneal dissectors, speculums, epithelial pupil markers in different sizes and curve pupil corneal dissectors

MANUAL INTRALAMELLAR KERATOPIGMENTATION IN CADAVER PIG EYES

This technique was carried out using the instruments specially designed for corneal tattooing previously described, different colors of micronized mineral pigments, and the keratopigmentation was performed in pig cadaver eyes to study and select the resulting colors (Figure 9.4).

After using the manual intralamellar keratopigmentation (MIK) technique pigmentation eyes were fixed in 10% formalin and were processed for histopathology. The sections of the corneas were stained with Hematoxylin-Eosin (H and E) and analysed to assess how deep the pigment was in the corneal stroma. The average depth of the pigment was 106 microns (Figure 9.5).

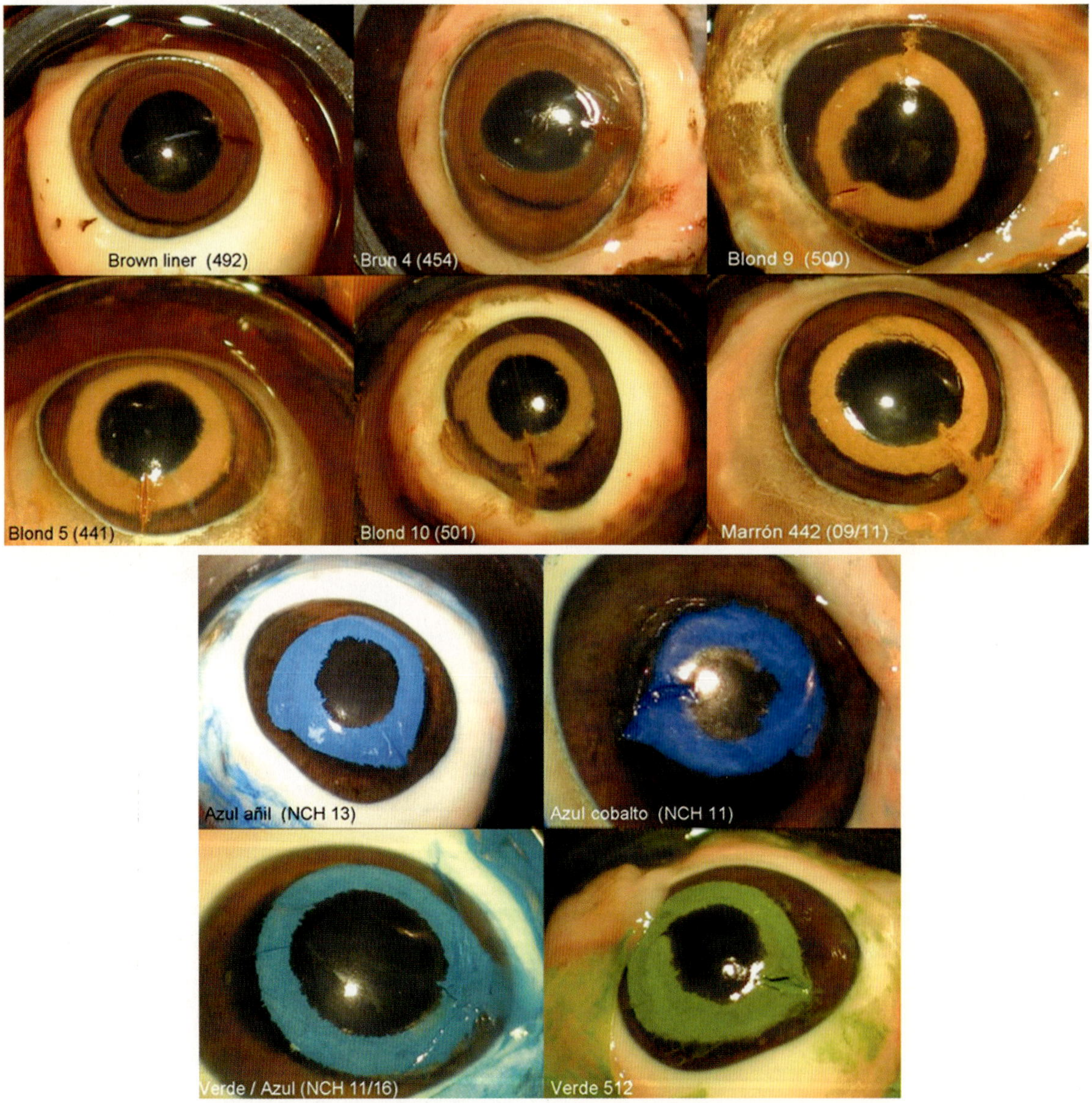

Fig. 9.4: Manual intralamellar keratopigmentation

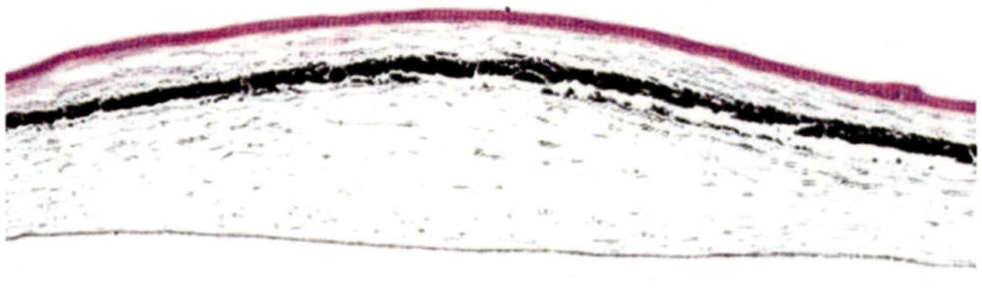

Fig. 9.5: Section of cornea stained with H and E. Magnification 400x

SUPERFICIAL AUTOMATED KERATOPIGMENTATION (SAK) IN PIG CADAVER EYES

To study the depth in the corneal stroma reached by the micropunctures performed for superficial keratopigmentation, many tests were carried out with almost all types of needles available in pig cadaver eyes. Then the eyes were processed for histopathology to measure the pigments depth.

The "maximum" depth refers to the maximum distance that the needle protrudes from the plastic cartridge, while the "minimum" refers to the minimum distance required to reach the cornea and pigment corneal tissue.

With this needles depth study we concluded that the correct depth to work with and at the same time have an adequated safety margin is the "minimum possible". The depth did not exceed 250 microns with any of the needles used in this test.

Human cornea thickness is normally between 500 and 550 microns, these values would be perfectly safe to pigment the cornea without the risk of perforation (Figures 9.6 to 9.8).

Another important aspect is that when the pigment is placed below the corneal epithelium, also favors its retention in the corneal stroma, because the pigment in the superficial transitional epithelium area fades due to the frequent cell regeneration on this area of the cornea.

Considering the data collected during this study we have decided to simplify the use of the different needles and we

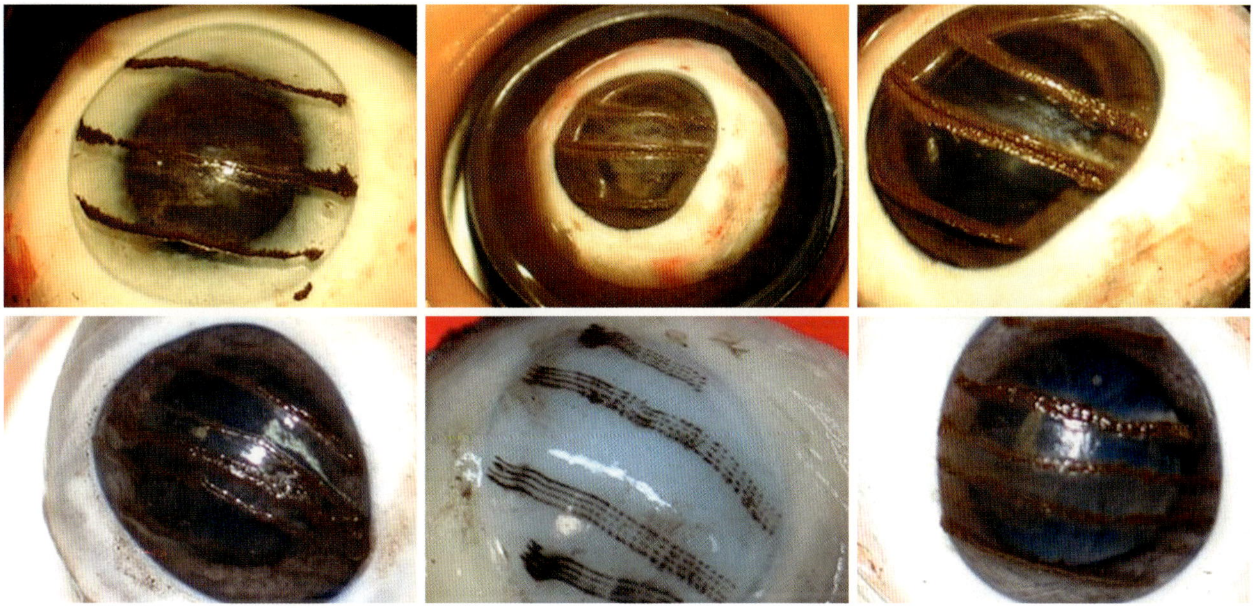

Fig. 9.6: Depth test with different needles in experimental cadaver eyes

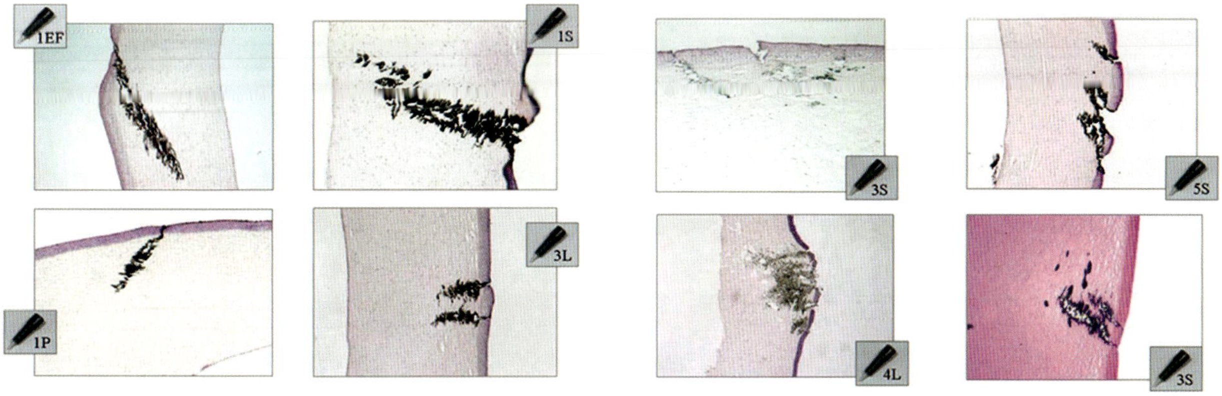

Fig. 9.7: Histological sections stained with H&E showing the maximum depth with different needles

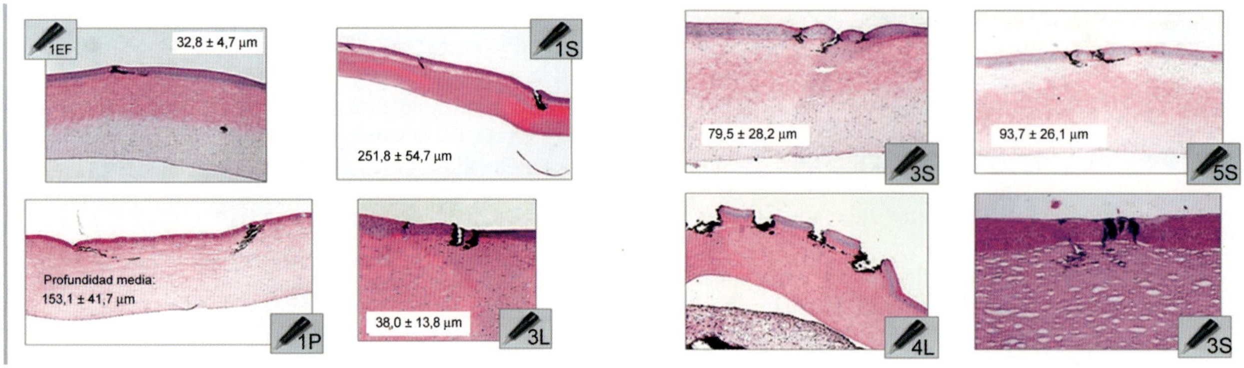

Fig. 9.8: Histological sections stained with H & E showing the minimum depth with different needles

have selected the most suitable depending on the area of the cornea that requires pigmentation:

- Needle #1: For small details and limbus area.
- Needle #5: For pupil and iris area.
- Needle #3: For general purposes.

Considering the suitable depth and the correct needle depending on the corneal area that requires pigmentation, the next step is to decide the color that better match the other eye. Therefore, another study was carried out in pig cadaver eyes to pigment and to reproduce the colors of a human iris (Figures 9.9 and 9.10).

Some colors were also mixed to get a more natural look and a more physiological cosmetic result (Figures 9.11 and 9.12).

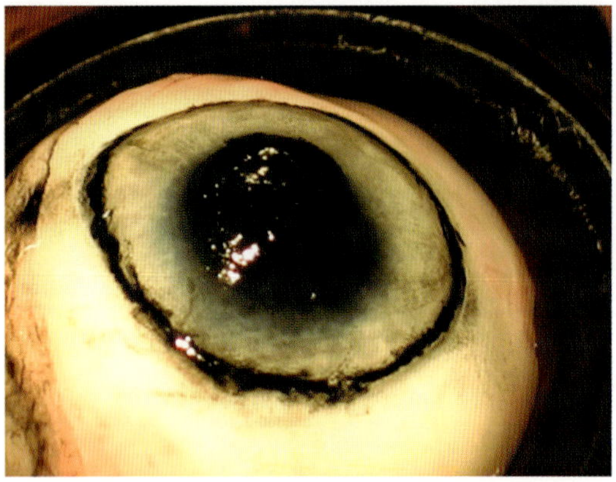

Fig. 9.9: Pupil + corneal limbus (Black)

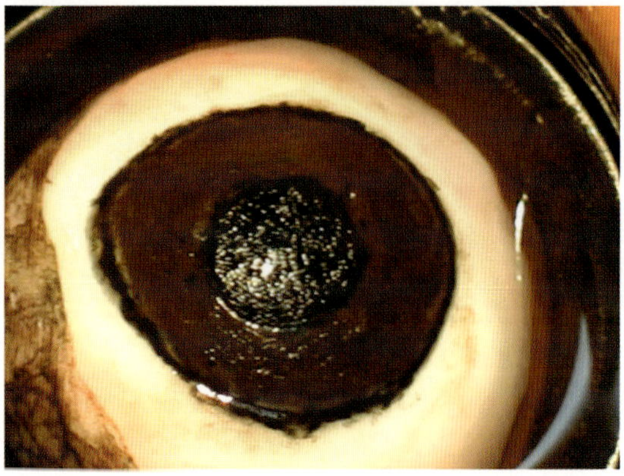

Fig. 9.10: Pupil + corneal limbus (Black) + Iris (Brown)

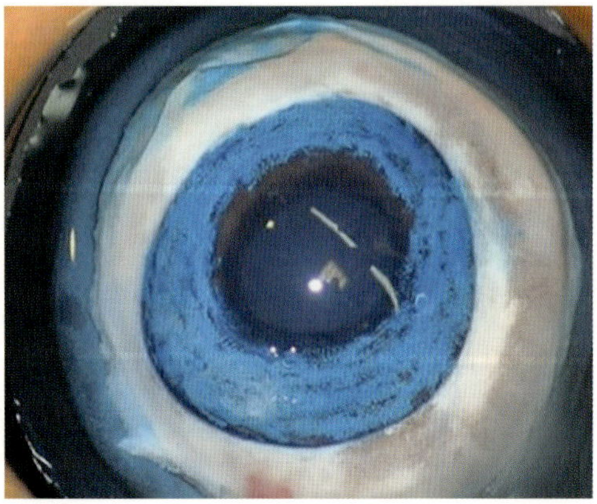

Fig. 9.11: Cobalt blue

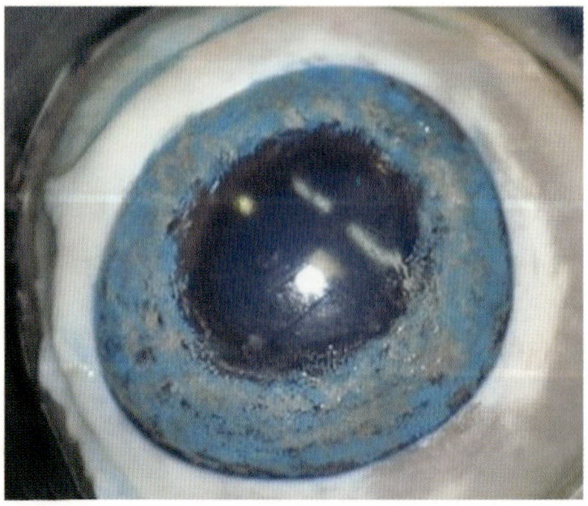

Fig. 9.12: Cobalt blue + Light gray + Dark gray

BIOCOMPATIBILITY AND TOLERANCE TESTS TO MICRONIZED MINERAL PIGMENTS FOR MANUAL INTRALAMELLAR KERATOPIGMENTATION (MIK) IN RABBITS

Objective

The purpose of this study was to determine the biocompatibility and tolerance to a series of micronized mineral pigments for keratopigmentation (corneal pigmentation or corneal tattooing), by using experimental animals. It is very important to test these pigments for keratopigmentation in animal models before moving to pilot studies in humans.

Methods

The animals (48 New Zealand rabbits) underwent a corneal pocket in only one eye, in which the micronized pigment was injected, using a 23 gauge irrigation cannula. Half of the animals were euthanized one month after the procedure and the other half 3 months after surgery for histopathological study. Signs of corneal and conjunctival inflammation were examined and/or pigment dispersion or discoloration (fading) were also looked in this study.

A circular corneal pocket was created in the central area of the cornea to mimic the pupil and another pocket was performed in the peripheral area to simulate the iris (Figure 9.13).

In this study four colors were tested: Black, Brown, Green and Blue (Figure 9.14).

Results

Three months after the injection of these different pigments, the clinical signs observed were the following Table 9.1).

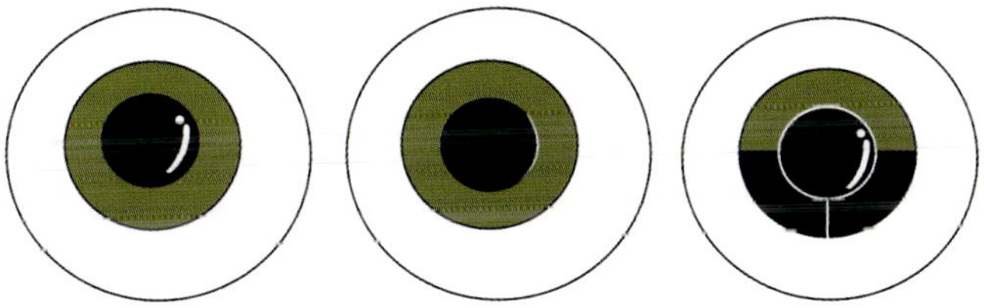

Fig. 9.13: These drawings represent the area of the cornea in which the pigmentation will be carried out

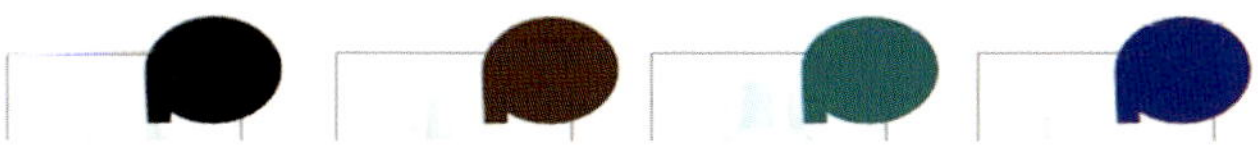

Fig. 9.14: Colors used for keratopigmentation in rabbits with MIK technique

The pigmented rabbit eyes showed the clinical results (Figures 9.15 to 9.17).

Table 9.1: Clinical results observed after 3 months of the keratopigmentation (MIK)

Pigment	*Clinical signs*		*Diffusion of pigment*
	Central KTP	*Peripheral KTP*	
Black	None	None	NO
Brown	Moderate inflammation	Moderate inflammation	NO
Green	None	Mild inflammation	NO
Blue	Mild inflammation	Moderate inflammation	NO

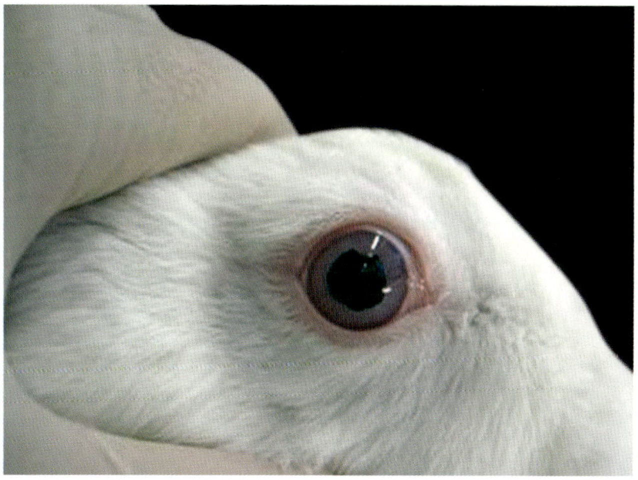

Fig. 9.15: Manual intralamellar keratopigmentation (MIK) with black pigment in the central area simulating the pupil

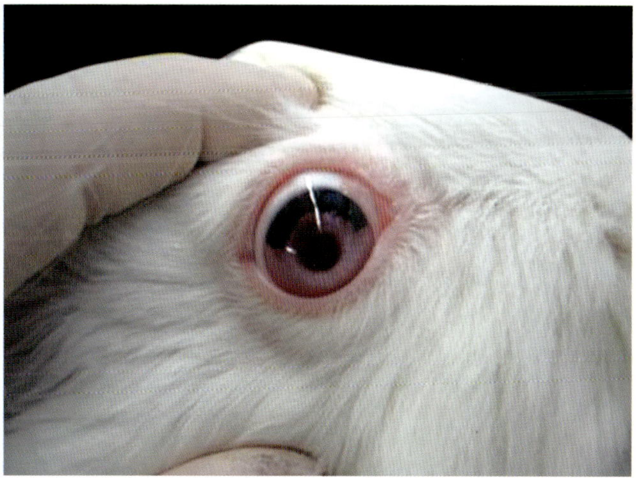

Fig. 9.16: Manual intralamellar keratopigmentation (MIK) with black pigment in the peripheral area simulating half inferior iris

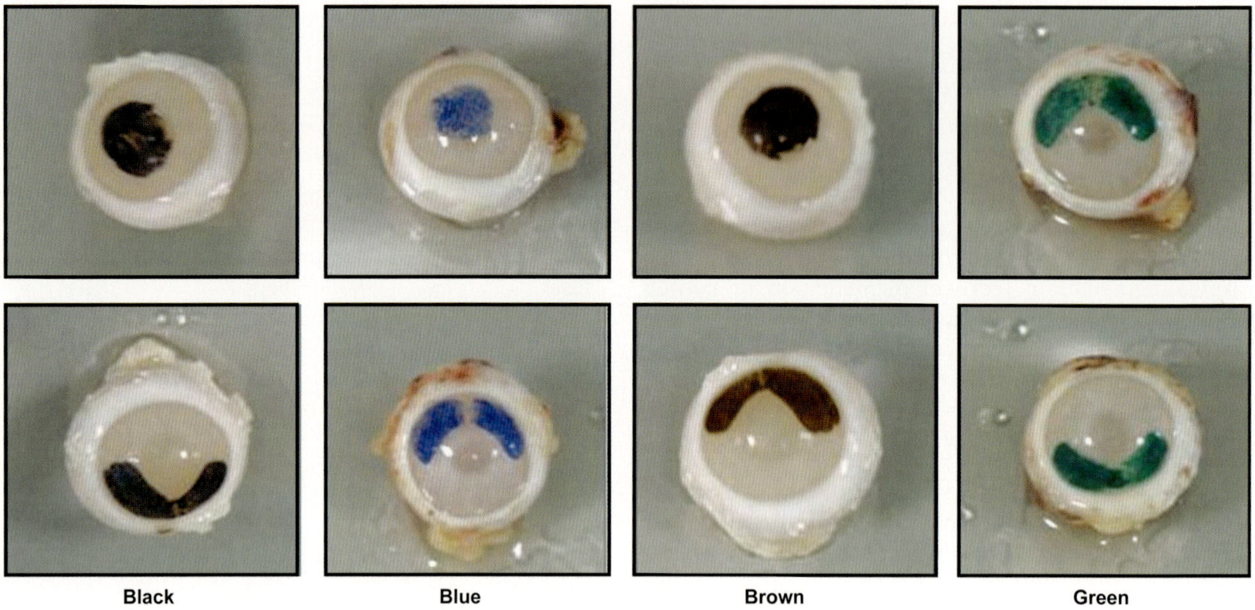

Fig. 9.17: Pigmented rabbit eyes after enucleation

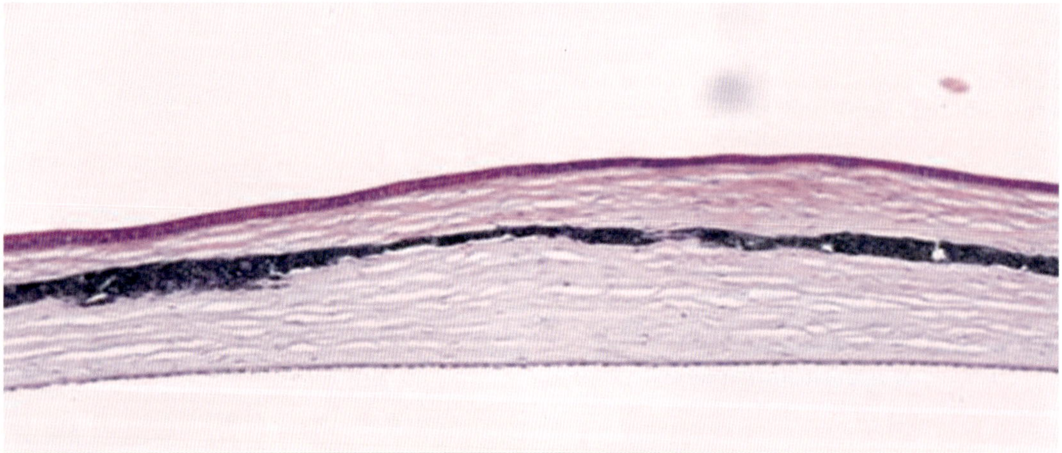

Fig. 9.18: Manual intralamellar keratopigmentation (MIK) technique in rabbits. No inflammation is observed with H and E stain. Magnification 100x

Histopathological examination of the studied corneas correlated with the previous results observed clinically. None inflammation (Figure 9.18) was observed with the black pigment, moderate inflammation with the brown pigment, mild inflammation with the blue, and none or mild inflammation with the green pigment.

SUPERFICIAL AUTOMATED KERATOPIGMENTATION (SAK) FOR KERATOPIGMENTATION IN AN ANIMAL MODEL

Objective

The purpose of this study is to evaluate "*in vivo*", using a rabbit model, the superficial automated technique for corneal micropigmentation.

Methods

18 New Zealand albino rabbits were used. Central corneal micropigmentation was performed to simulate the pupil, using permanent Black pigment and needle 1 in nine rabbits. Peripheral corneal micropigmentation was performed to simulate the iris, using Permanent Black pigment with needle 5 in the other nine (Figures 9.19 and 9.20).

Results

Seven months after surgery there was no inflammatory response and no signs of corneal neovascularization was observed in any of the animals. With the correct parameters and the depth of the needles used, no ocular perforations or other surgical complications occurred.

The visual and cosmetic appearance of the corneal micropigmentation was excellent. A minimal fading of the pigmentation was noticed 7 months after the surgery (Figures 9.21 and 9.22).

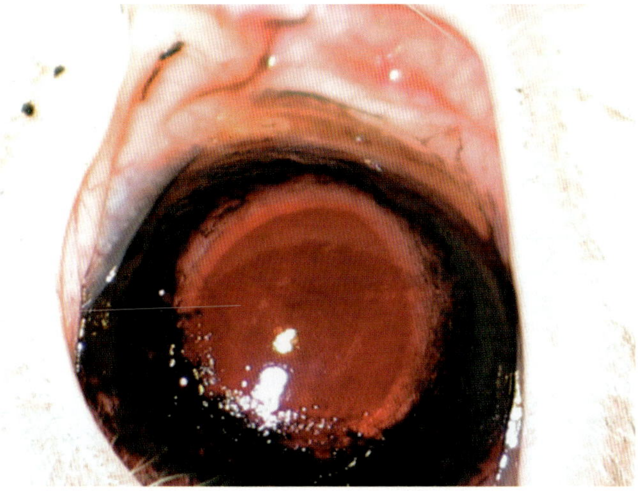

Fig. 9.19: Peripheral corneal micropigmentation (iris simulation). Immediately postsurgery

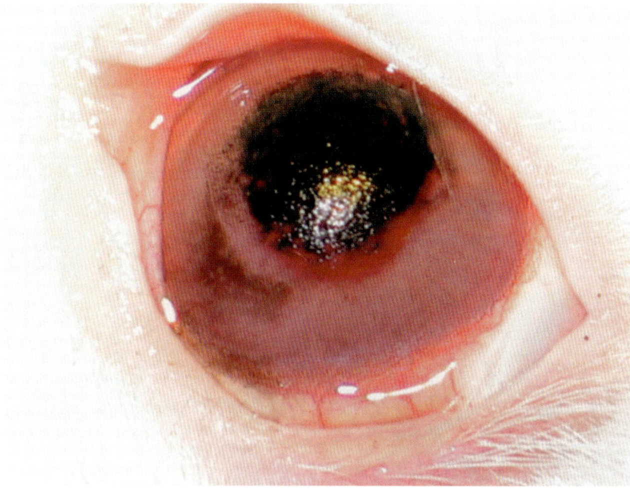

Fig. 9.20: Central corneal micropigmentation (pupil simulation). Immediately postsurgery

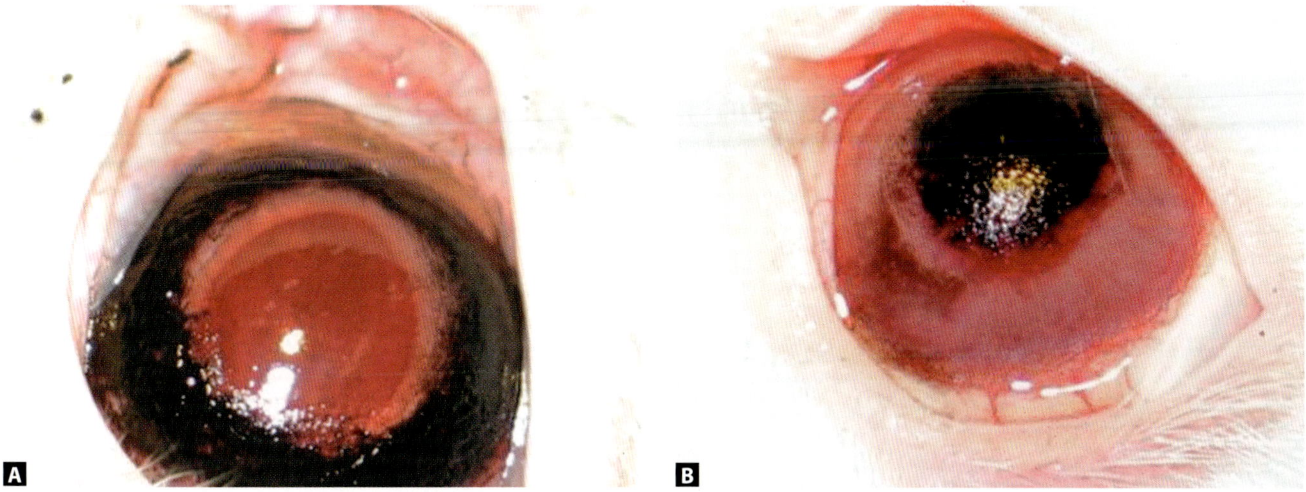

Figs 9.21A and B: Peripheral corneal micropigmentation (iris simulation). Two months postsurgery

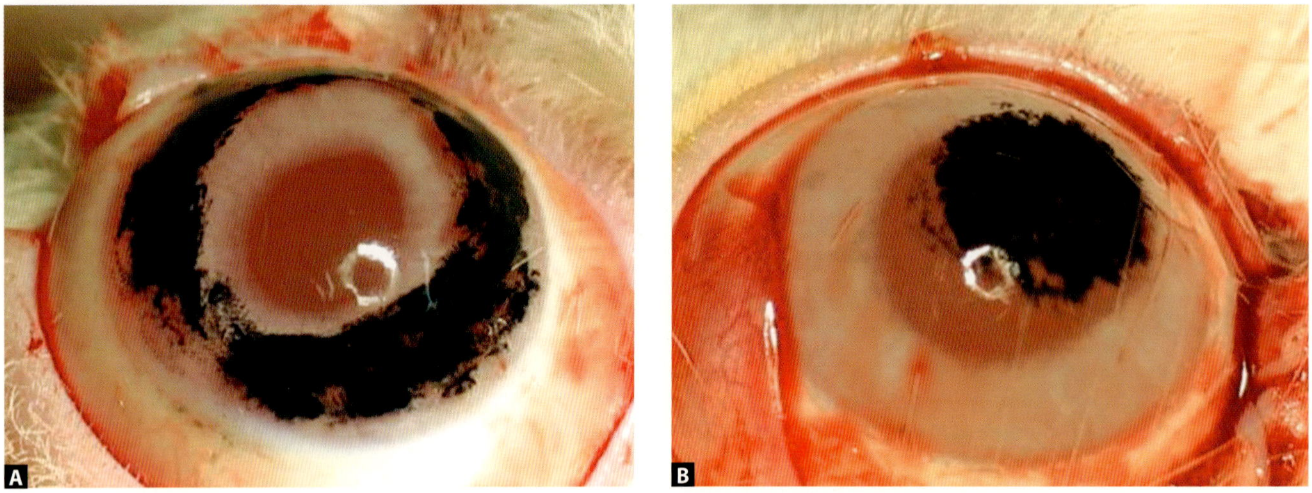

Figs 9.22A and B: Central corneal micropigmentation (pupil simulation). Seven months postsurgery

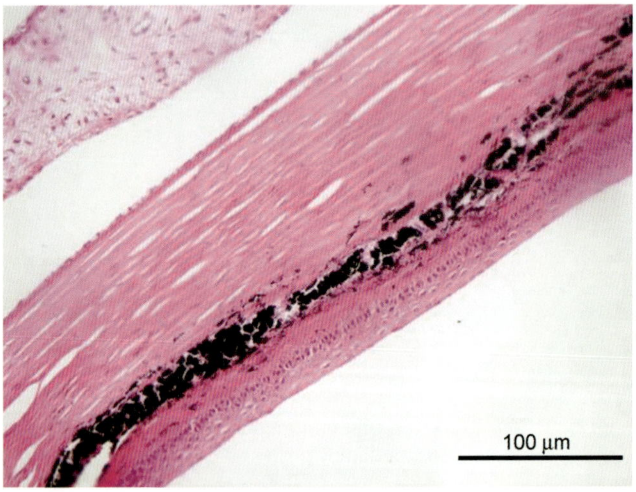

Fig. 9.23: Peripheral corneal SAK (iris simulation). H and E stain (Original magnification 400x)

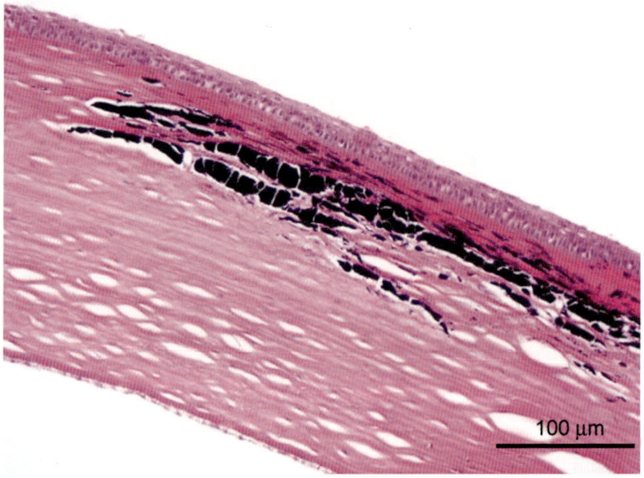

Fig. 9.24: Central corneal SAK (pupil simulation). H and E stain (Original magnification 400x)

Histopathology

Histopathology of the analysed corneas was similar to the clinical results observed. The studied corneas presented a few inflammatory cells within the stroma but there were no evidence of neovascularization. The location of the pigment was predominantly in the superficial third of the corneal stroma, and no diffusion the pigment was noticed (Figures 9.23 and 9.24).

Conclusion

The results obtained after the superficial micropigmentation technique in rabbits corneas were excellent. This results showed that keratopigmentation could be also considered for human pigmentation.

BIOCOMPATIBILITY AND TOLERANCE TESTS TO MICRONIZED MINERAL PIGMENTS FOR KERATOPIGMENTATION IN RABBITS USING PHYSIOLOGICAL COLORS

Objectives

- To study biocompatibility and tolerance of mixed micronized mineral pigments from a clinical and a histopathological perspective.
- To study the range of colors available for a more physiological cosmetic result, using micronized mineral pigments in a suitable experimental model, not only for cosmetic reasons but also for therapeutic purposes.

Procedure

Experimental model of 28 eyes belonging to 14 adult New Zealand albino rabbits were used. A corneal intralamellar tunnel was performed to inject the pigment inside those tunnels. The steps were as follows:

- A 5 mm pupillary area was marked with a surgical marker.
- A radial incision was performed with a surgical blade, up to a depth of approximately 200 microns.
- An intrastromal dissection of approximately 50% of the corneal thickness was performed using an 8 mm intrastromal corneal dissector (corneal CPK spiral dissector, Epsilon, Irvine CA, USA) to simulate the iris (180° clockwise and 180° counterclockwise) respecting the pupillary area (5 mm) and trying to make a single (connected) 360° tunnel.
- The tunnel was extended with a 10 mm dissector and the selected color was injected using a 1 mL syringe and a 23 gauge irrigation cannula.
- The incision was closed without stitches (Figures 9.25 and 9.26).

Follow-up

- The animals were examined under slit lamp 1 week, 1 month, 2 months and 3 months after surgery.
- At 3 months after surgery, the animals were sacrificed and eyes enucleated for histopathology.

Pigments

The keratopigmentation was performed using micronized mineral pigments. These pigments are registered with the Spanish Drug Agency (AEMPS) and comply with the Resolution of the Council of Europe (RasAP). The colors used were light blue, green, bluish brown and greenish brown. The pigments were mixed and dissolved in sterile saline solution (BSS) to achieve more physiological colors and to mimic the normal color of a human iris.

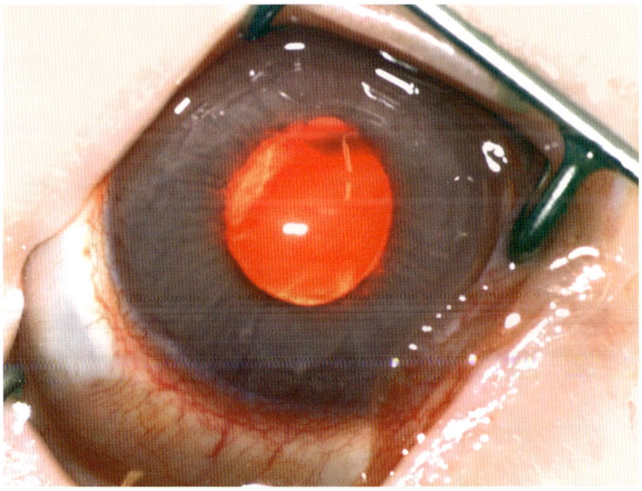

Fig. 9.25: New Zealand Albino Rabbit eye before keratopigmentation

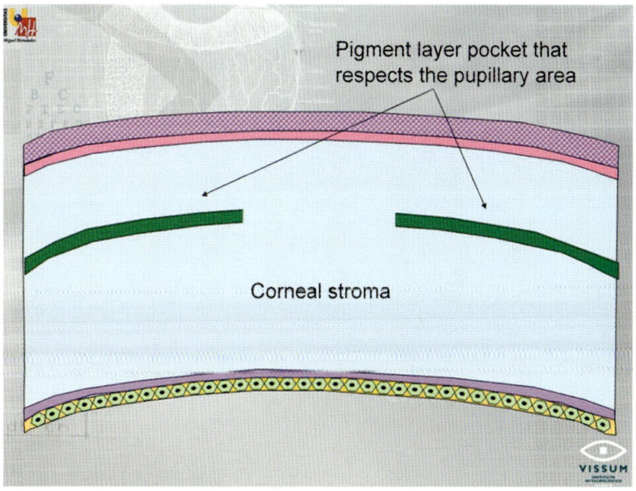

Fig. 9.26: Intrastromal technique of corneal dissector

Clinical Results

Three months after the injection of the different pigments, the clinical examination of the pigmented eyes was performed. No signs of conjunctival hyperemia, or swelling, or neovascularization were observed.

The pigmented rabbit eyes had the following aspect 3 months after the surgery (Figures 9.27A to D:

The histopathological examination of the corneas correlates very well with the clinical results observed, showing neither swelling, nor neovascularization (Figures 9.28A and B).

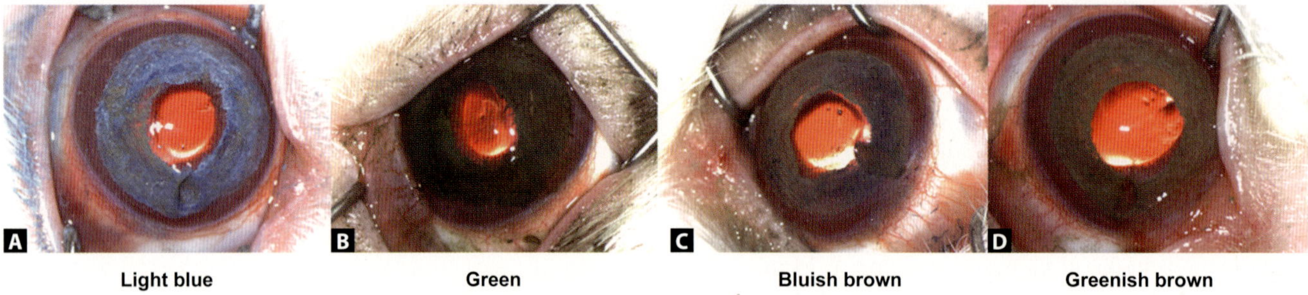

Figs 9.27A to D: Pigmented rabbit eyes after 3 months of follow-up. The colors used were more physiologic and the technique used was a complete tunnel

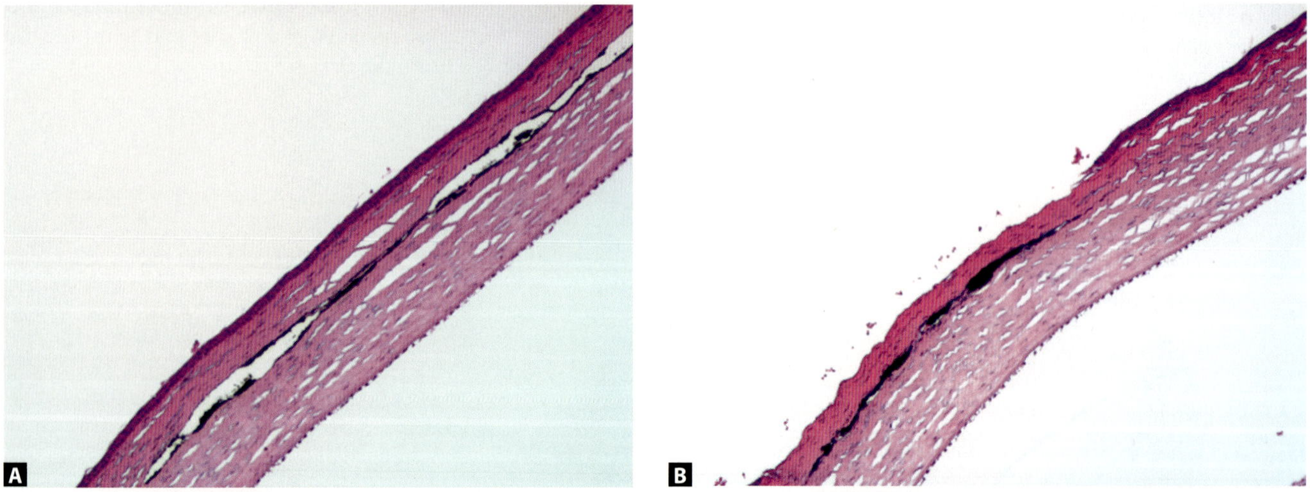

Figs 9.28A and B: Intrastromal micropigmentation: No inflammation is observed. Hematoxylin-Eosin staining. Magnification 100x.

REPRODUCTION OF THE EYE OF A PATIENT

In this case, we try of reproduce the normal iris of a patient in an experimental pig cadaver eye using both Manual Intralamellar Keratopigmentation (MIK) and Superficial Automated Keratopigmentation (SAK) techniques.

MIK technique was carried out with only one incision at 12 o'clock using an helicoidal corneal dissector (Epsilon, USA). Then the pigment was injected in the tunnel using a light blue color (Figures 9.29 and 9.30).

After MIK, SAK technique was performed circumferentially along the pupil area to simulate the morphology of the iris. A light grey pigment was also used in the same way for the gray details of the eye. To complete the pigmentation, light brown dots were performed to achieve a more natural look.

For a more natural look, the light blue pigment was applied using a zig zag maneuver around all the corneal limbus to achieve a darker blue tone in the external part of the iris.

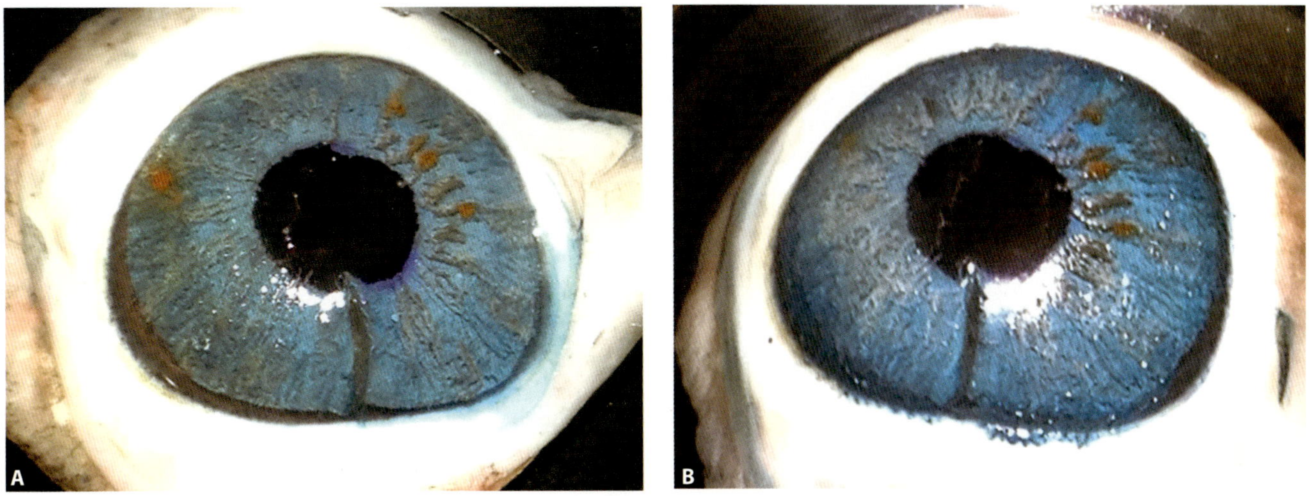

Figs 9.29A and B: Reproduction of blue eye of a patient in an experimental eye

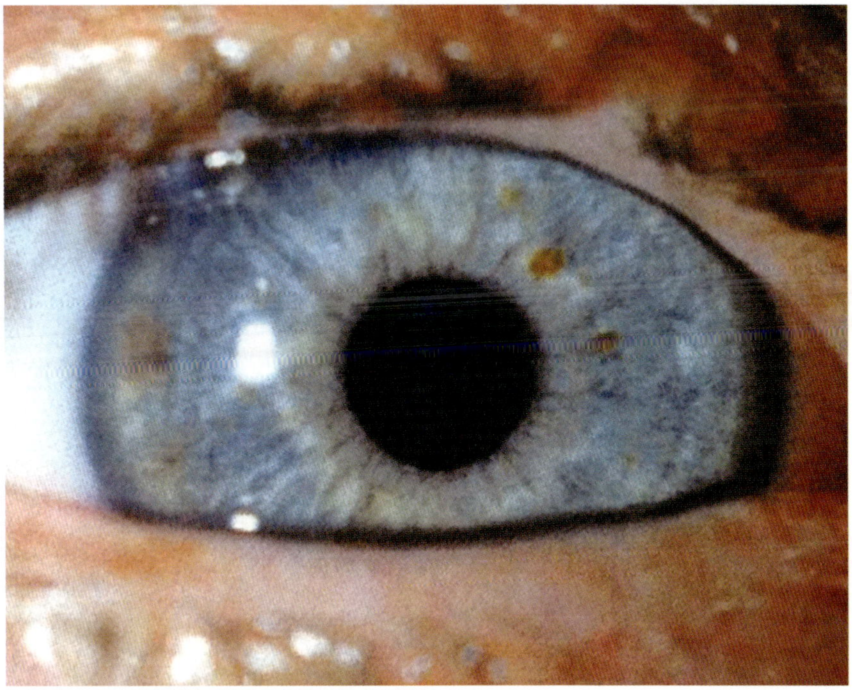

Fig. 9.30: Normal blue eye of a patient

SAME COLOR AND DIFFERENT TECHNIQUES

In this case, we used a blue pigment intralamellarly with MIK technique in the left half and the same color in the right half but with superficial technique (SAK) following a radial pattern.

The most important conclusion of this experiment is that the intensity of a color can change if the pigment is applied intrastromally or superficially. This result is consistent with all the colors tested.

This experiment was important to determine that the selection of the pigment color should be different if MIK or SAK will be performed (Figures 9.31A to C).

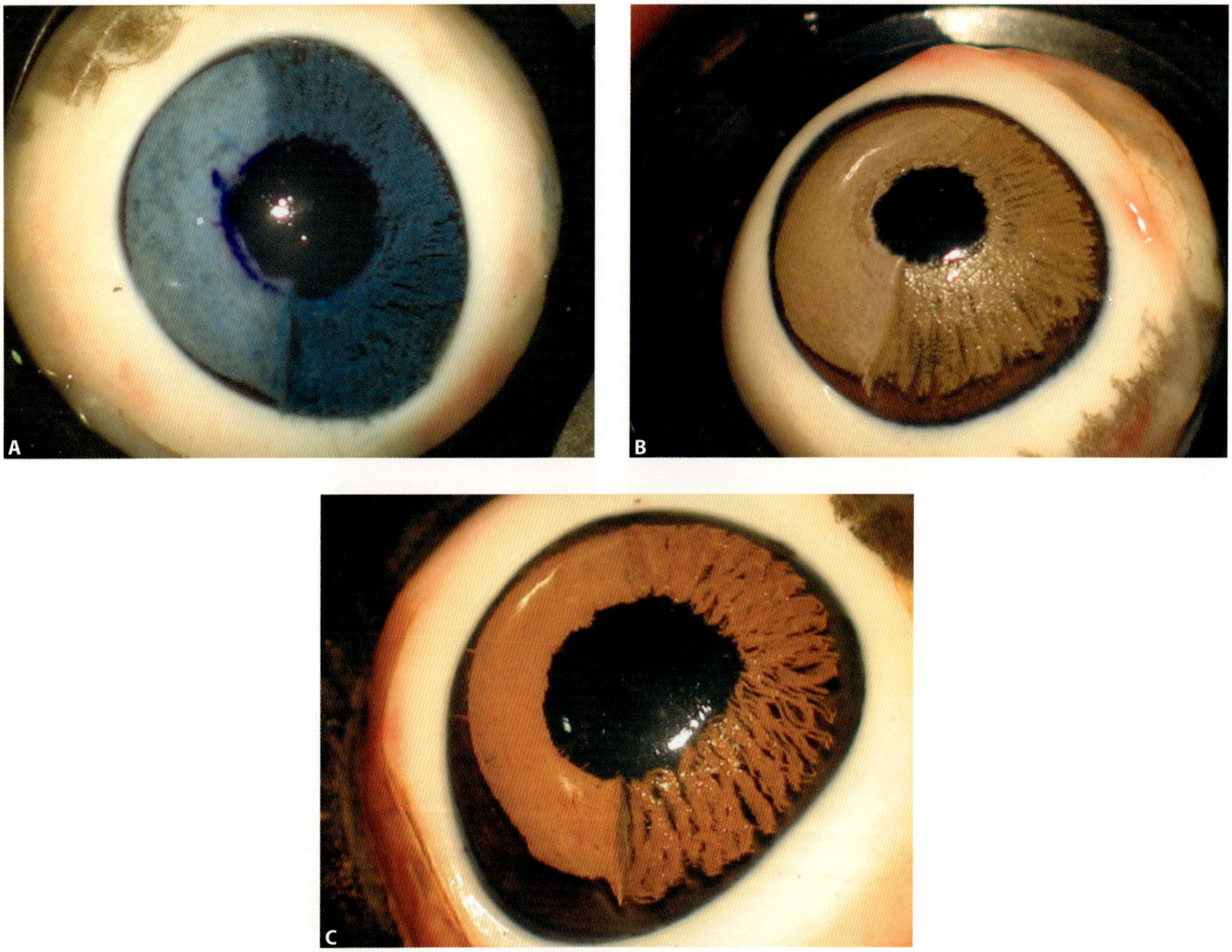

Figs 9.31A to C: Blue, gray and light brown colors applied intralamellarly (MIK) on the left half and using the superficial technique (SAK) on the right half. In all of them we can appreciate the left half with MIK more light color than the right half with SAK

Section 3

Clinical Atlas of Keratopigmentation

Editors: Jorge L Alió, Mohamed El Bahrawy

Clinical Atlas of Keratopigmentation

10

PART I: COSMETIC THERAPEUTIC KERATOPIGMENTATION

SUPERFICIAL AUTOMATED KERATOPIGMENTATION (SAK)

CASE 1

Clinical Histroy

A 15-year-old male with high myopia and history of right eye retinal detachment, presented with a visual acuity of perception of light on his right eye and 0.3 (decimal value) on his left eye.

Preoperative Data

On slit lamp examination, there was a right eye corneal opacity with band keratopathy and traumatic severe iris defects. Fundus examination showed the retinal detachment treated with silicone oil. Preretinal fibrosis and atrophic retinopathy were also observed. The examination of the left eye was within normal limits (Figure 10.1).

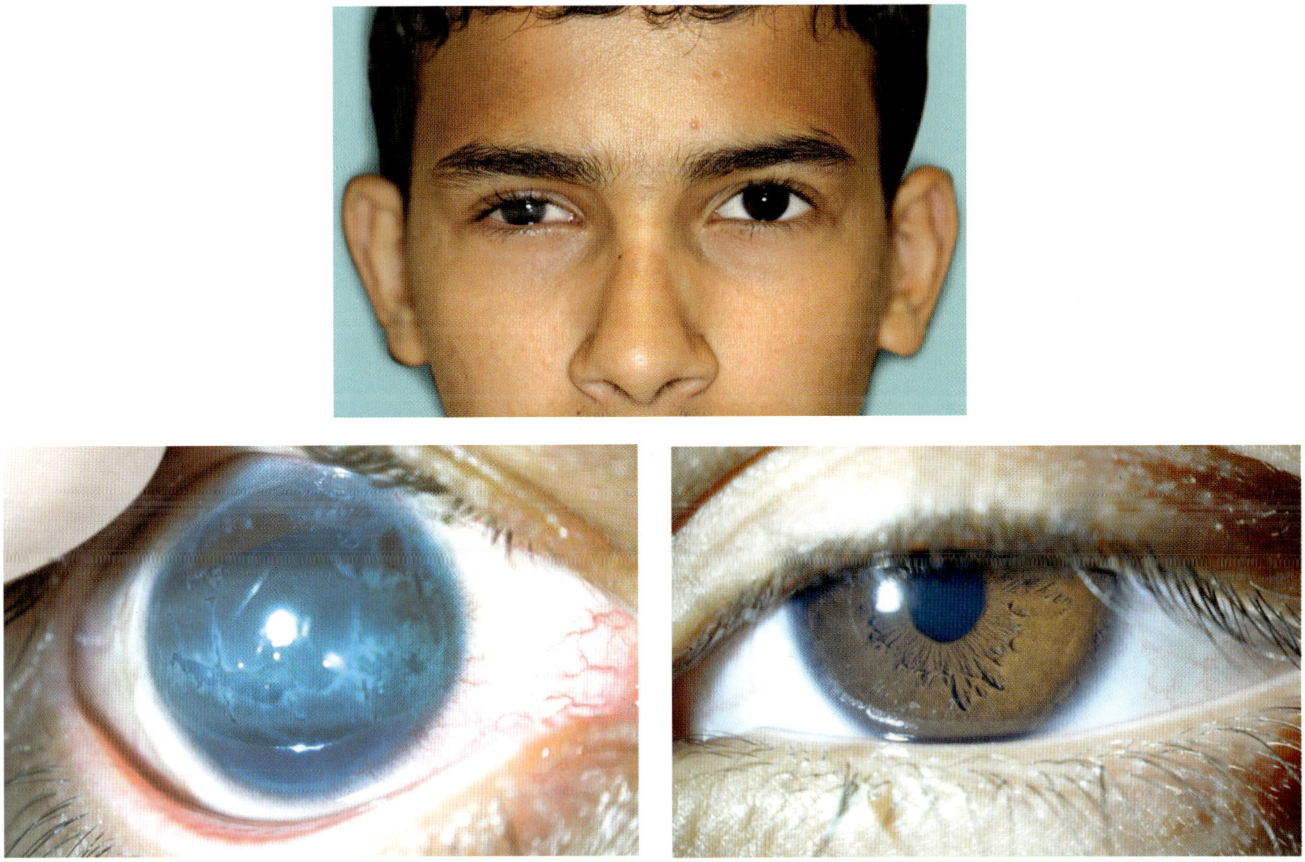

Fig. 10.1: (Above) Cosmetic appearance of both eyes; (Below) Normal left eye and band keratopathy of right eye

Surgical Technique

Superficial keratopigmentation technique:

Iris: Brown (VEMP 200) using needle number 3

Pupil: Black (VEMP 100) using needle number 1

Left eye phakic intraocular implantation on the same setting.

Postoperative Results

Excellent cosmetic appearance with minimal hyperemia but no further complications (Figure 10.2).

Follow-up and Comments

On follow-up appointments, it was observed that the pigmented cornea mimics very well the color of his left eye, but the pupil was slightly blurred (Figure 10.3).

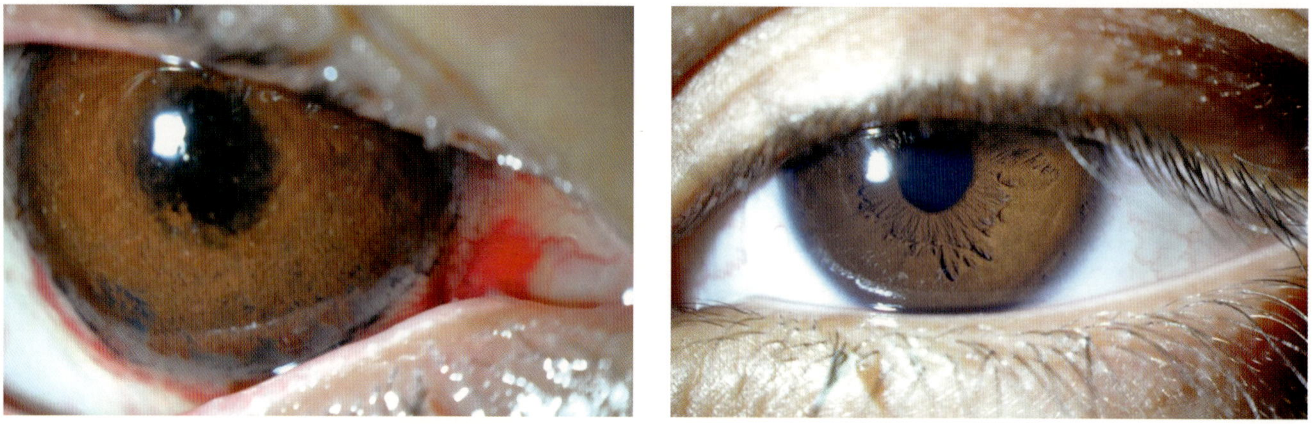

Fig. 10.2 : Postoperative results. Cosmetic appearance of both eyes

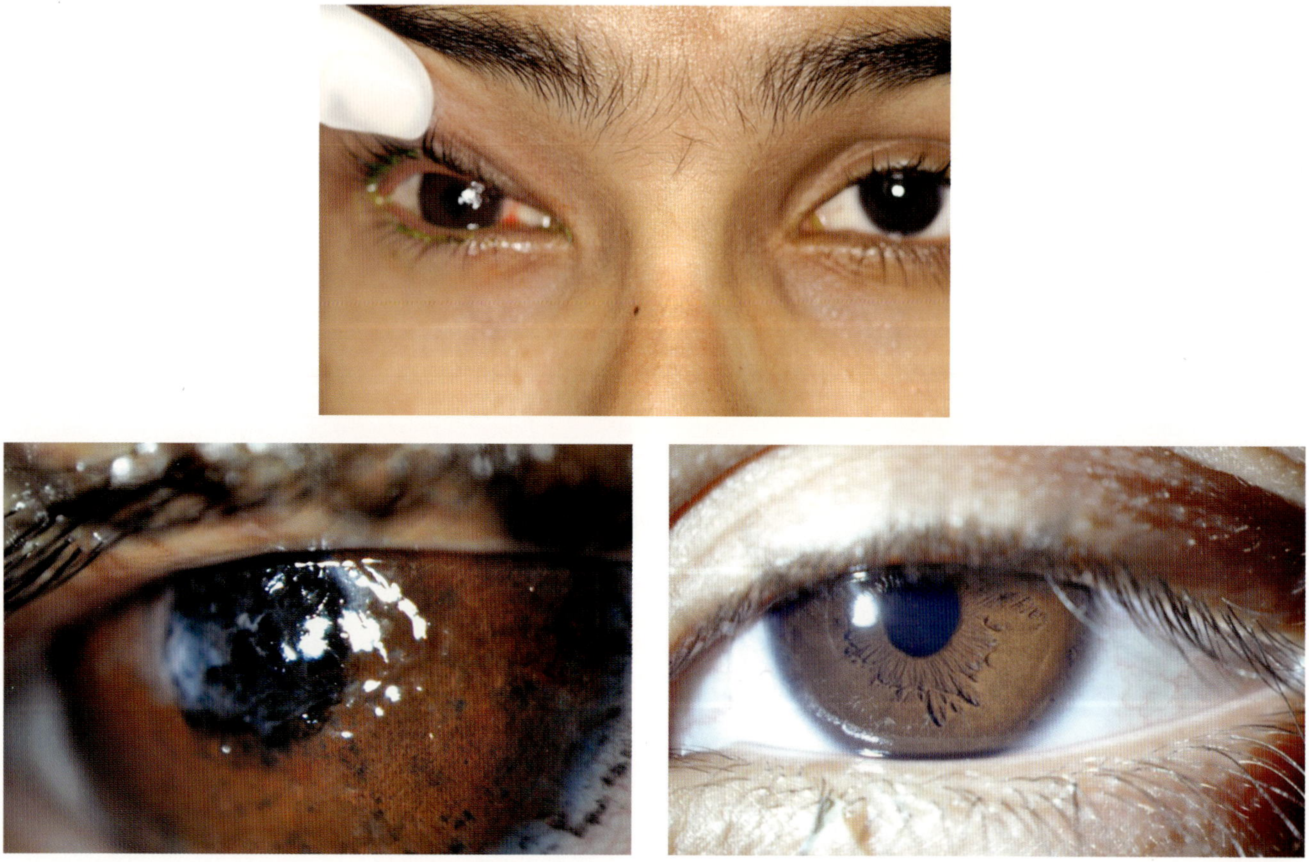

Fig. 10.3: Cosmetic results one month after the surgery

CASE 2

Clinical Histroy

A 33-year-old male with a history of trauma in his left eye, presented with a previous corneal tattooing and was interested in improving the cosmetic appearance of the corneal pigmentation

Preoperative Data

Slit-lamp examination showed a left band keratopathy with discoloration and fading of the previous pigmentation. His visual acuity was 1,0 (decimal value) and no perception of light for right and left eyes repectively (Figure 10.4).

Surgical Technique

Superficial technique: Using black carbon (VEMP 110) for the pupil area (marked using a calliper at 3,75 mm) and brown pigment (VEMP 200) to mask the rest of the band keratopathy.

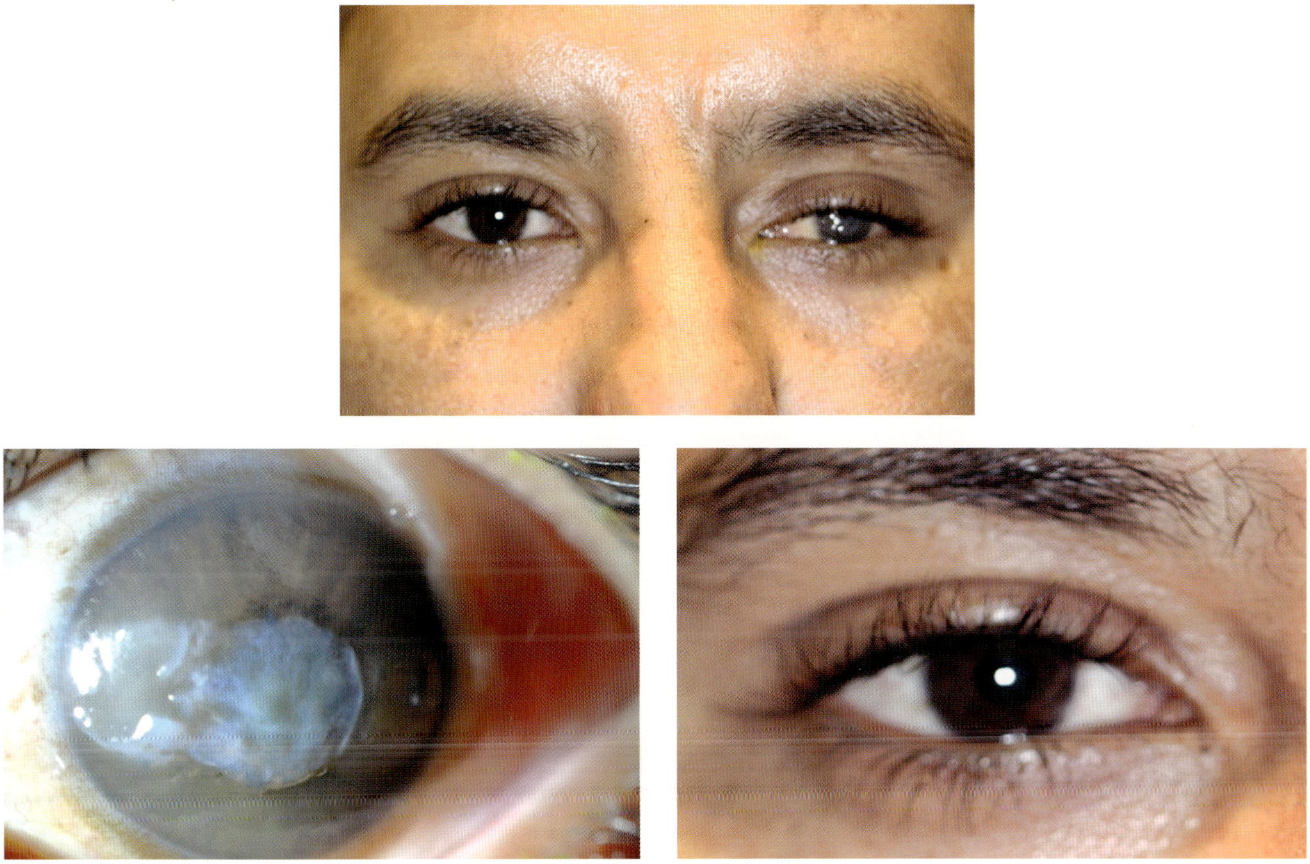

Fig. 10.4: Ocular examination: (Above) Cosmetic appearance of both eyes; (Below) Left corneal opacity

Postoperative Results

Minimal edema with excellent cosmetic appearance. Upper lid ptosis correction was recommended.

Follow-up and Comments

- On one month follow-up, pigment dispersion and discoloration was observed and repigmentation was recommended
- A second pigmentation was performed with alcohol assisted deepithelialization. The pupil diameter was marked at 3 mm and the pupil area pigmented with a black pigment. The rest was pigmented using a brown pigment
- The last examination demonstrated an excellent cosmetic result (Figure 10.5).

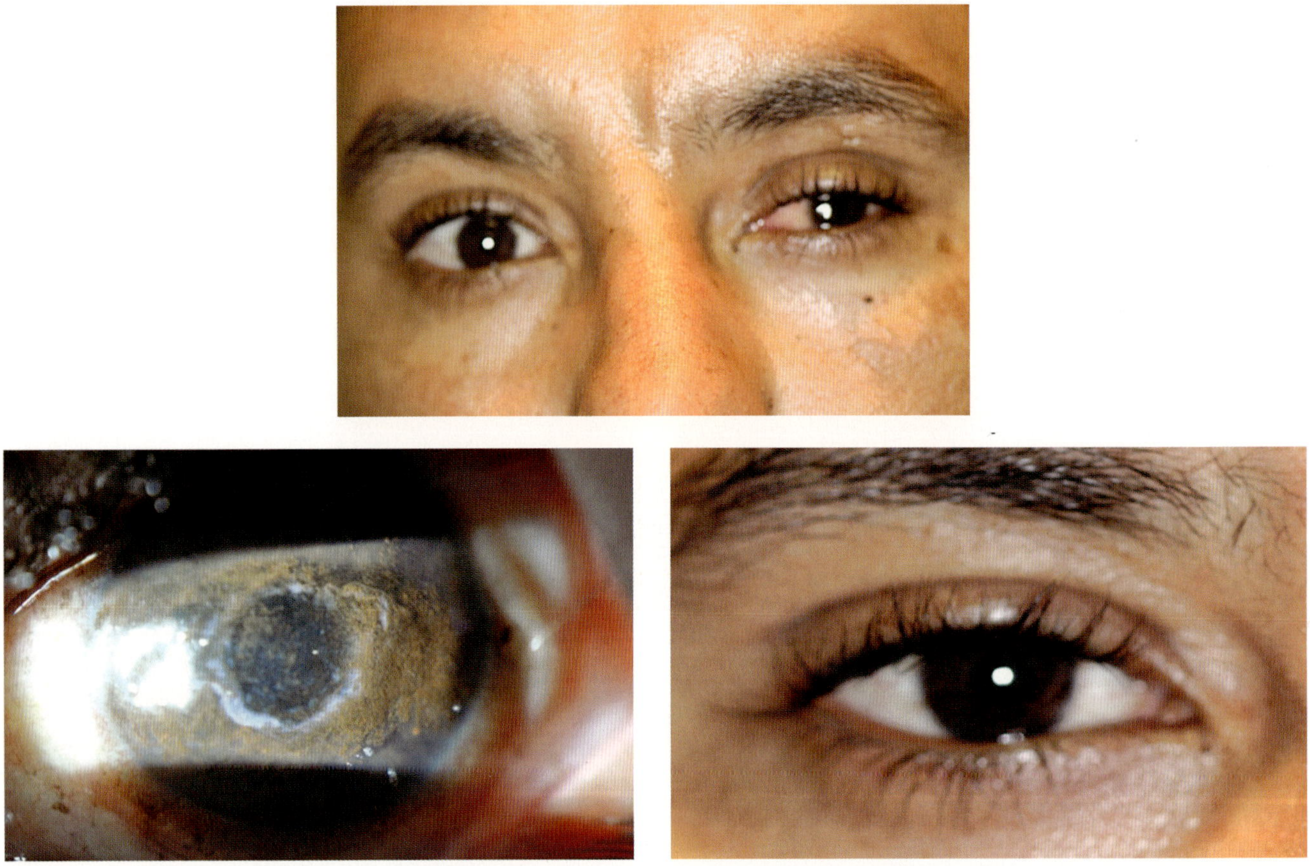

Fig. 10.5: Final results after superficial corneal staining

CASE 3

Clinical History

A 72-year-old female with high myopia and a previous complicated cataract surgery, subsequent endophthalmitis, presented with a secondary glaucoma and a left blind eye.

Preoperative Data

On examination, the right eye was pseudophakic. The left eye was aphakic and had a calcified corneal opacity (band keratopathy), with a dilated fixed pupil. Visual acuity was no perception of light on that side. Funduscopy showed areas of myopic atrophy (Figure 10.6).

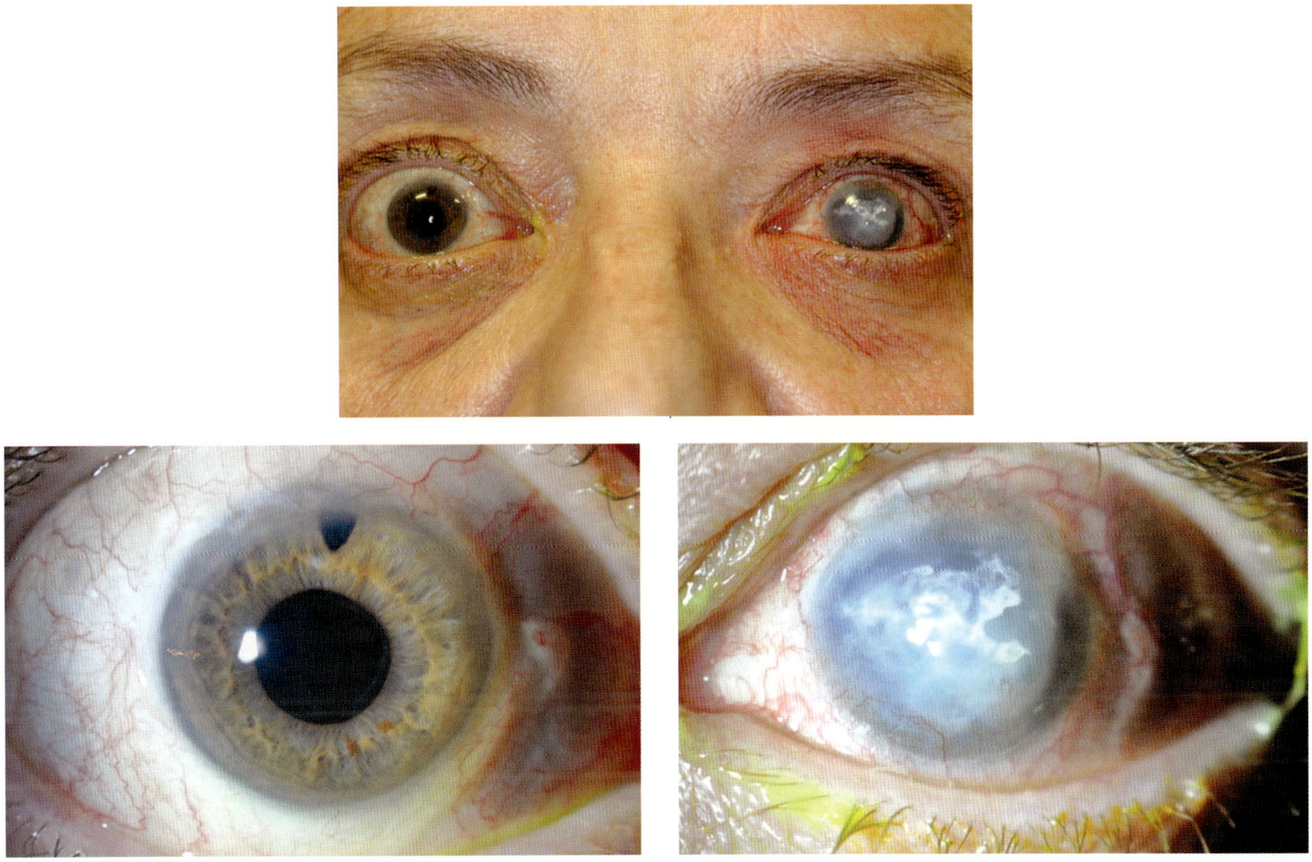

Fig. 10.6: Ocular examination: (Above) Cosmetic appearance of both eyes; (Below) Clear cornea on right eye and corneal calcification of left eye

Surgical Technique

Superficial keratopigmentation using greenish brown color (VEMP 501) combined with cyclodiode photocoagulation at the same surgical session

Postoperative Results

Excellent cosmetic results with a regular distribution of the pigment.

Follow-up and Comments

Fading of the color was observed after a few years and a second superficial keratopigmentation was performed. The colors used were green (VEMP 500) and brown (VEMP 410) to simulate the iris, and black (VEMP 130) for the pupil area. A few months after the surgery, the cosmetic appearance was good with a minimal degree of conjunctival injection (Figure 10.7).

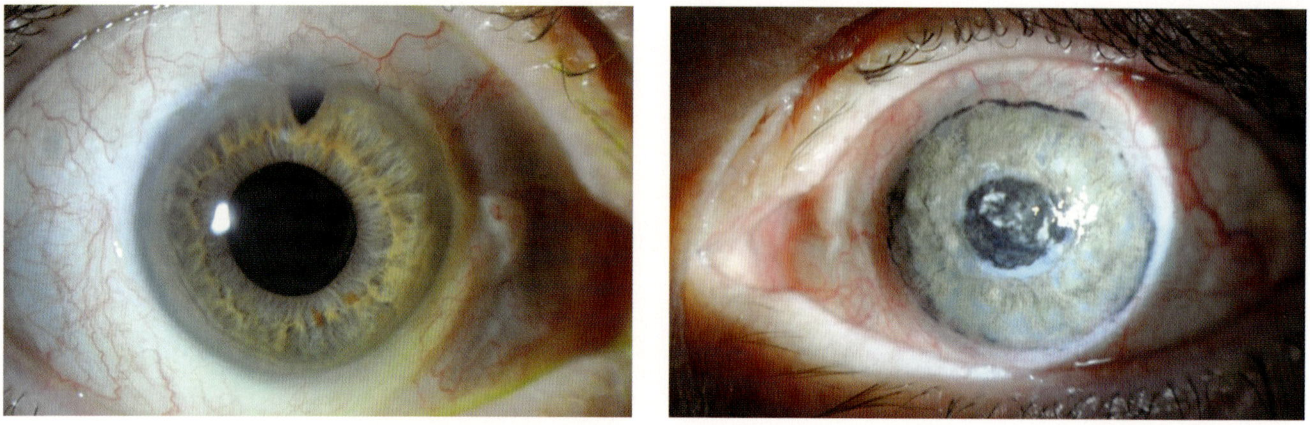

Fig. 10.7: Postoperative results. (Right) Clear cornea on right eye; (Left) Left eye after superficial keratopigmentation

CASE 4

Clinical Histroy

A 32-year-old middle eastern male patient, presented with a white opaque cornea due to previous trauma and a right exotropia. He also developed an intolerance to cosmetic contact lenses and a cosmetic shell was recommended.

Preoperative Data

The patient presented with a right eye total chalky white calcification, a 260 degrees limbal stem cell deficiency, and a right exotropia of 35 to 40 PD. The visual acuity was no perception of light.

Both eyes showed megalophthalmos; left eye horizontal corneal diameter was 12.5 mm and a pupil of 3.5 mm (Figure 10.8).

Surgical Technique

Superficial keratopigmentation technique using multiple needles for the iris area and a single needle for the pupil area and the limbus. The colors used were brown (VEMP 200) for

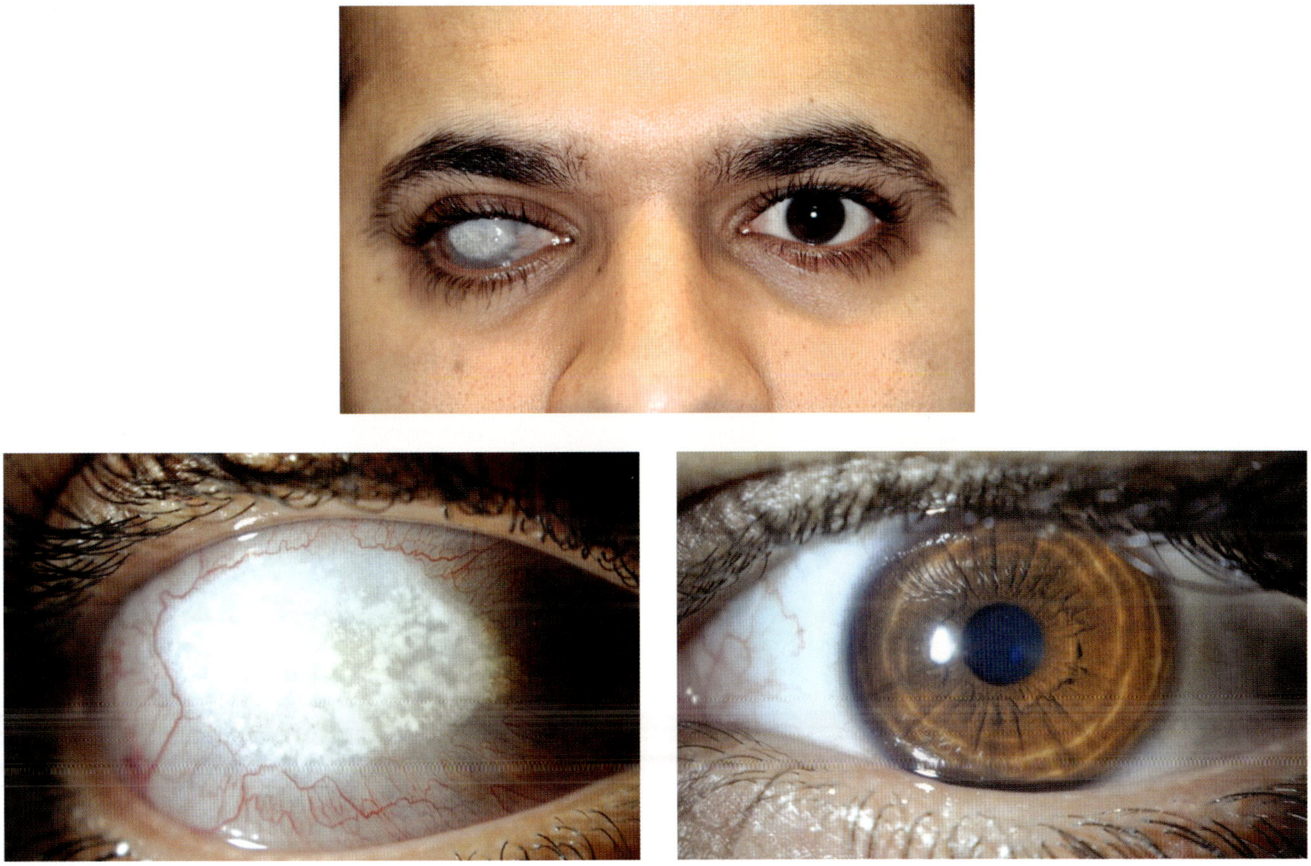

Fig. 10.8: Ocular examination: (Above) Cosmetic appearance of both eyes; (Below) Normal left eye and corneal calcification on right eye

the iris area and black (VEMP 100) for the pupil area. The exotropia was corrected at the same time.

Postoperative Results

One day postoperatively, patient did not experience any pain and no complications were observed except for a minimal degree of postoperative conjunctival injection (Figure 10.9).

Follow-up and Comments

- Three months after surgery, the patient was completely satisfied with the results. The simulated iris and pupil were well-pigmented with a small conjunctival area incorrectly pigmented (inferotemporal grayish black trace)
- One year after surgery, the pigmentation pattern was regular and stable. Another superficial keratopigmentation might be required in 4 to 5 years to treat the possible discoloration (Figure 10.10).

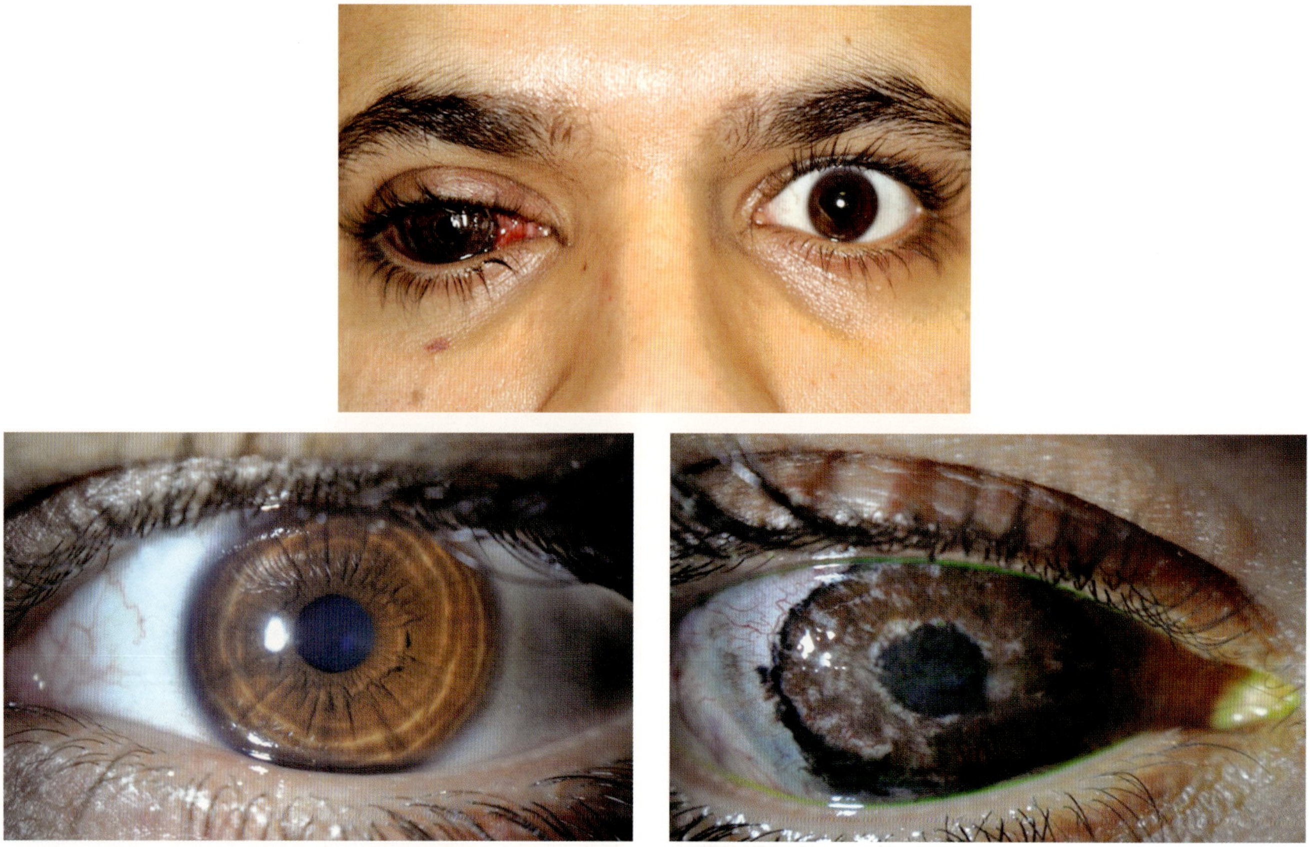

Fig. 10.9: Postoperative results. (Above) Cosmetic appearance of both eyes; (Below) Keratopigmentation on right eye, and normal examination on left eye

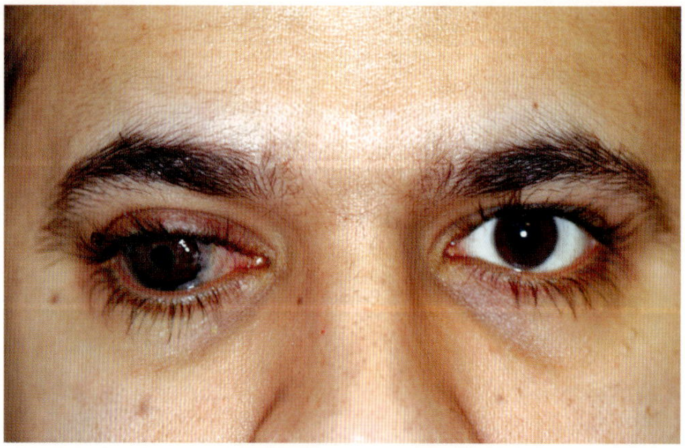

Fig. 10.10: Cosmetic results 3 months after surgery

CASE 5

Clinical History

A 36-year-old female with history of right eye trauma.

Preoperative Data

On examination right eye presented with a diffuse corneal opacity and visual acuity was no perception of light on her right eye (Figure 10.11).

Surgical Technique

Superficial keratopigmentaion technique, using brown (VEMP 290) with needle number 3 for the iris area and black (VEMP 190) with needle number 1 for the pupil area and limbus.

Postoperative Results

First visit postoperatively: Excellent result after superficial pigmentation (Figure 10.12).

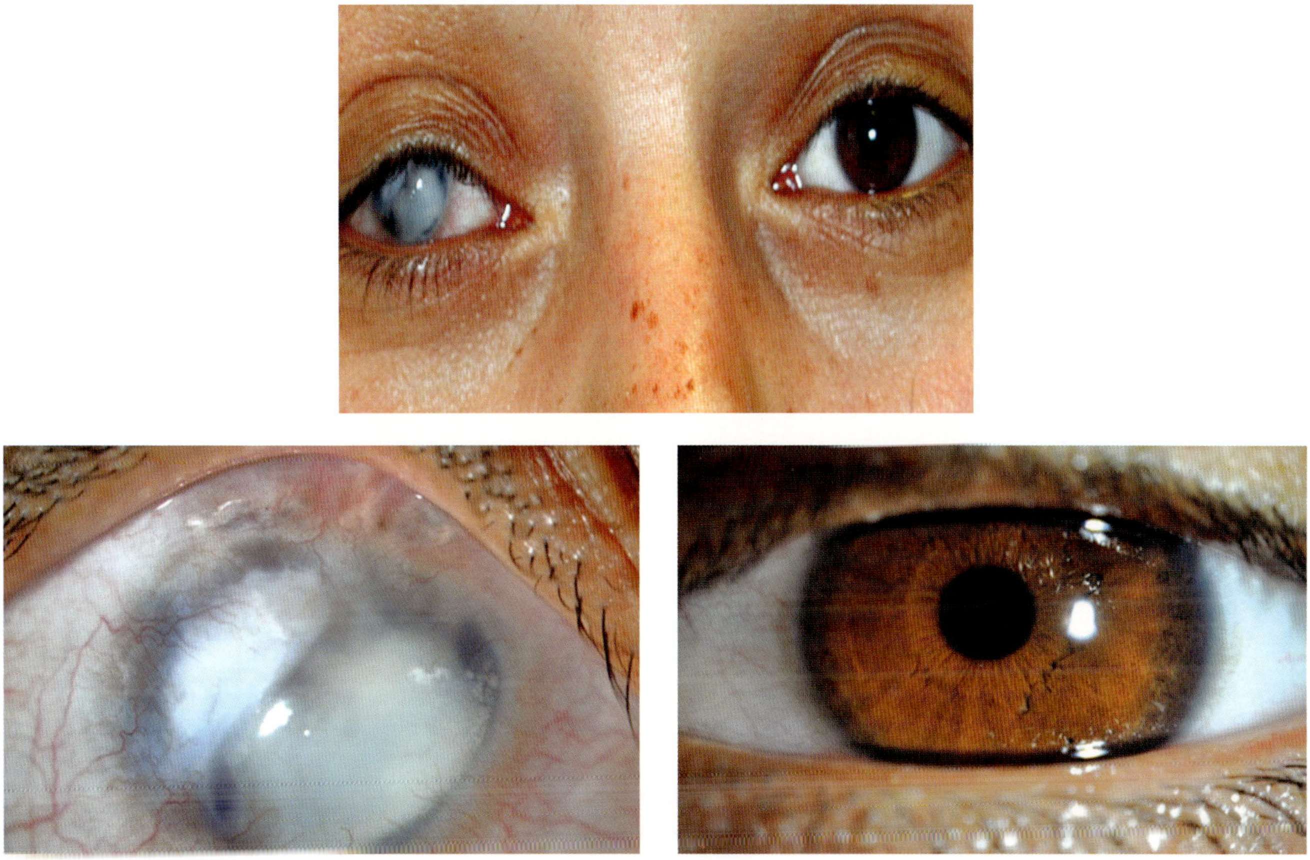

Fig. 10.11: (Above) Cosmetic appearance of both eyes; (Below) Slit-lamp examination of left normal eye and right eye corneal opacity

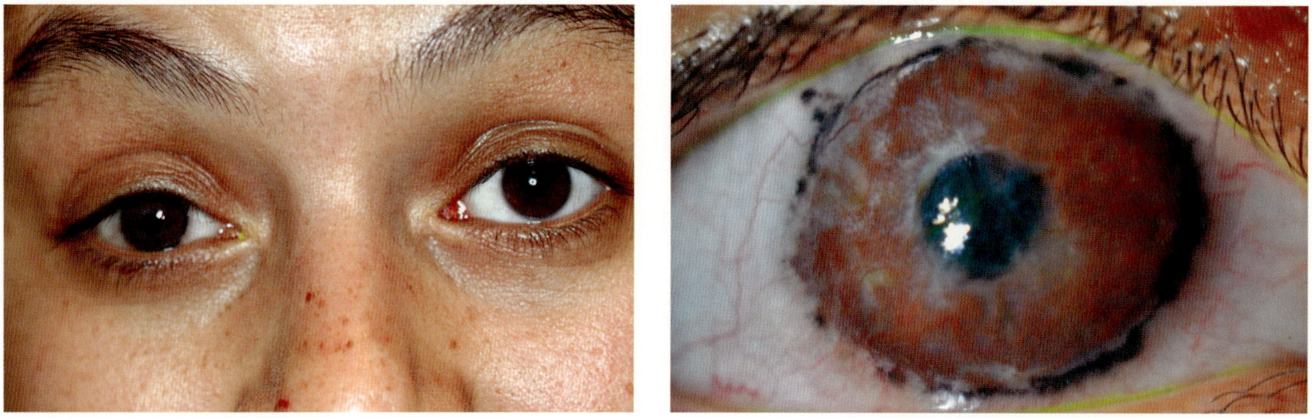

Fig. 10.12: Postoperative results. (Right) Slit-lamp examination of pigmented eye; (Left) Cosmetic appearance eyes of both eyes

Follow-up and Comments

Three months after surgery, it was recommended to repigment some areas to improve the cosmetic appearance to fill some defects.

A second procedure was performed using the same superficial technique and the same pigments. After this second procedure, excellent cosmetic results were achieved with high patient satisfaction (Figure 10.13).

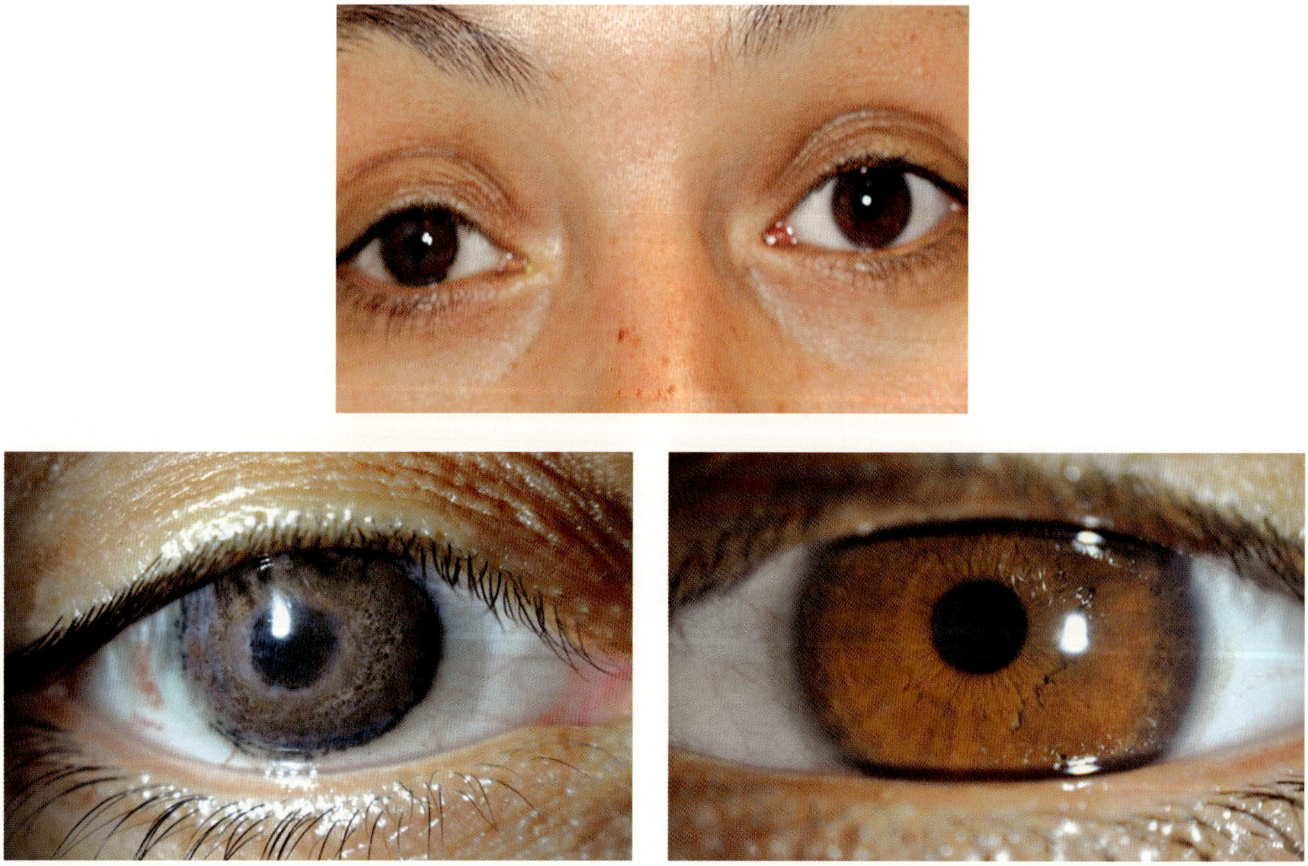

Fig. 10.13 : Final cosmetic results

CASE 6

Clinical History

A 38-year-old female underwent a right eye complicated cataract extraction surgery.

Preoperative Data

Patient presented with right eye totally opacified cornea and the visual acuity was no perception of light. The examination on her left eye was unremarkable with visual acuity of 1.0 (decimal) (Figure 10.14).

Surgical Technique

Superficial keratopigmentation technique was performed with multiple needles to simulate the iris and a single needle for the pupil area. The colors used were prepared green (VEMP 591) with brown (VEMP 290) for the iris area and black (VEMP 190) for the pupil area. Cyclodiode-photocoagulation was also performed at the same surgical session.

Postoperative Results

Postoperatively, the patient was safisfied with the cosmetic results, and did not present any major postoperative symptom or complication. Cosmetic evaluation was very good except for lack of adequate limbal pigmentation (Figure 10.15).

Follow-up and Comments

Three months after the surgery, the final color was slightly darker compared to the other eye. The limbus was also poorly marked.

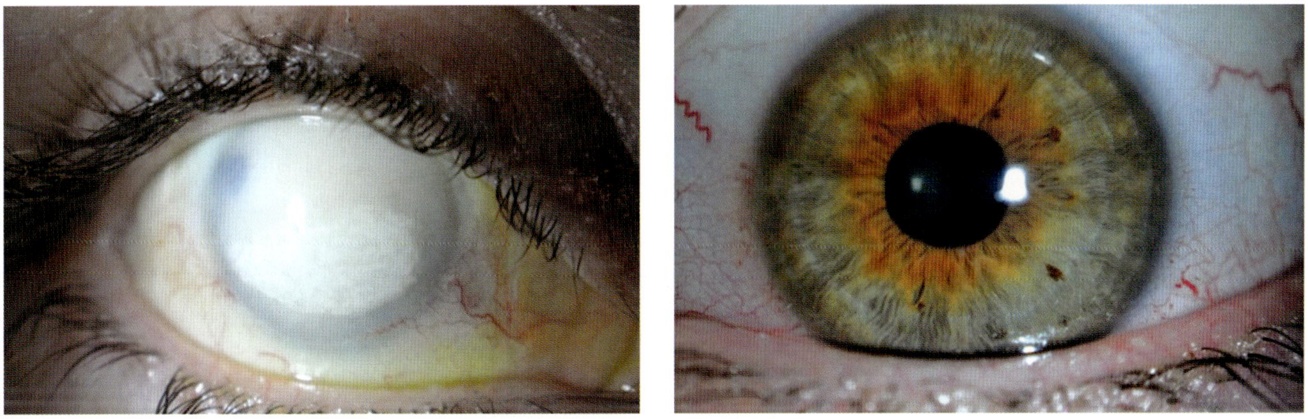

Fig. 10.14: Slit-lamp examination of both eyes. Right eye corneal opacification and normal left eye

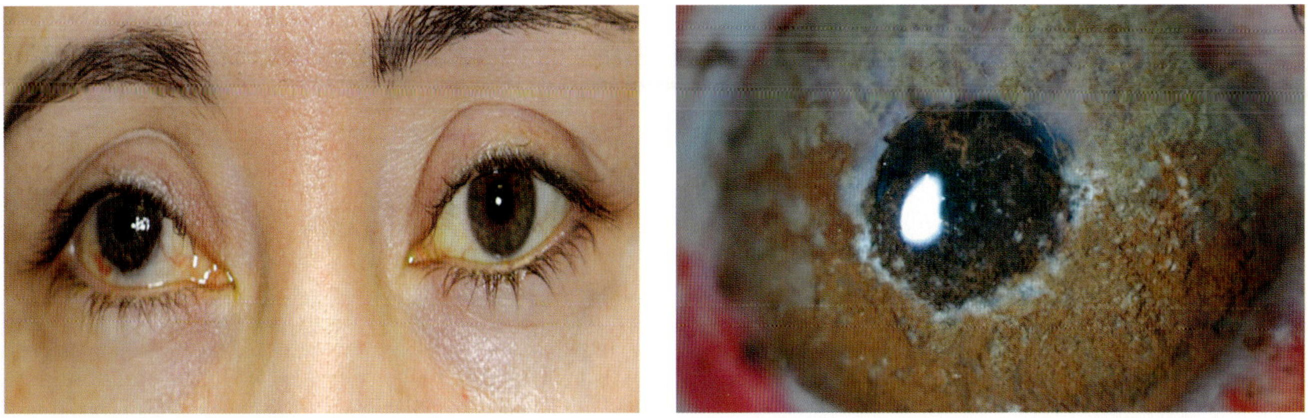

Fig. 10.15: Postoperative results. Cosmetic appearance of both eyes (left) and keratopigmentation pattern detailed (right)

A second keratopigmentation surgery was performed to enhance the cosmetic appearance. Cyclodiode photocoagulation was repeated at the same time, using brown (VEMP 499) with brown (VEMP 495) for iris and black (VEMP 190) for pupil.

One month after the surgery, the cosmetic result was greatly improved (Figure 10.16).

Two years after the surgery, the pupil area was irregular, distorted and blurred (Figure 10.17), therefore a third tattooing was performed. This keratopigmentation procedure was done using a superficial technique with needle number 3 and colors clear brown (VEMP 410) and green (VEMP 500) for the iris area, and needle number 1 and color black (VEMP 100) for pupil area and limbus.

Postoperative cosmetic appearance was excellent with good patient safisfaction (Figure 10.18).

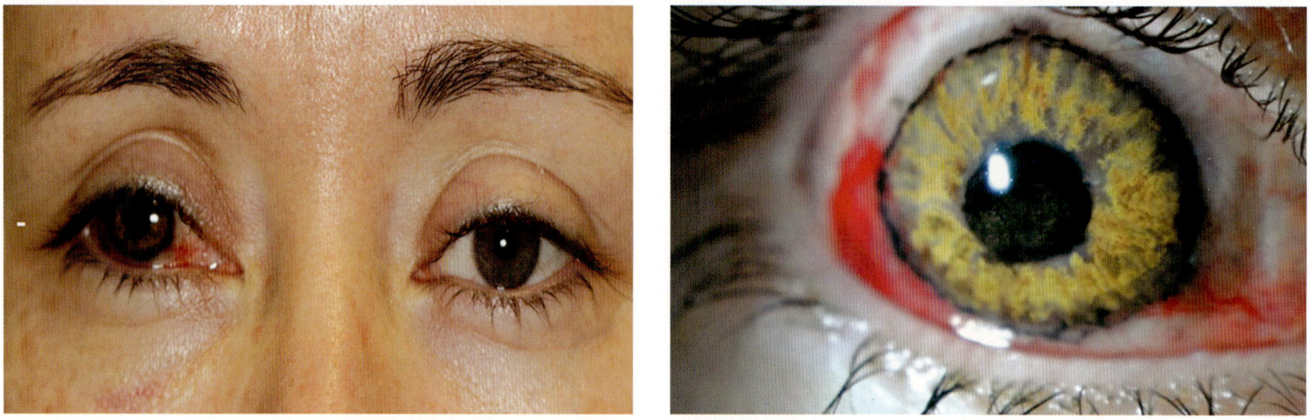

Fig. 10.16 : Examination after second keratopigmentation

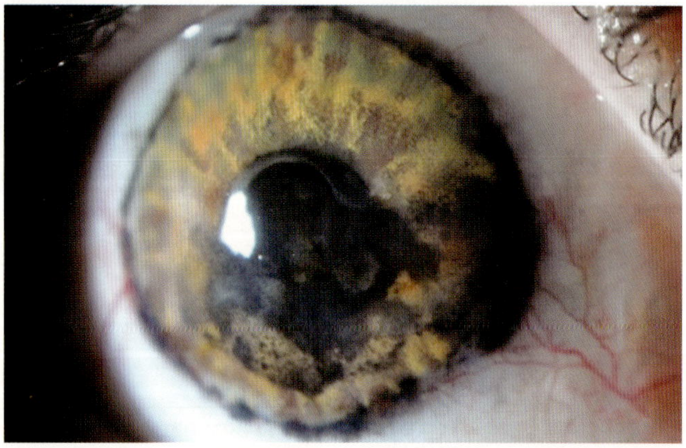

Fig. 10.17: Pupillary distortion, two years after the first keratopigmentation

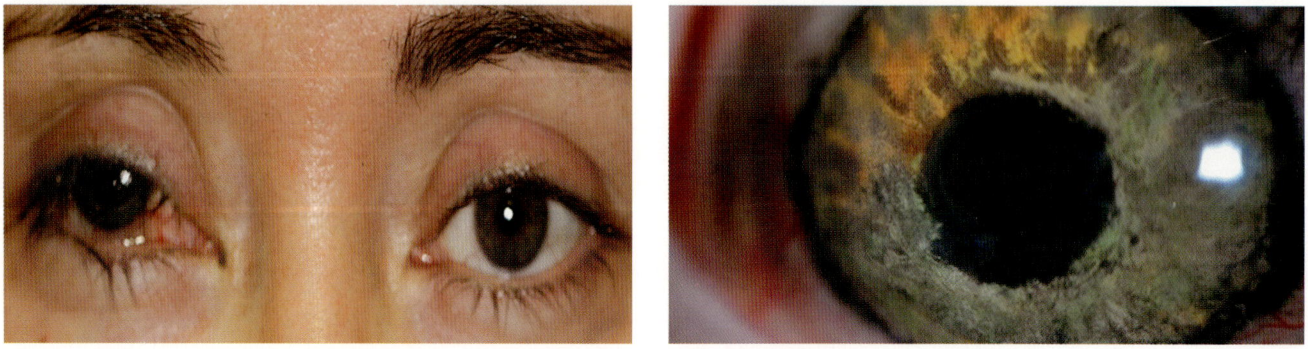

Fig. 10.18: Postoperative result after the third keratopigmentation surgery

CASE 7

Clinical History

A 30-year-old male with history of left eye traumatic cataract, retinal detachment, progressive corneal opacity and extensive superficial calcification presented with a visual acuity of no perception of light. His right eye was under topical treatment for glaucoma with intraocular pressures under control and a visual acuity of 1.0 (decimal).

Preoperative Data

This patient was interested in a permanent cosmetic solution because cosmetic contact lenses were slightly uncomfortable for him (Figure 10.19).

Surgical Technique

Superficial keratopigmentation technique, with multiple needles to mimic the iris and a single needle for the pupil area and the limbus. The colors used were gray blue (VEMP 691) for the iris area and black (VEMP 190) for the pupil area. A squint surgery was performed to correct the exotropia at the same time.

Postoperative Results

First visit postoperatively: Patient was satisfied with the cosmetic result. No pain or any other complication was observed, except for a minimal postoperative conjunctival injection. The blue color of the simulated iris was slightly different from the healthy eye, and the pupil was blurred

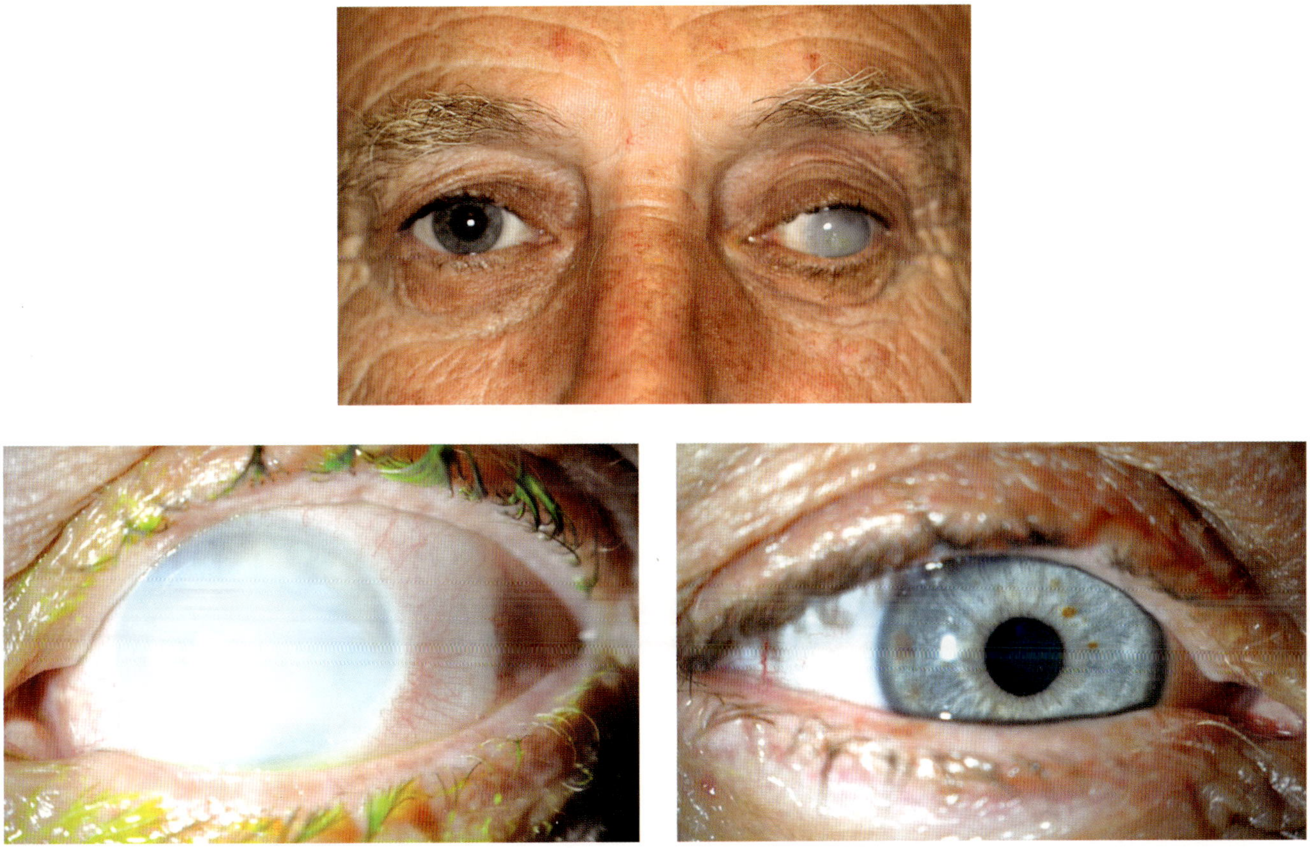

Fig. 10.19: Slit-lamp examination (Above): Cosmetic appearance of both eyes; (Below) Normal right eye and corneal calcification on left eye

and not well defined. Therefore, a second superficial keratopigmentation was performed to retouch the pupil area and the limbus with the black color and using a greenish tone for the iris area (Figure 10.20).

Follow-up and Comments

A second superficial keratopigmentation was performed using light green and grayish green (VEMP 591).

Three months after the surgery, the patient was satisfied with the cosmetic result, and one year after the surgery the outcomes remained without changes (Figure 10.21).

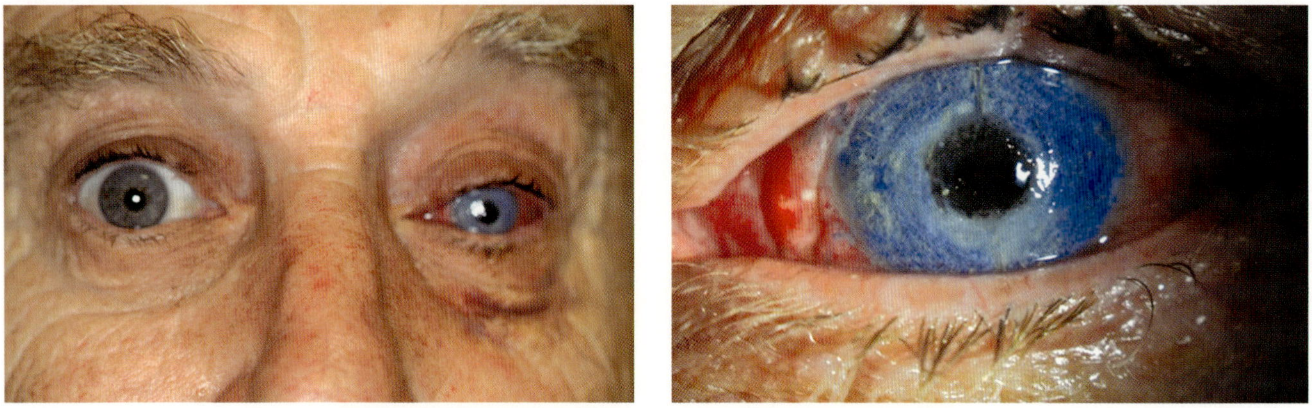

Fig. 10.20: Postoperative results. (Right) Slit-lamp examination after keratopigmentation; (Left) Cosmetic appearance of both eyes

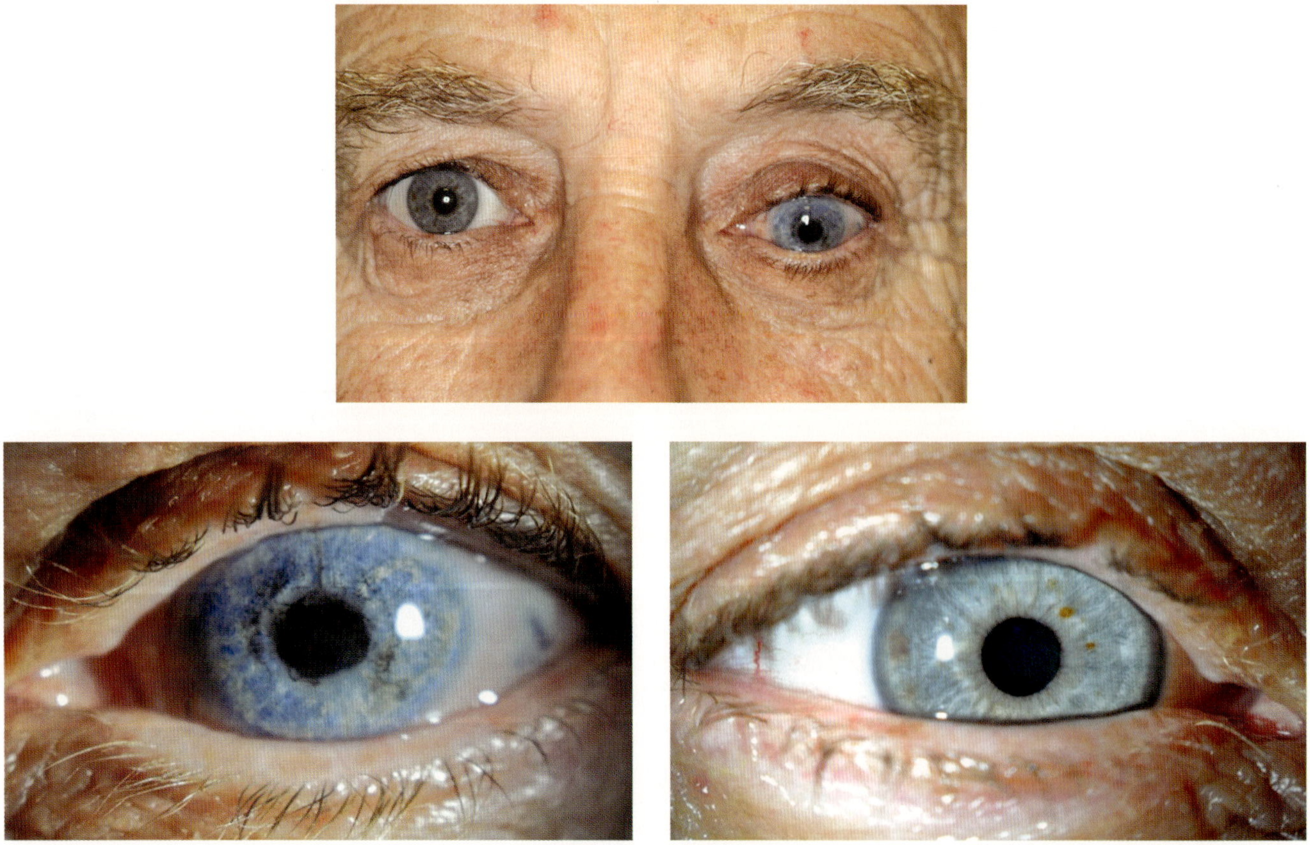

Fig. 10.21: Cosmetic results 3 months after surgery

MANUAL INTRALAMELLAR KERATOPIGMENTATION

CASE 8

Intolerable diplopia eliminated by keratopigmentation.

Clinical History

A 30-year-old male, with previous history of squint surgery at the ages of 4 and 23 years old, presented with diplopia. He commented that the diplopia worsened after the eye alignment. His visual acuity was 1.0 (decimal) in both eyes.

Preoperative Data

Refraction and orthoptic examination was performed to correct the diplopia using prisms. Unfortunately, it was impossible to improve his condition, and a more permanent solution using keratopigmentation was considered to treat the double vision.

Surgical Technique

Manual intrastromal keratopigmentation technique was performed using the VISSUM intrastromal micropigmentation dissectors to create the intralamellar tunnels. The pupil area was marked at 4 mm of diameter and using brown (VEMP 290) pigment.

Postoperative Results

First visit postoperatively: Patient expressed satisfaction with the relief of the visual disability symptoms with no pain or any other complications. Cosmetic evaluation showed a very good pupil profile (Figure 10.22).

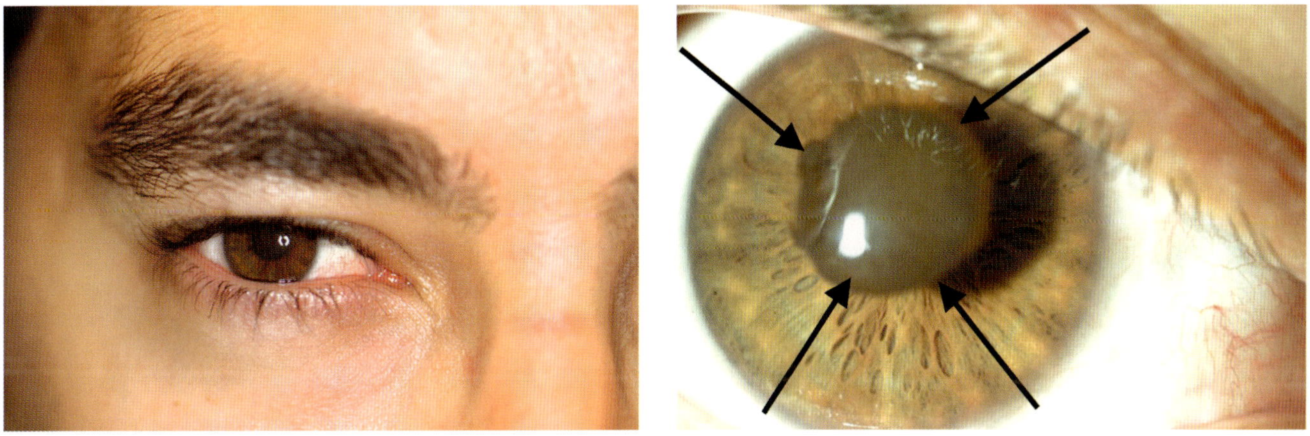

Fig. 10.22: Postoperative results. (Right) Slit-lamp biomicroscopy of keratopigmentation pattern; (Left) Cosmetic appearance of right eye. (Arrows indicates the limits of the keratopigmentation pattern)

Follow-up and Comments

On 6 months follow-up, Patient was still satisfied with his results, and the cosmetic evaluation showed pigment slightly blurred at the edges due to peripheral pigment dispersion, with slight stromal corneal opacity, but with stable pupil diameter in high, medium and low mesopic conditions. This case has been the subject of long-term follow-up (Figure 10.23).

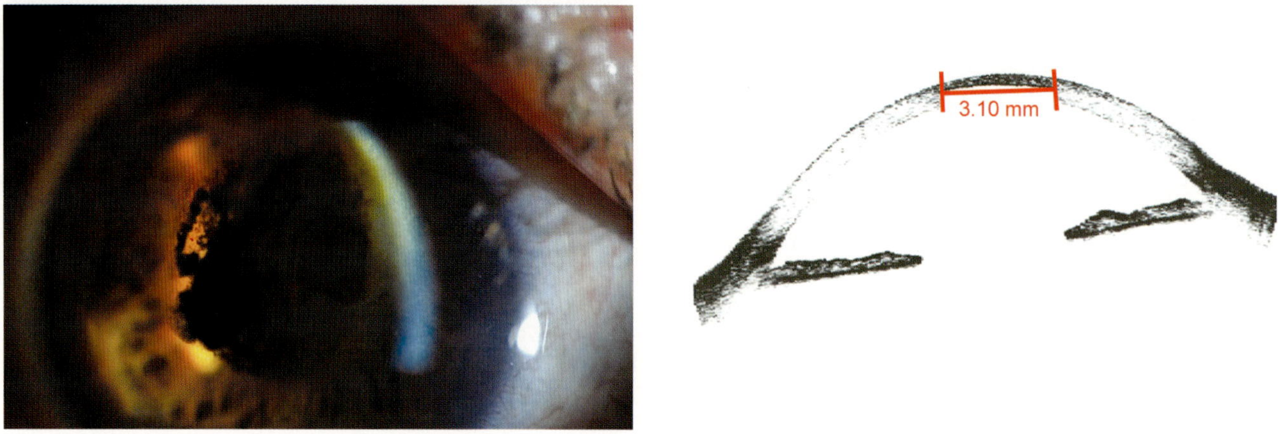

Fig. 10.23: On 6 months follow-up: (Right) Anterior segment OCT of pigmented pupil; (Left) Peripheral pigment dispersion

COMBINED SUPERFICIAL AUTOMATED KERATOPIGMENTATION (SAK) AND MANUAL INTRALAMELLAR KERATOPIGMENTATION (MIK)

CASE 9

Clinical History

A 30-year-old male with history of trauma on his left eye and several operations with poor outcomes, presented with a left blind eye and a severe corneal opacity.

Preoperative Data

On examination, his left eye cornea was opacified (white) and deformed with a full-thickness traumatic scar and pseudophakia. The visual acuity was 1.2 (decimal) and hand movements in right and left eyes respectively (Figure 10.24).

Surgical Technique

Superficial and manual intrastromal techniques using dark brown (VEMP 290) and black (VEMP 190) pigments to simulate the iris and the pupil, with strabismus and ptosis surgery simultaneously.

Postoperative Results

Moderate to severe postoperative inflammation with conjunctival injection and insufficient pupil pigmentation (Figure 10.25).

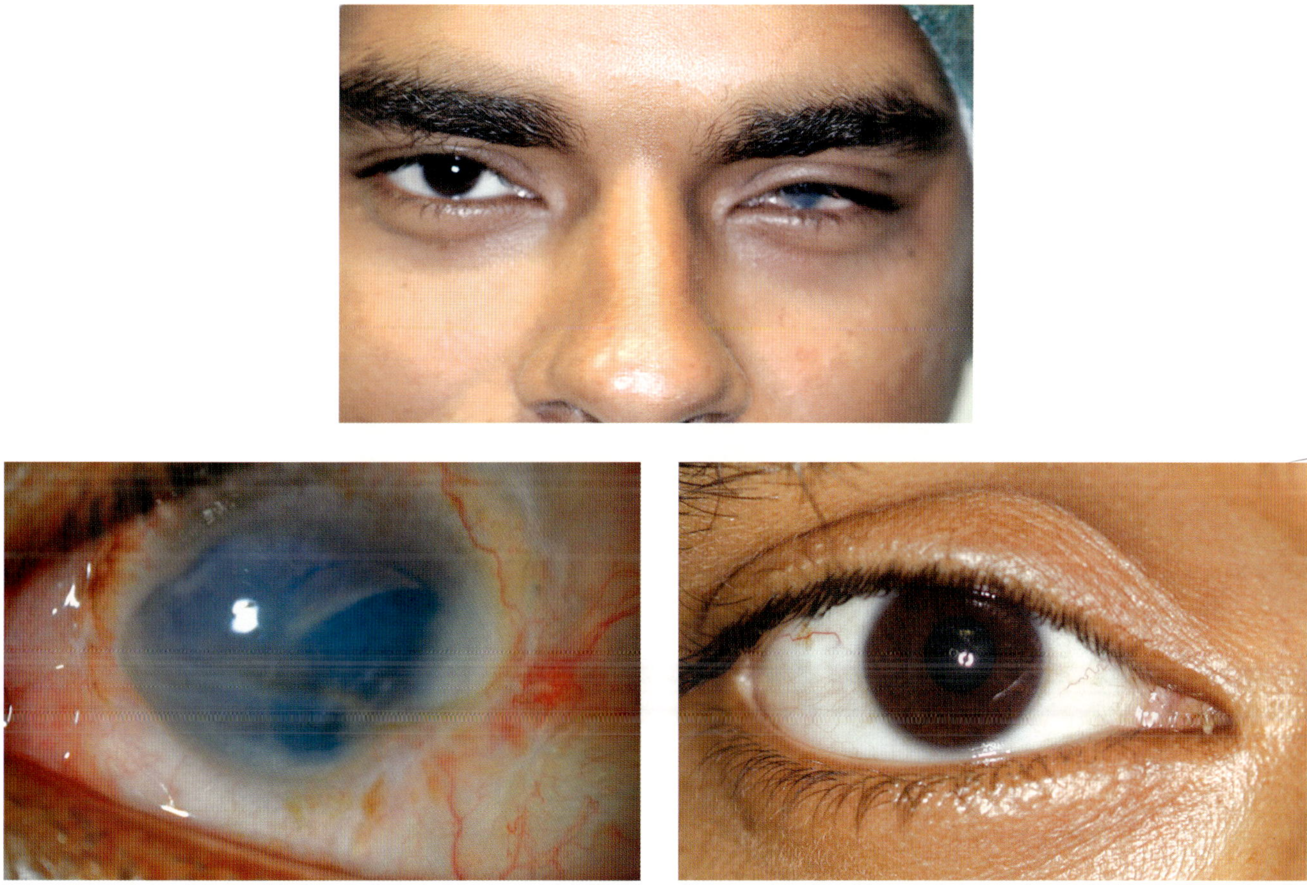

Fig. 10.24: Slit-lamp examination: (Above) Cosmetic appearance of both eyes; (Below) Normal right eye and corneal opacity of left eye

Follow-up and Comments

A second keratopigmentation surgery was performed, completing pupil profile using the same colors.

After the surgery the cosmetic appearance was excellent, and the enophthalmus was treated with an intraorbital filler injected in the retrobulbar space.

Then a third surgery using the superficial keratopigmentation technique was done to pigment the pupil again, using a black (VEMP 190) pigment (3.5 mm for the pupil diameter). The iris area was also pigmented using brown (VEMP 290).

Final result: Excellent cosmetic appearance and great patient satisfaction (Figure 10.26).

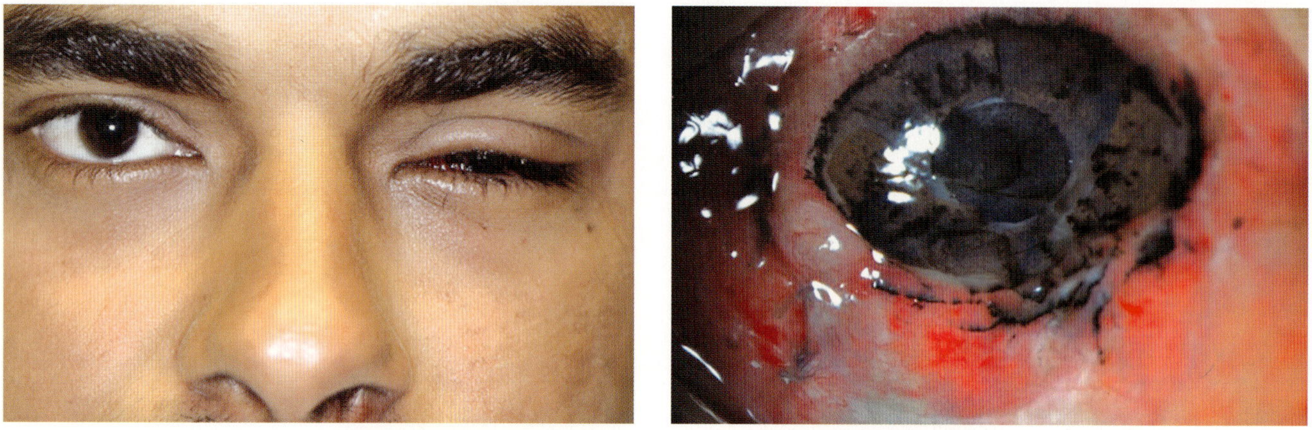

Fig. 10.25: Postoperative results. (Right) Slit-lamp examination; (Left) Cosmetic appearance of both eyes

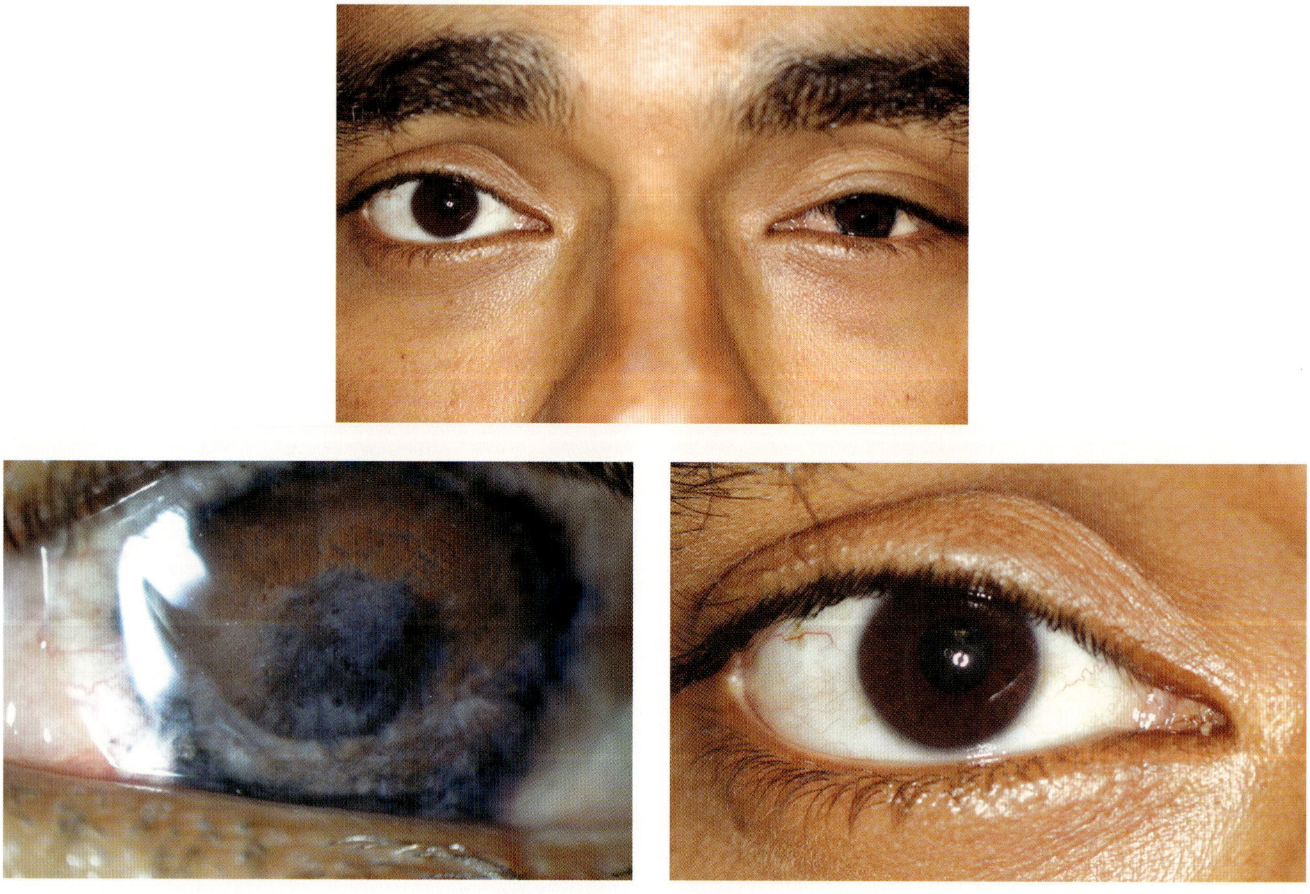

Fig. 10.26: Final cosmetic result

CASE 10

Clinical Histroy

A 37 years old female patient with a history of bilateral cytomegalovirus endophthalmitis, followed by corneal ulceration.

Right eye had undergone in another center cataract extraction surgery and left eye underwent keratoplasty with no improvement of vision. She was asking for cosmetic surgery

Preoperative Data

On examination, bilateral corneal opacity with no perception of light in both eyes, and severe exotropia was also observed (Figure 10.27).

Surgical Technique

Combined superficial and intrastromal techniques: Starting with brown (VEMP 290) color then green brown (VEMP 591)

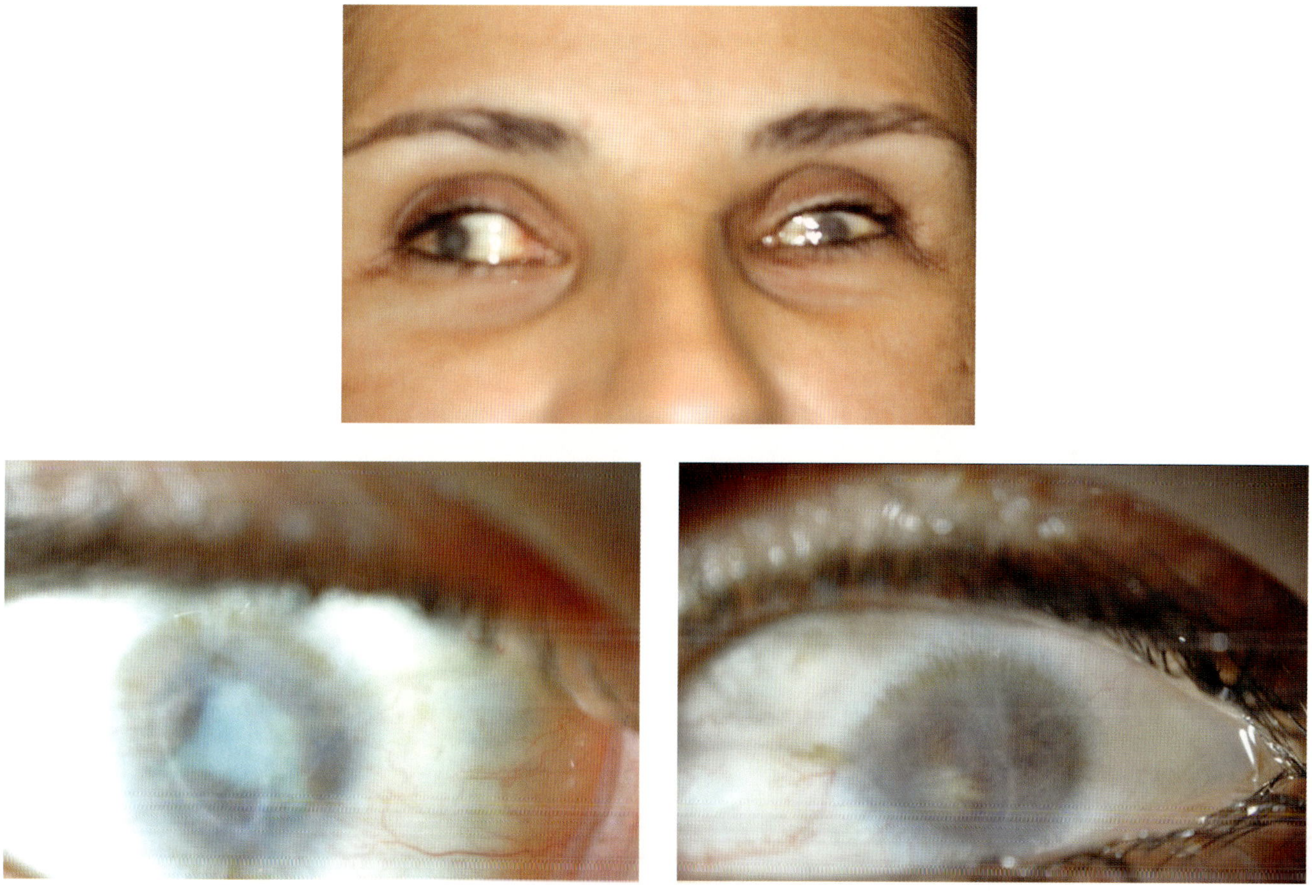

Fig. 10.27: Slit-lamp biomicroscopy: (Above) Cosmetic appearance of both eyes; (Below) Bilateral corneal opacity

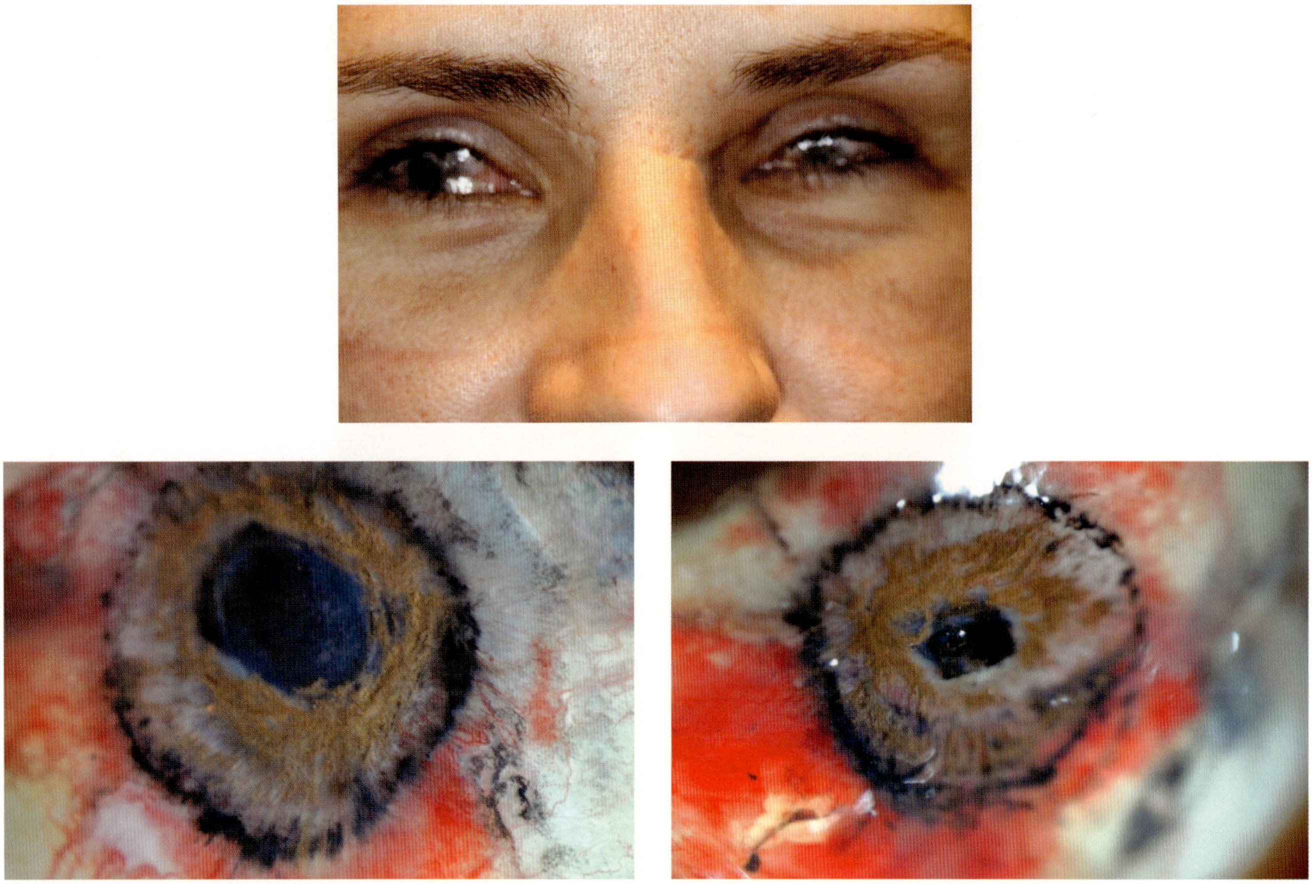

Fig. 10.28: Outcomes following the second surgery

and black (VEMP 190), with simultaneous strabismus and intraocular injection of silicone in both eyes.

Postoperative Results

- *Right eye:* good appearance with small iris defect at the limbus
- Left eye: Conjunctival chemosis, with stable pigmentation

Follow-up and Comments

- *Second surgery at 3 months:* Pigmentation enhancement was performed with brown (VEMP 290) and black and more silicone injection was done in both eyes
- One year later the pigmentation showed good aspect with light pigment dispersion (Figure 10.28).

CASE 11

Clinical History

A 60-year-old female with history of left eye endophthalmitis at the age of 9 years old.

Preoperative Data

On examination, her left eye presented with a complete corneal opacity and her visual acuity was no perception of light. However, the visual acuity of the right eye was normal (decimal 1.0) (Figure 10.29).

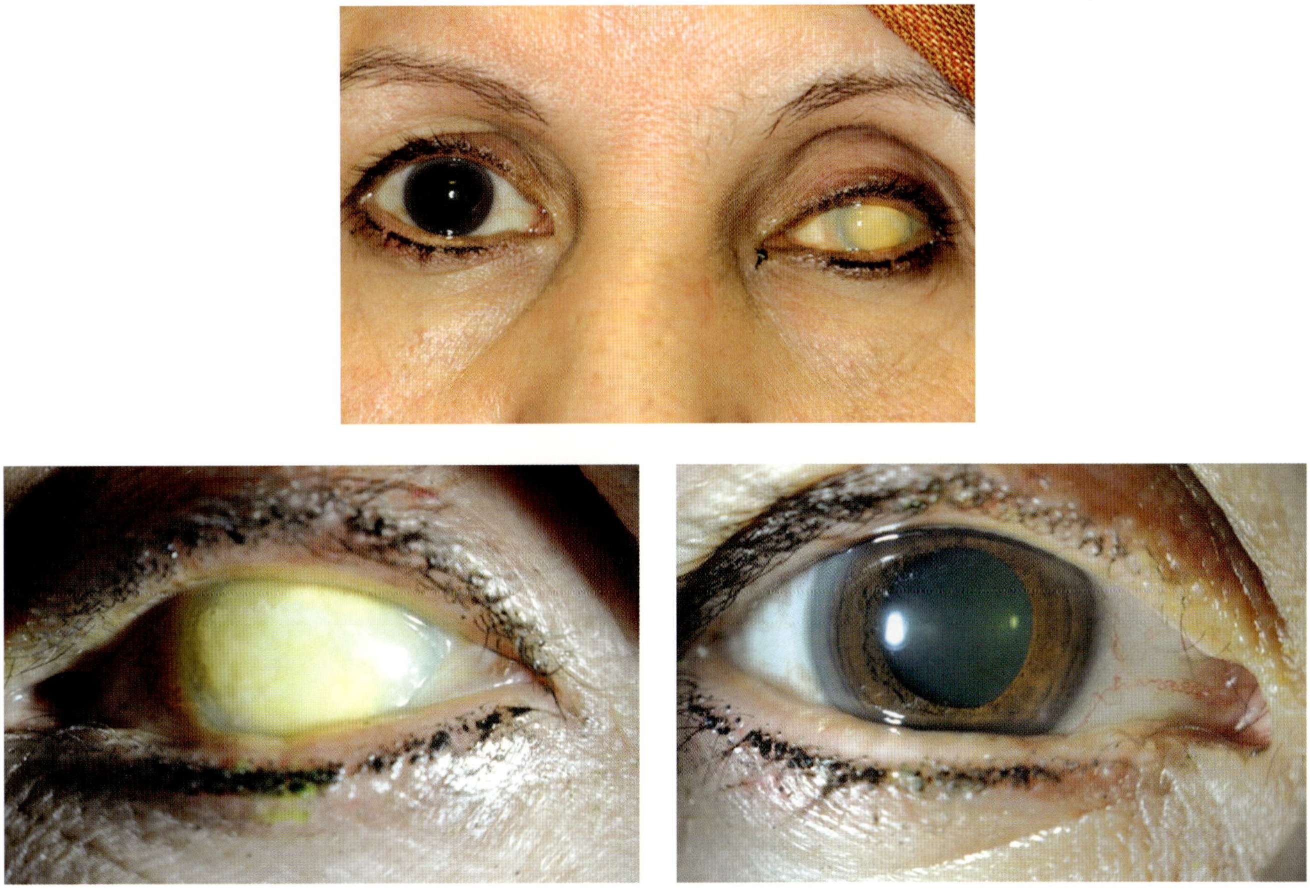

Fig. 10.29: Slit-lamp examination: (Above) Cosmetic appearance of both eyes; (Below) Normal appearance of her right eye and corneal calcification on her left eye

Surgical Technique

Manual intrastromal keratopigmentation combined with the superficial keratopigmentation technique, using black (VEMP 110) for the pupil area and brown (VEMP 200) for the iris area.

Postoperative Results

Good outcomes with regular distribution of the pigments.

Follow-up and Comments

On follow-up, a regular and stable pigmentation was observed, with no dispersion of the pigments. Postoperatively, it was recommended to increase the orbital volume with a filler to improve the cosmetic appearance (Figure 10.30).

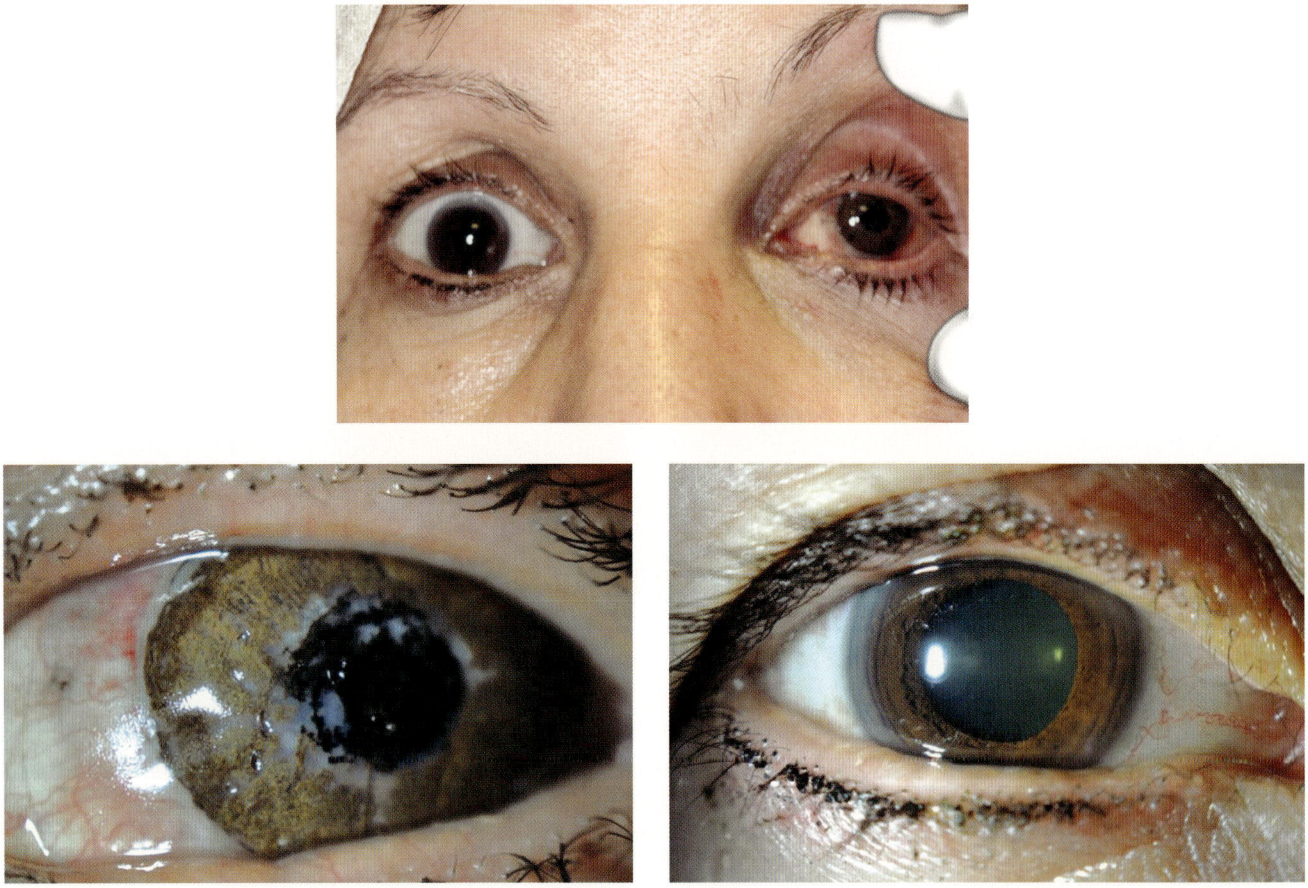

Fig. 10.30: Cosmetic result one month after surgery

CASE 12

Clinical Histroy

A 44 years old female patient, with a history of left eye car accident trauma at the age of 13, she underwent emergency repair but with gradual decrease of visual acuity and worsening of the cosmetic appearance

Preoperative Data

On examination, left eye complete corneal opacity, neovessels, and no anterior chamber details. Retroillumination indicates atrophic iris (Figure 10.31).

Surgical Technique

Superficial keratopigmentation with combined manual intrastromal techniques:

- *Iris:* Brown (VEMP 200) using needle number 3
- *Pupil:* Black (VEMP 100) using needle number 1 set at 7 mm

With anterior segment reconstruction and sulcus suturing of intraocular lens simultaneous strabismus surgery.

Postoperative Results

Good aspect with mild inflammation (Figure 10.32).

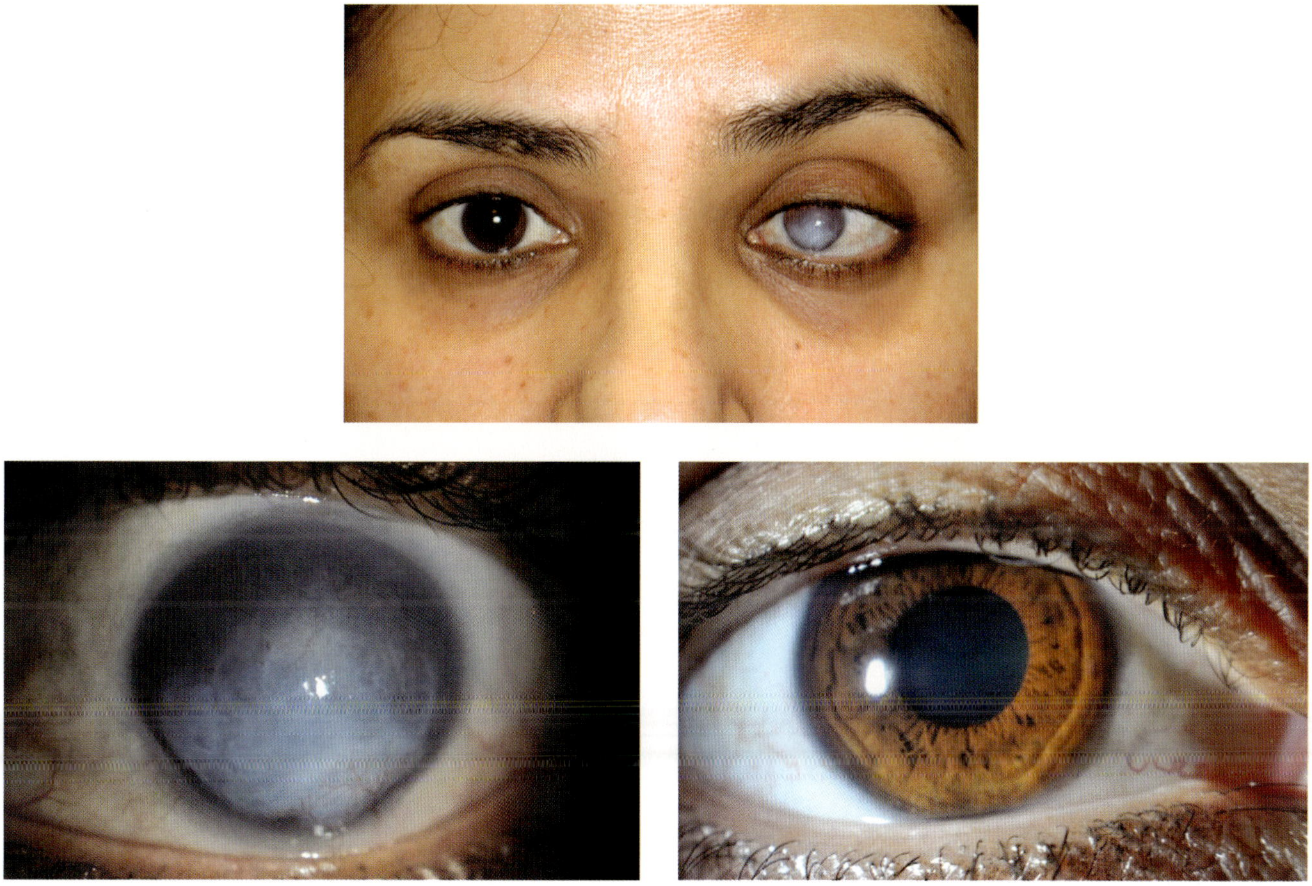

Fig. 10.31: Slit-lamp biomicroscopy: (Above) Cosmetic appearance of both eyes; (Below) Normal right eye and corneal calcification of left eye

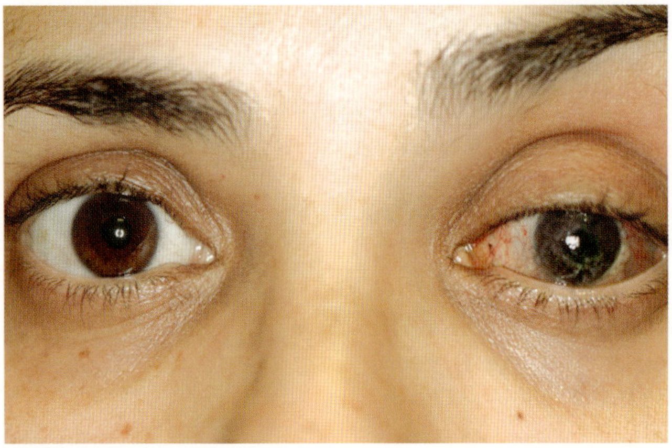

Fig. 10.32 : Postoperative results. Cosmetic appearance of both eyes

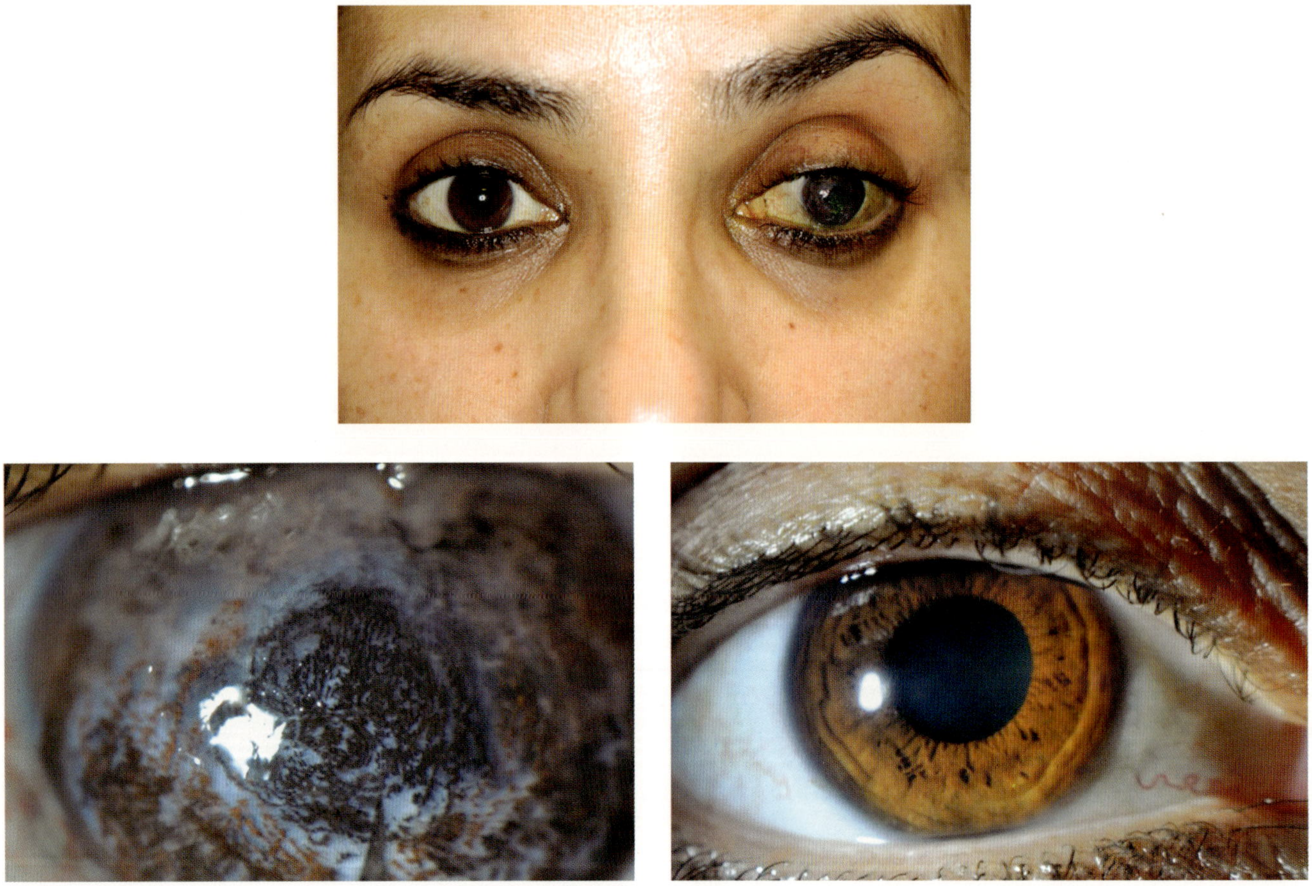

Fig. 10.33: One month follow-up cosmetic results

Follow-up and Comments

On follow-up at one month: Discreet area of pigmentation dispersion a little poor area of paralimbal pigmentation, otherwise good surface (Figure 10.33). Patient was advice to consider pigment retouch with ptosis surgery for further improvement of cosmetic appearance

CASE 13

Clinical History

A 43-year-old male with history of trauma and poor vision on his left eye since then.

Preoperative Data

On examination, a phthisis bulbi and band keratopathy was observed in his left eye. The visual acuity was 1.0 (decimal) and no perception of light, for right and left eyes respectively (Figure 10.34).

Surgical Technique

A combination of manual intrastromal and superficial keratopigmentation techniques were performed, using brown (VEMP 291) with needle 3 for the iris area and black (VEMP 191) with needle 1 for the pupil area.

Postoperative Results

Acceptable results with a moderate conjunctival injection. However, the pupil was slightly bigger and distorted compared to the other eye (Figure 10.35). Therefore, a second keratopigmentation was done to improve the cosmetic appearance.

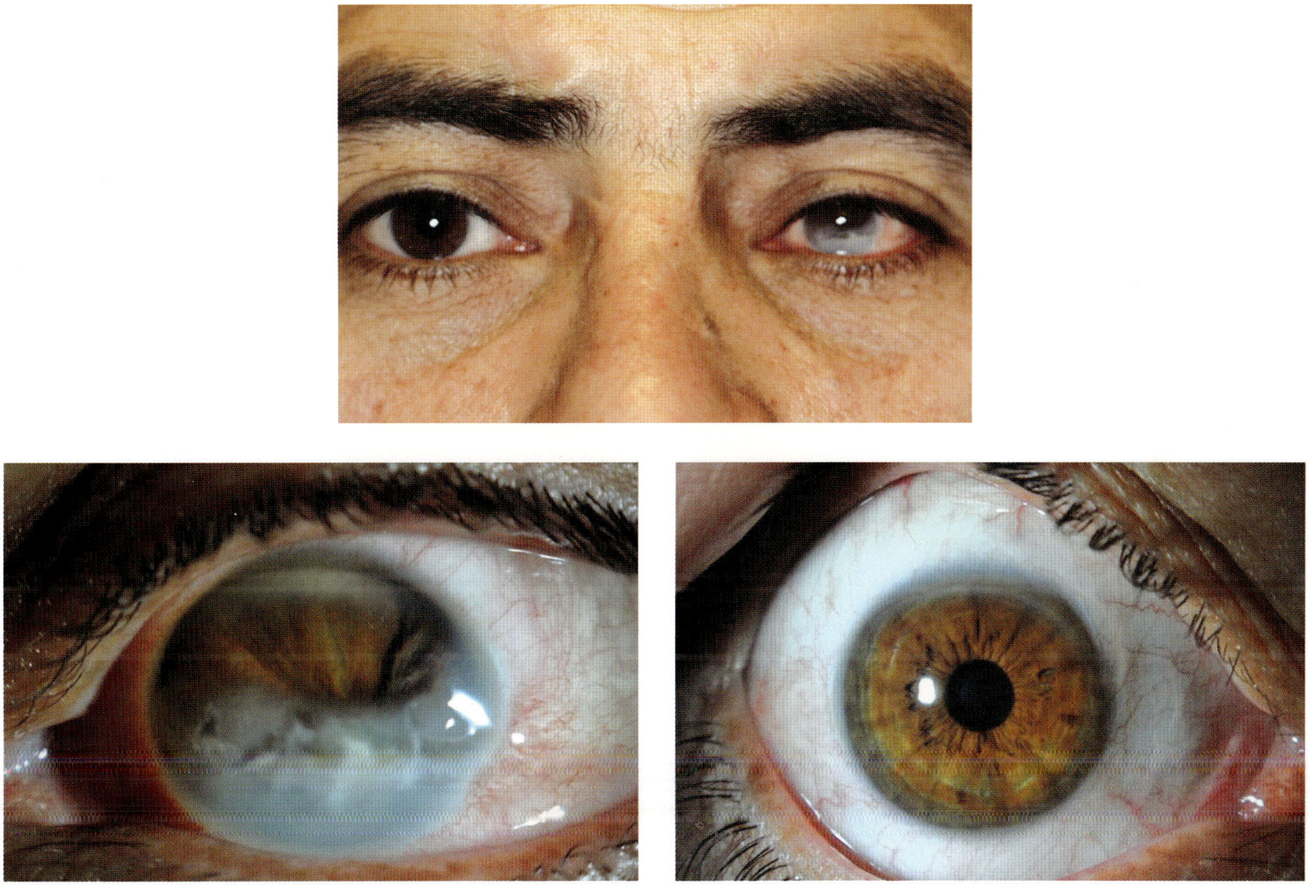

Fig. 10.34: Slit-lamp examination: (Above) Cosmetic appearance of both eyes; (Below) Normal right eye and traumatized left eye

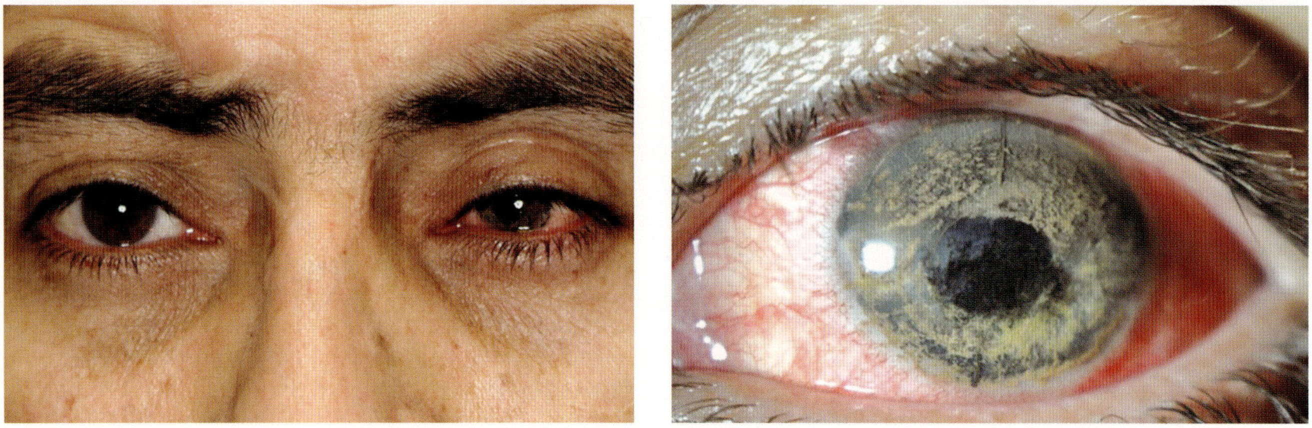

Fig. 10.35: Postoperative results. (Right) Slit-lamp biomicroscopy after keratopigmentation; (Left) Cosmetic appearance of both eyes

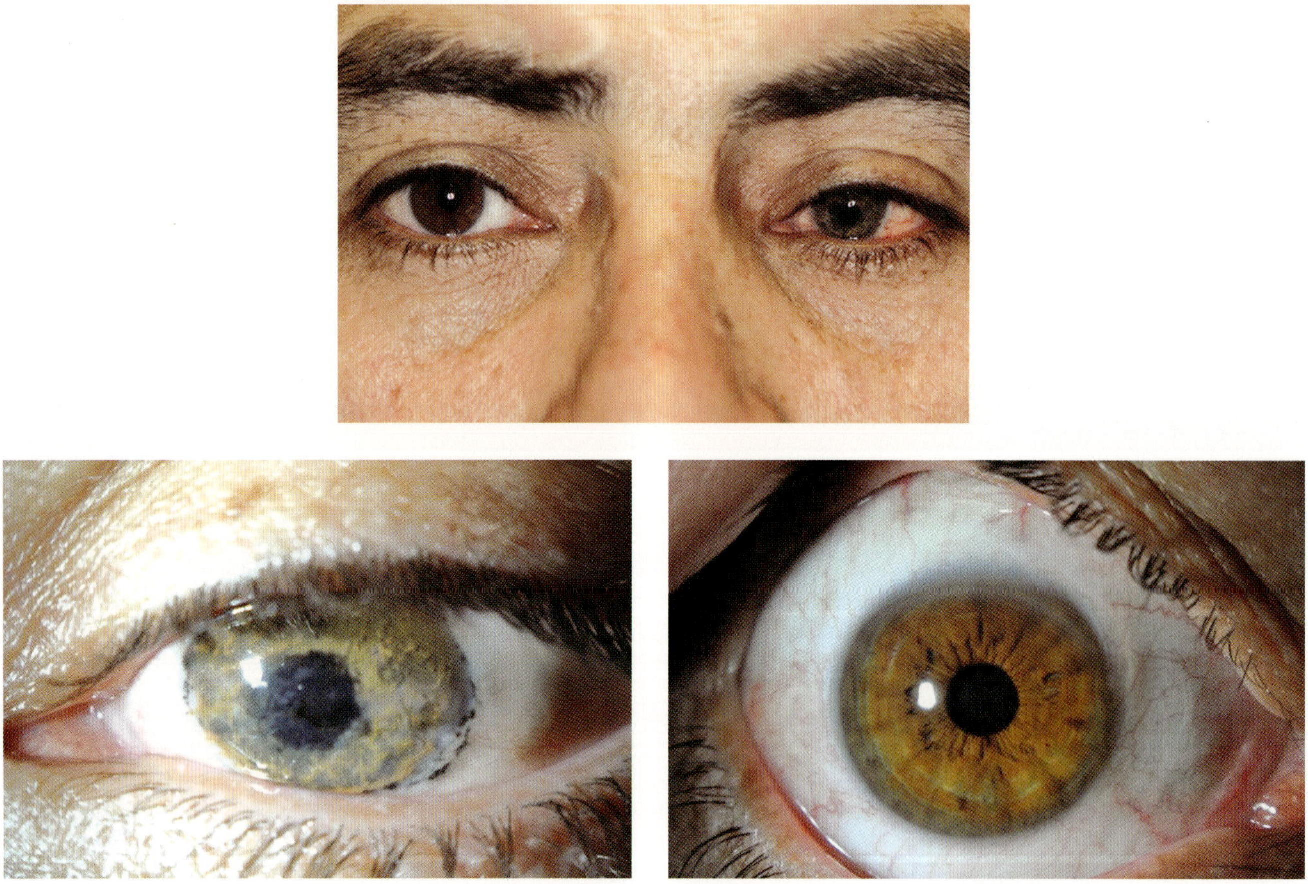

Fig. 10.36: Final cosmetic result

Follow-up and Comments

A second surgery was carried out to reform the pupil area, marking the pupil at 4 mm of diameter and using black (VEMP 191) to pigment the area again.

After the second surgery, the pupil was excentric inferonasally and the iris was lighter than the other eye.

Six months after the operation, the appearance was good with a minimal conjunctival injection (Figure 10.36).

CASE 14

Clinical Histroy

A 73 years old male patient with complicated right eye cataract surgery for which he underwent vitrectomy surgery with poor outcome and intraocular infection (endophthalmitis) ending in pthysis bulbi with severe cosmetic imbalance.

Preoperative Data

On examination, right eye complete corneal opacity with conjunctival hyperemia, enophthalmos and no perception of light. Right eye was cataractous with visual acuity of 0.7; for which he underwent uneventful cataract surgery (Figure 10.37).

Surgical Technique

Combined manual intrastromal and superficial techniques

- *Iris:* Brown (VEMP 290) using needle number 3
- *Pupil:* Black (VEMP 190) using needle number 1.

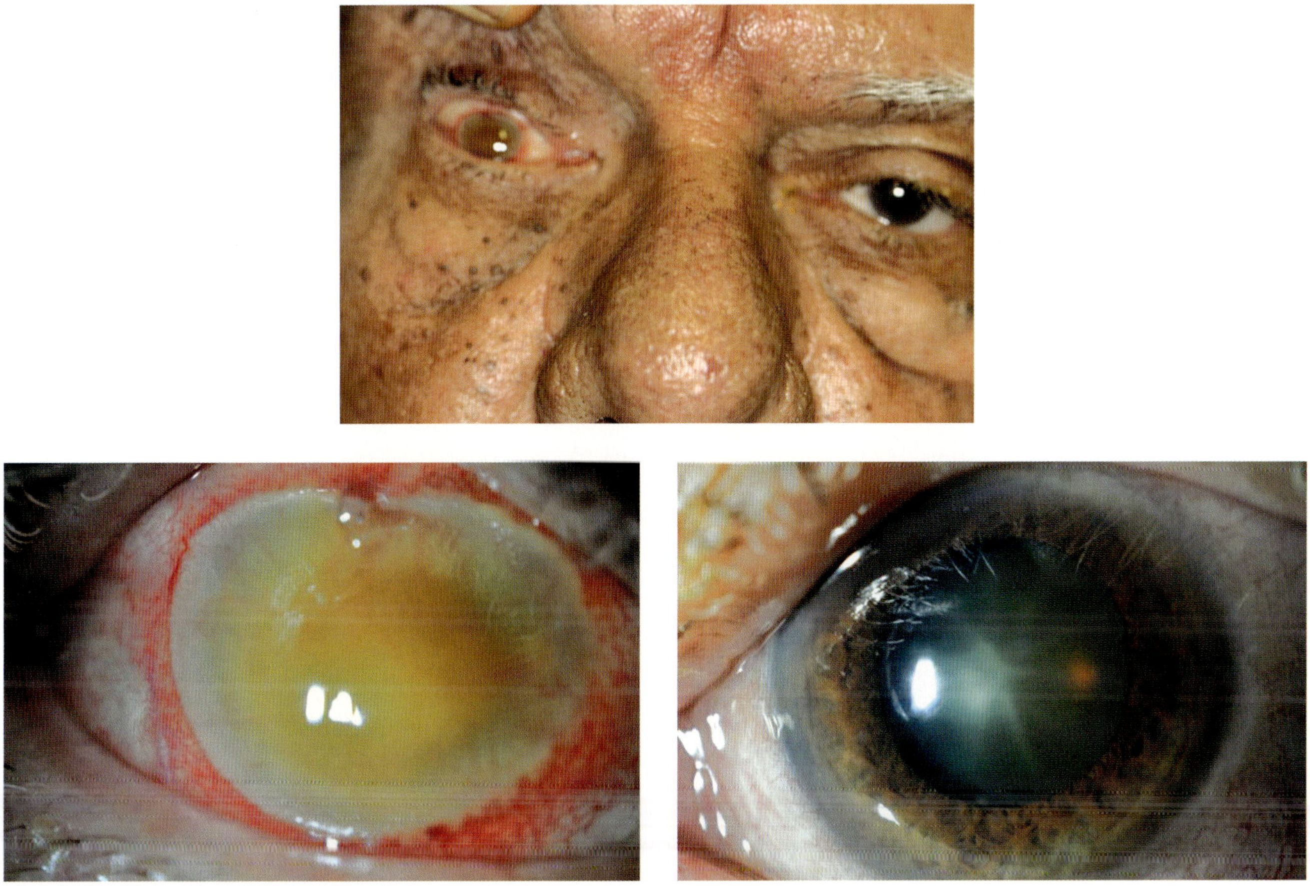

Fig. 10.37: Slit-lamp biomicroscopy: (Above) Cosmetic appearance of both eyes; (Below) Normal left eye and opacified right eye

Postoperative Results

Patient highly satisfied with results, with minimal hyperemia and excellent results, and he was advised to under ptosis surgery for more improvement of the cosmetic appearance

Follow-up and Comments

On follow-up, stable pigmentation, with very good aspect and high patient satisfaction (Figure 10.38).

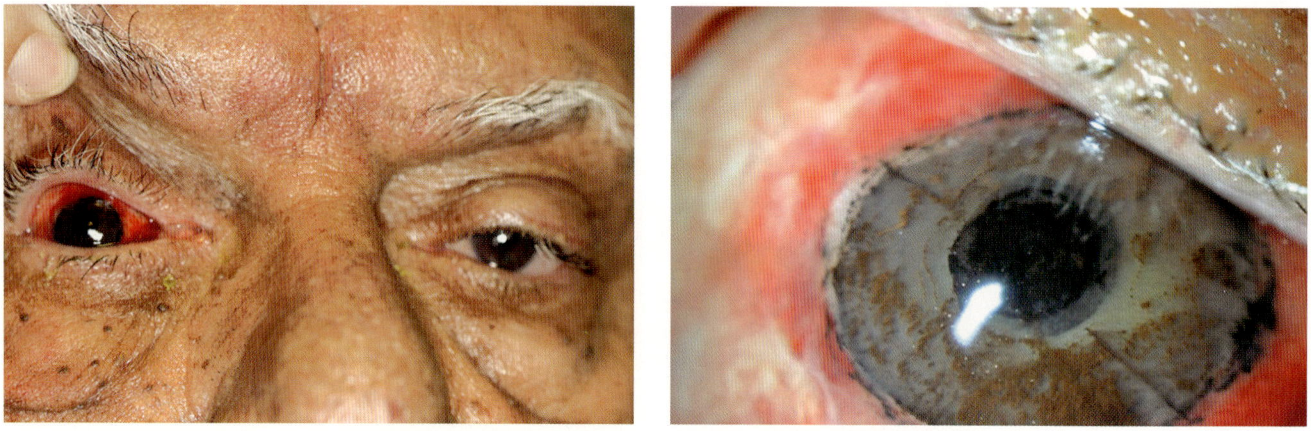

Fig. 10.38: One month follow-up cosmetic results

FEMTOSECOND-ASSISTED KERATOPIGMENTATION (FAK) (INCLUDING COMBINED TECHNIQUES)

CASE 15

Clinical History

A 34-year-male with history of left congenital cataract surgery at the age of 7, and history of trauma on the same eye,10 years before without re-intervention.

Preoperative Data

On examination, his left cornea was opacified and there was a traumatic iris defect between 10-12 o'clock (Figure 10.39).

Surgical Technique

Femtosecond-assisted keratopigmentation using greenish brown (VEMP 591) and black (VEMP 190) pigments.

Postoperative Results

Very good results, with minimal conjunctival injection (Figure 10.40).

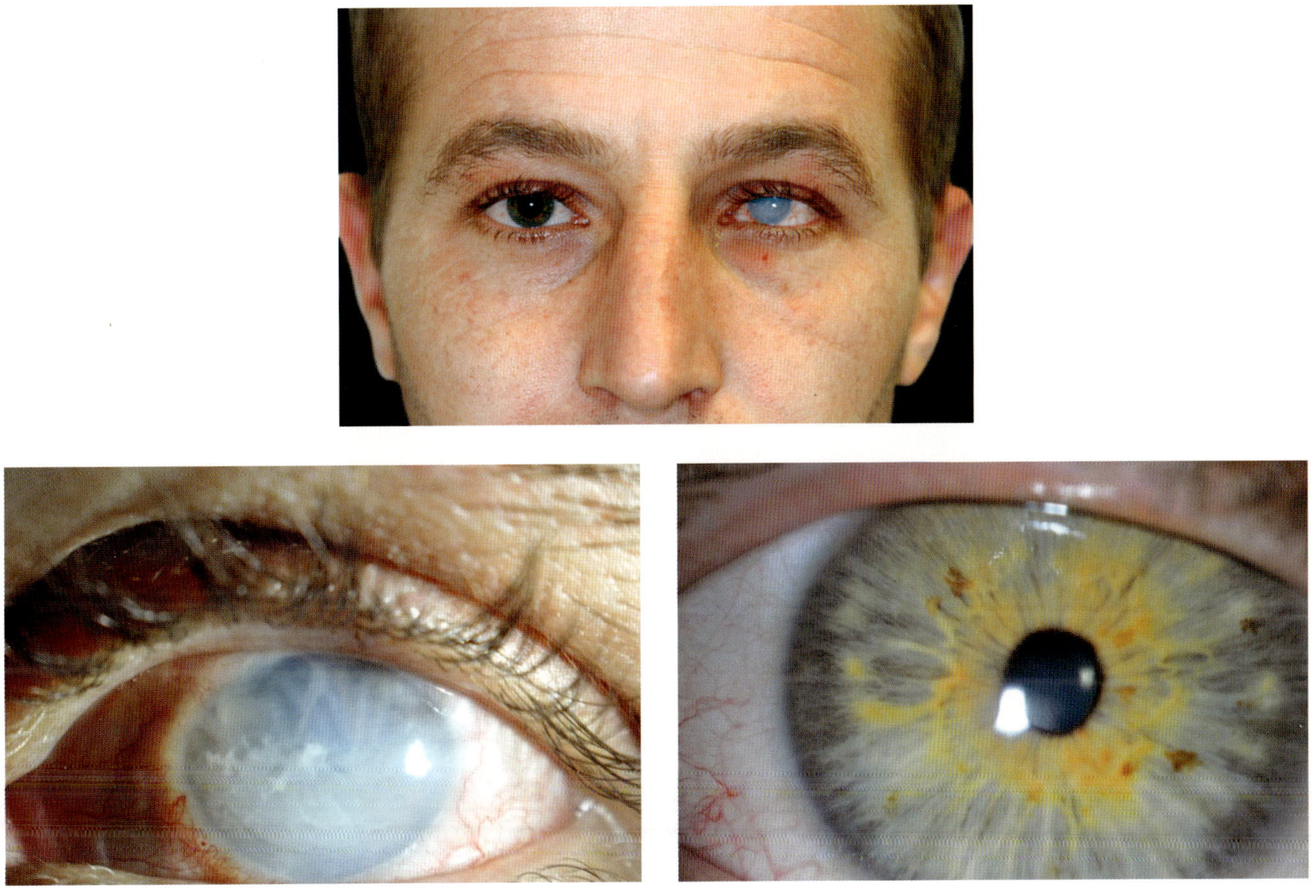

Fig. 10.39: Slit-lamp examination: (Above) Cosmetic appearance of both eyes; (Below) Normal right eye and corneal opacity of left eye

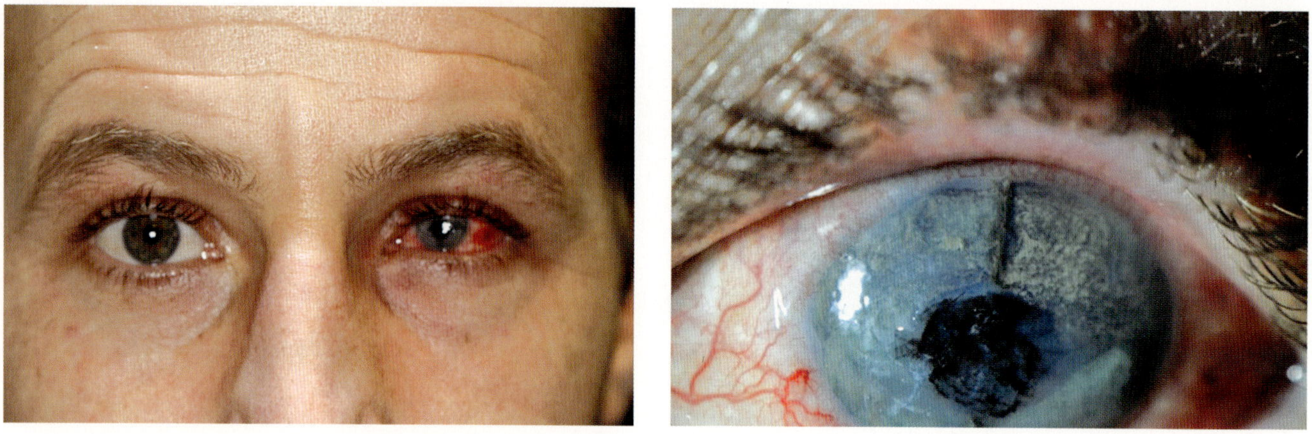

Fig. 10.40: Postoperative results. (Right) Slit-lamp examination after keratopigmentation; (Left) Cosmetic appearance of both eyes

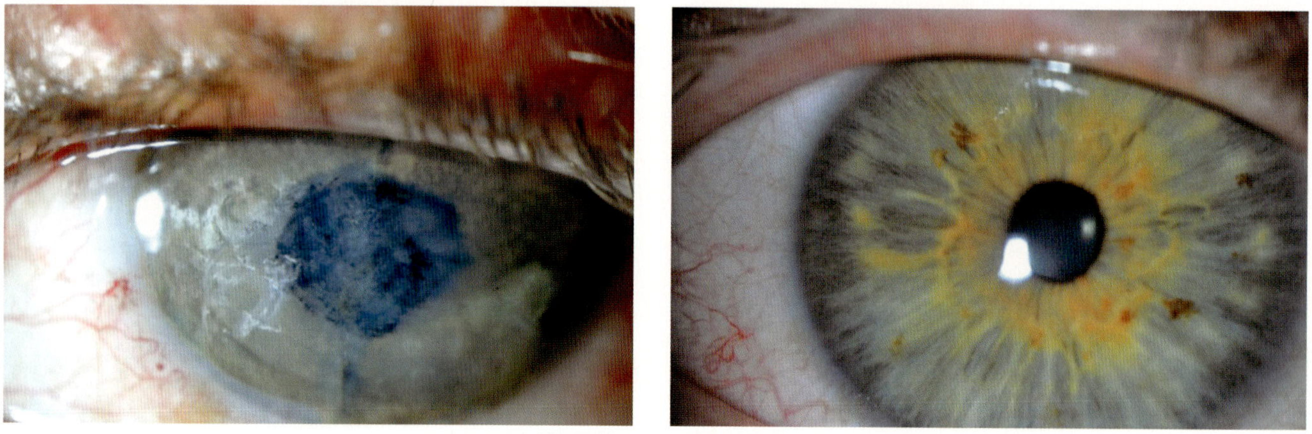

Fig. 10.41: Final cosmetic result

Follow-up and Comments

On follow-up, a slight fading of the pigmentation pattern was observed, but the cosmetic result was still very good (Figure 10.41), however he might need a re-pigmentation of the pupil and iris area in the future.

CASE 16

CLINICAL HISTORY

A 64-year-old female underwent bilateral cataract surgery in the past. There was a complication on her right eye that required further surgery. She underwent a right vitrectomy and silicone oil injection.

Preoperative Data

On examination, her right eye cornea was decompensated with several Descemet's membrane folds. This was the vitrectomized eye with silicone oil. Her visual acuity was hand movements on that side (Figure 10.42).

Surgical Technique

Femtosecond-assisted keratopigmentation technique, using a brown (VEMP 200) color to mimic the iris. The intralamellar tunnel was created with this measures: 4.5 mm for the inner diameter of the tunnel and 9.5 mm for the outer diameter.

Manual intrastromal technique was also performed to recreate the pupil using a black (VEMP 100) color.

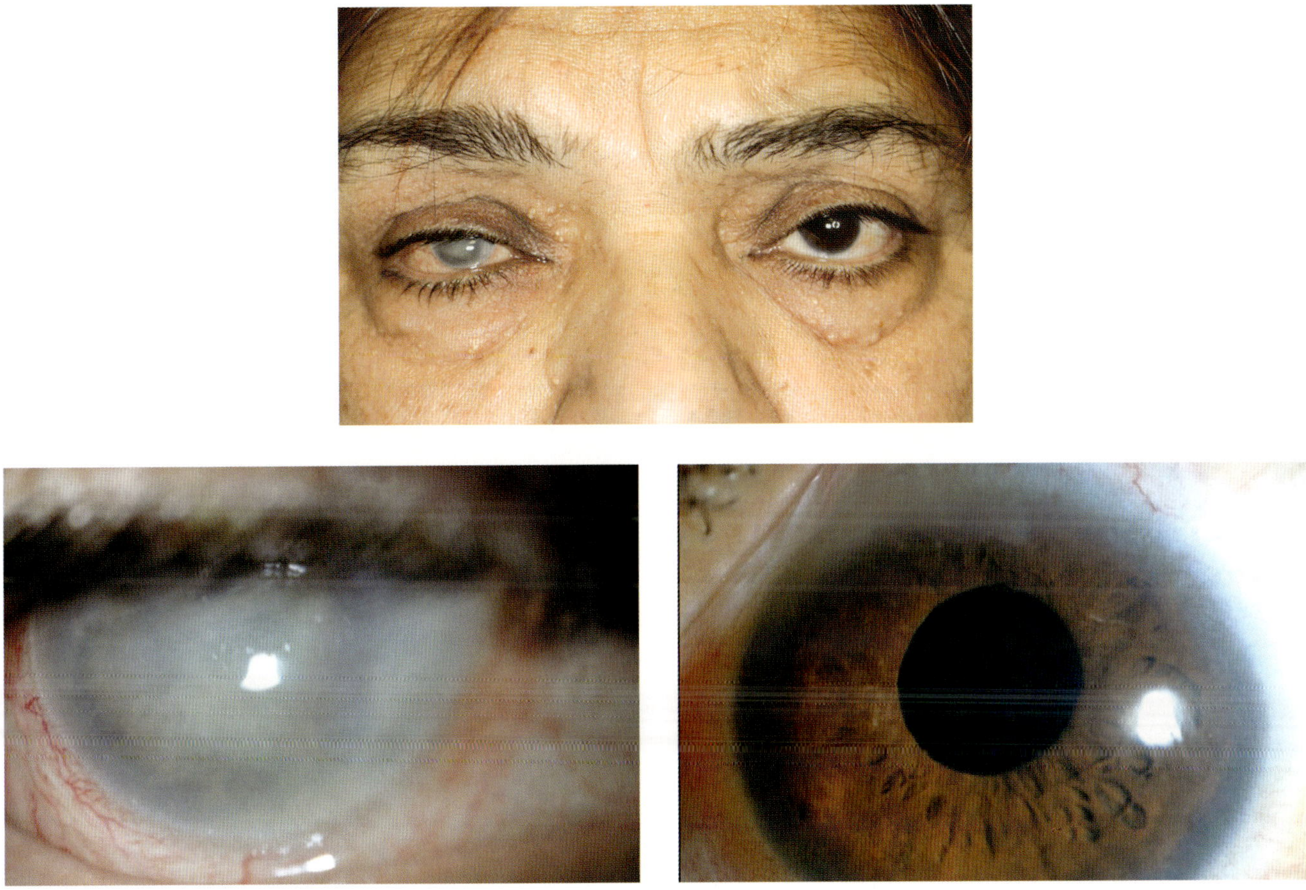

Fig. 10.42: Slit-lamp examination: (Above) Cosmetic appearance of both eyes; (Below) Normal left eye and corneal opacity of right eye

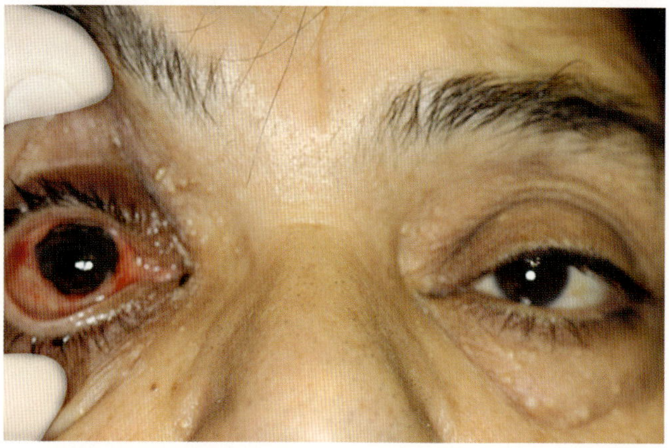

Fig. 10.43: Postoperative results. Cosmetic appearance of both eyes

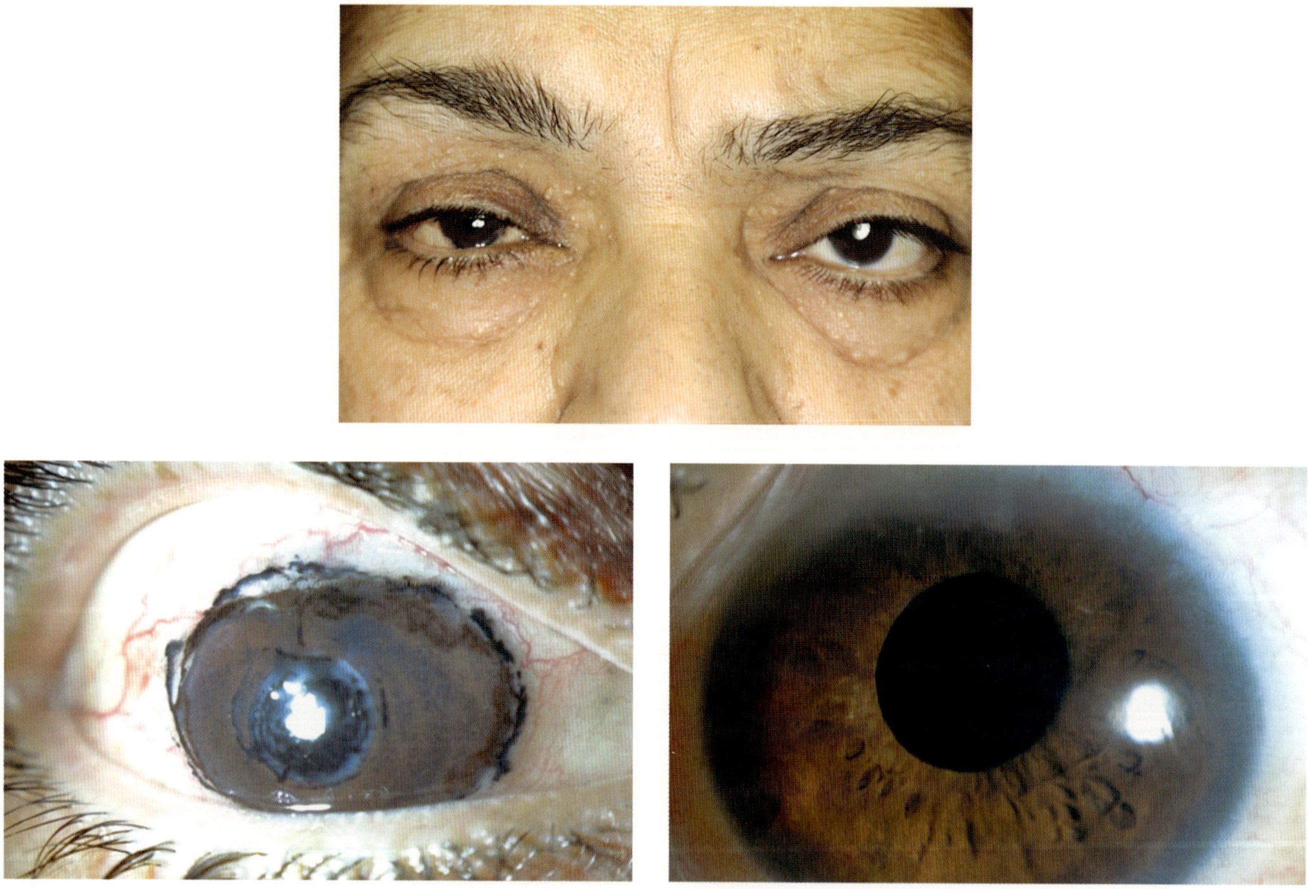

Fig. 10.44: Cosmetic result 3 months after surgery

Postoperative Results

Minimal inflammation with excellent cosmetic appearance (Figure 10.43).

Follow-up and Comments

The patient was highly satisfied with stable and a regular pigmentation of the cornea (Figure 10.44).

CASE 17

Clinical History

A 59-year-old high myopic male, who had a left eye retinal detachment, and therefore a left vitrectomy 15 years ago, presented with a left eye corneal opacity.

Preoperative Data

On examination, there was a neovascularized corneal opacity on his left eye, phthisis bulbi and the visual acuity was no perception of light. There was also a nuclear cataract with a reduced visual acuity on his right eye and a cataract surgery was performed (Figure 10.45).

Surgical Technique

Femtosecond-assisted keratopigmentation technique, using brown (VEMP 290) for the iris area and black (VEMP 190) for the pupil area.

The femtosecond settings were 9.5 mm of diameter for the outer limit of the tunnel and 4.5 mm of diameter for the inner edge of the tunnel. An strabismus surgery was also carried out.

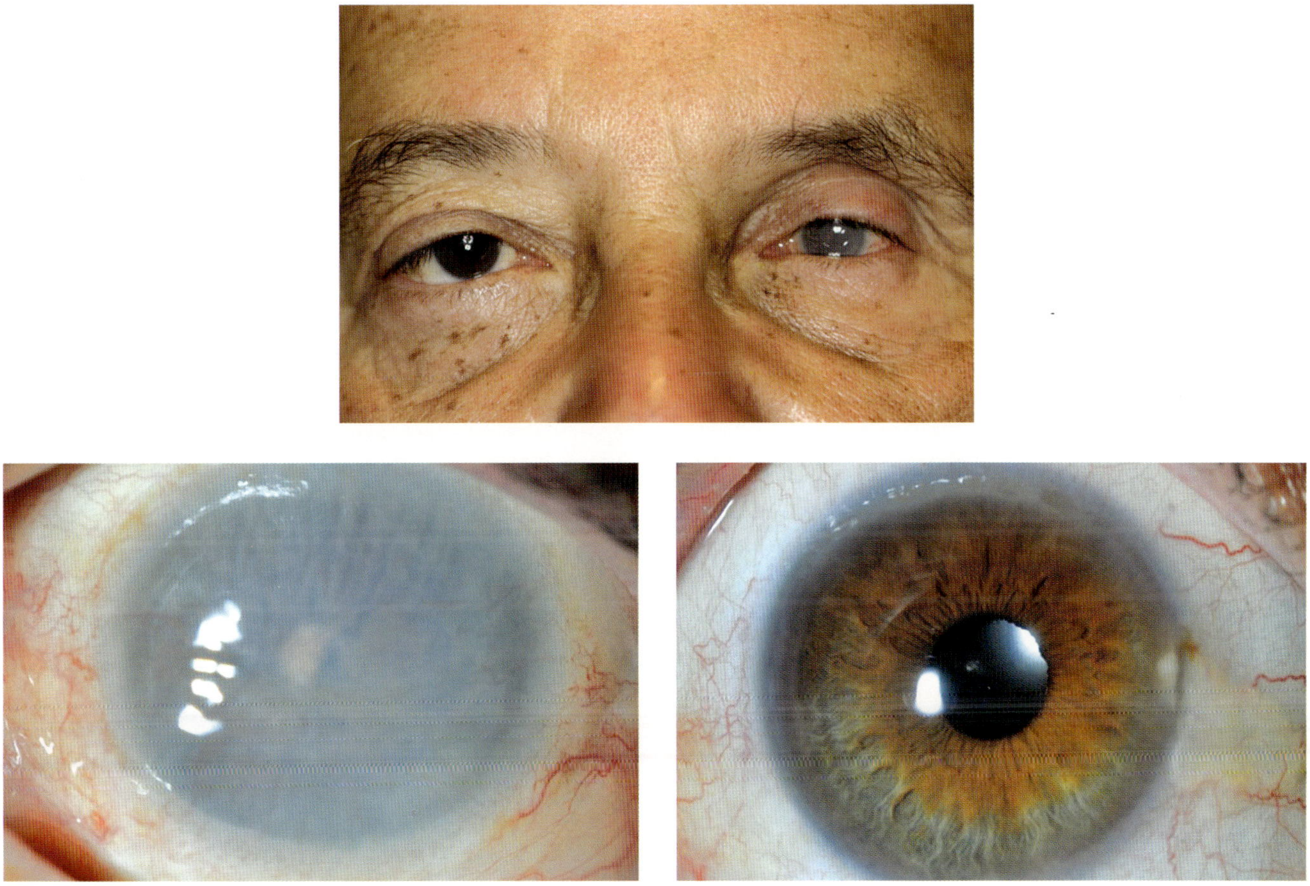

Fig. 10.45: Slit-lamp examination: (Above) Cosmetic appearance of both eyes; (Below) Normal right eye and corneal opacification of left eye

Postoperative Results

Moderate inflammation with excellent cosmetic appearance and good disposition of the pigments inside the intralamellar tunnel.

Follow-up and Comments

Excellent cosmetic results, the final visual acuity was 0,8 (decimal) and no perception of light for right and left eyes respectively (Figure 10.46).

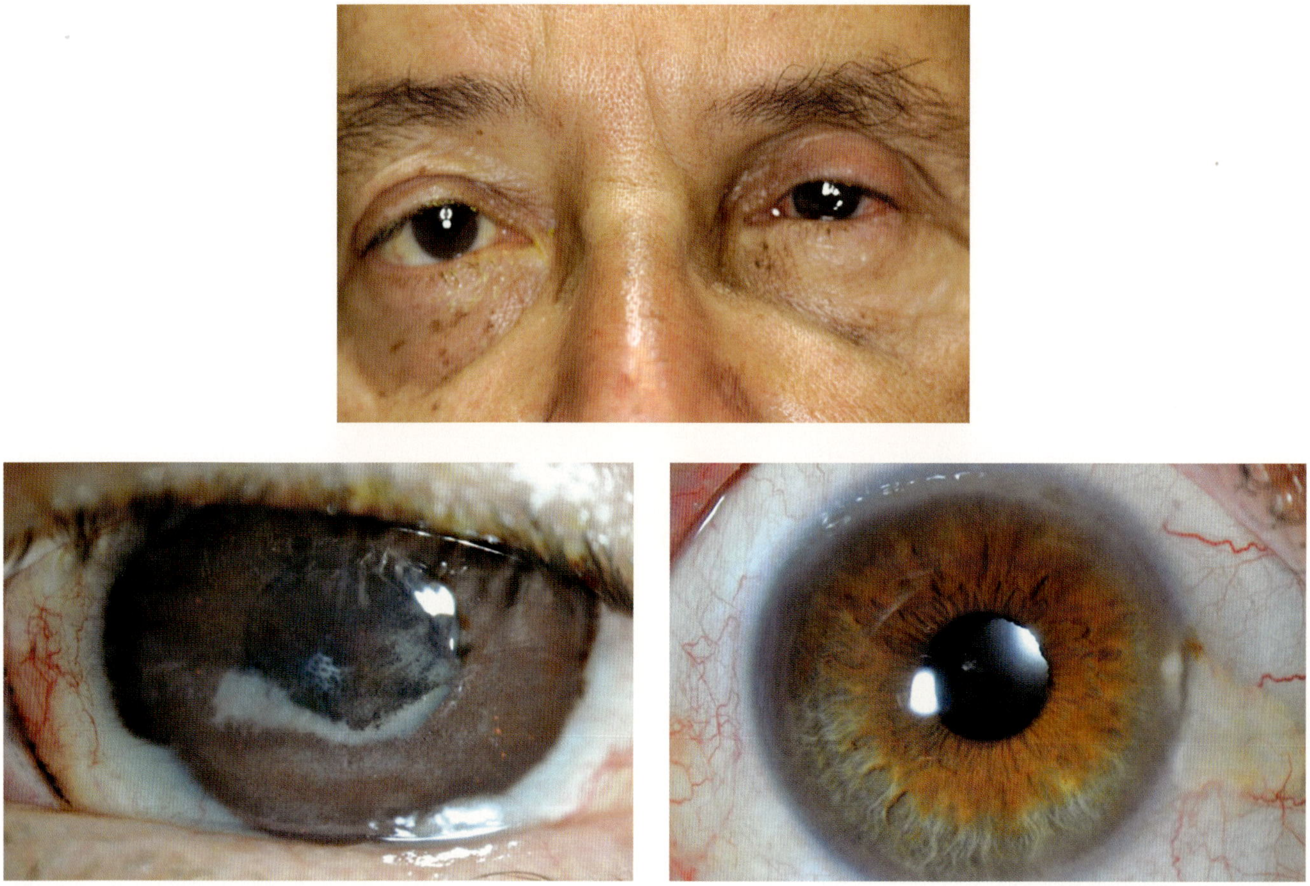

Fig. 10.46: Cosmetic results 3 months after surgery.

CASE 18

Clinical History

A 26-year-old male with history of right eye car accident 2 years before his presentation.

Preoperative Data

On examination, patient presented with an adherent dense corneal opacification, a distorted and affected pupil and a traumatic cataract. His visual acuity was no perception of light on that side (Figure 10.47).

Surgical Technique

Superficial and femtosecond-assisted keratopigmentation techniques: The pupil was marked at 3.5 mm of diameter and colored using needle 3 and black (VEMP 190) pigment. The limbus was also colored with the same pigment and brown (VEMP 290) was used for the iris area using needle 5.

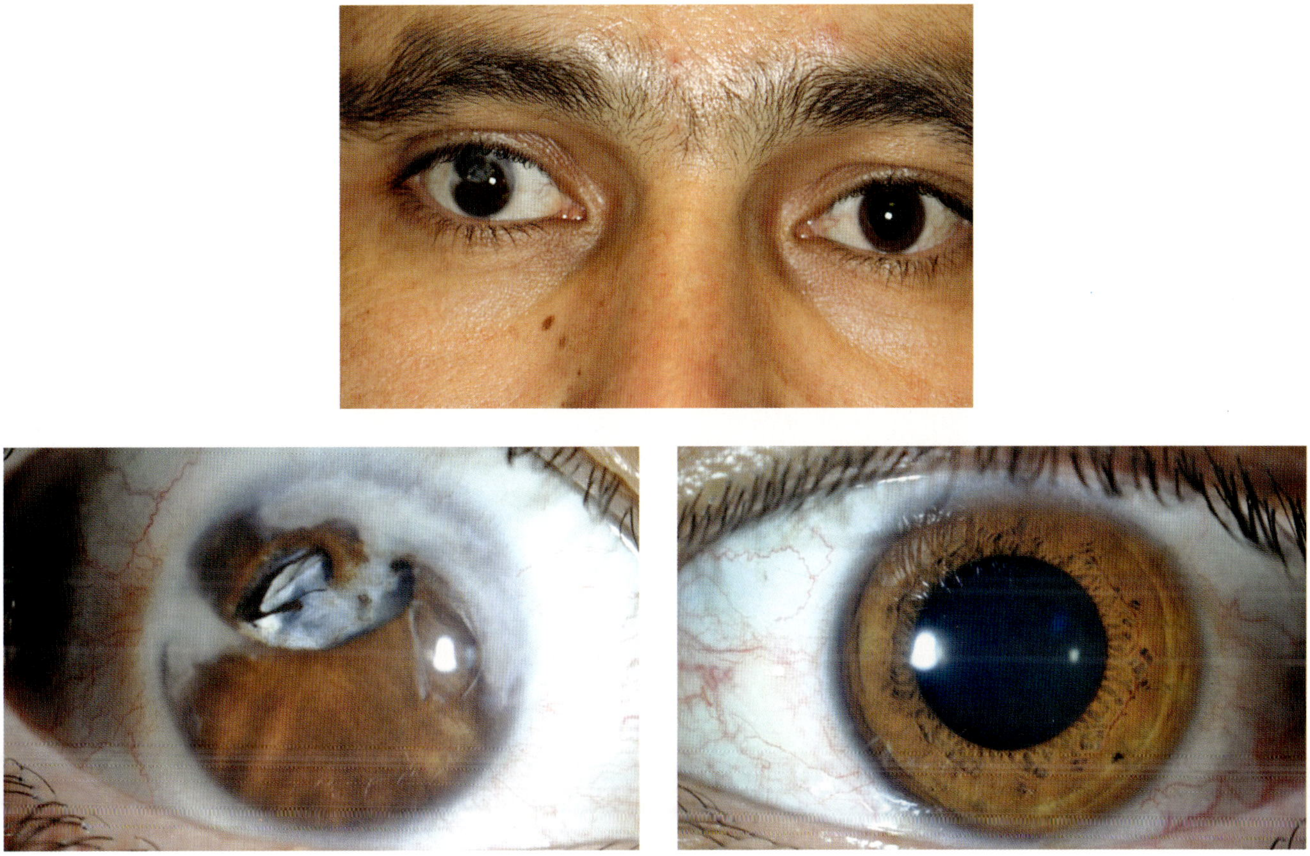

Fig. 10.47: Slit-lamp examination: (Above) Cosmetic appearance of both eyes; (Below) Normal left eye and right traumatic eye

Postoperative Results

First visit postoperatively: Patient presented with moderate hyperemia and excellent cosmetic appearance (Figure 10.48).

Follow-up and Comments

Excellent results. An strabismus surgery was carried out at this stage (Figure 10.49).

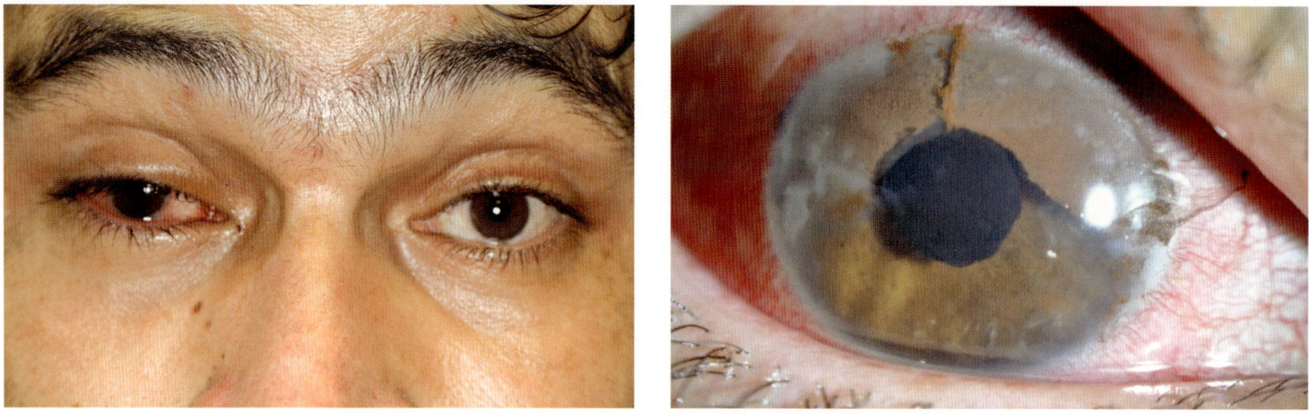

Fig. 10.48: Postoperative results. (Right) Slit-lamp view after keratopigmentation; (Left) Cosmetic appearance of both eyes

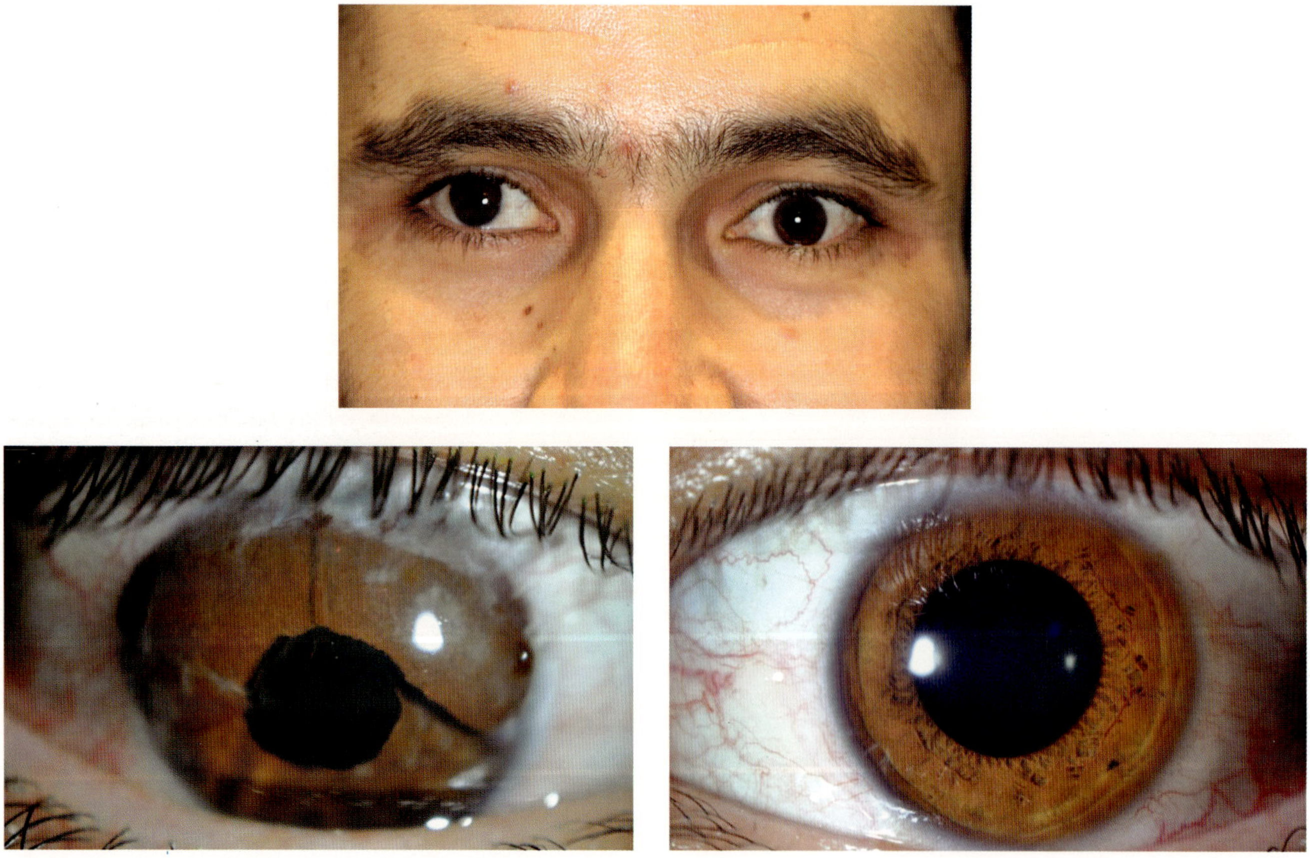

Fig. 10.49: Cosmetic results 3 months after surgery

CASE 19

Clinical History

A 15-year-old female with history of right eye spike injury at the age of 1 year.

Preoperative Data

On examination, corneal opacity, neovascularization and traumatic iris atrophy was observed in her right eye. The visual acuity was count finger at 10 cm and 1.0 (decimal) for right and left eyes respectively (Figure 10.50).

Surgical Technique

Femtosecond-assisted keratopigmentation technique, using brown (VEMP 290) pigment. The tunnel was created with an external diameter of 9.5 mm and an internal diameter of 4 mm, at 300 microns of depth and the incision at 90 degrees, assisted by manual intrastromal dissection after the femtosecond laser was applied.

PTK at 50 microns of depth was also performed to correct her band keratopathy.

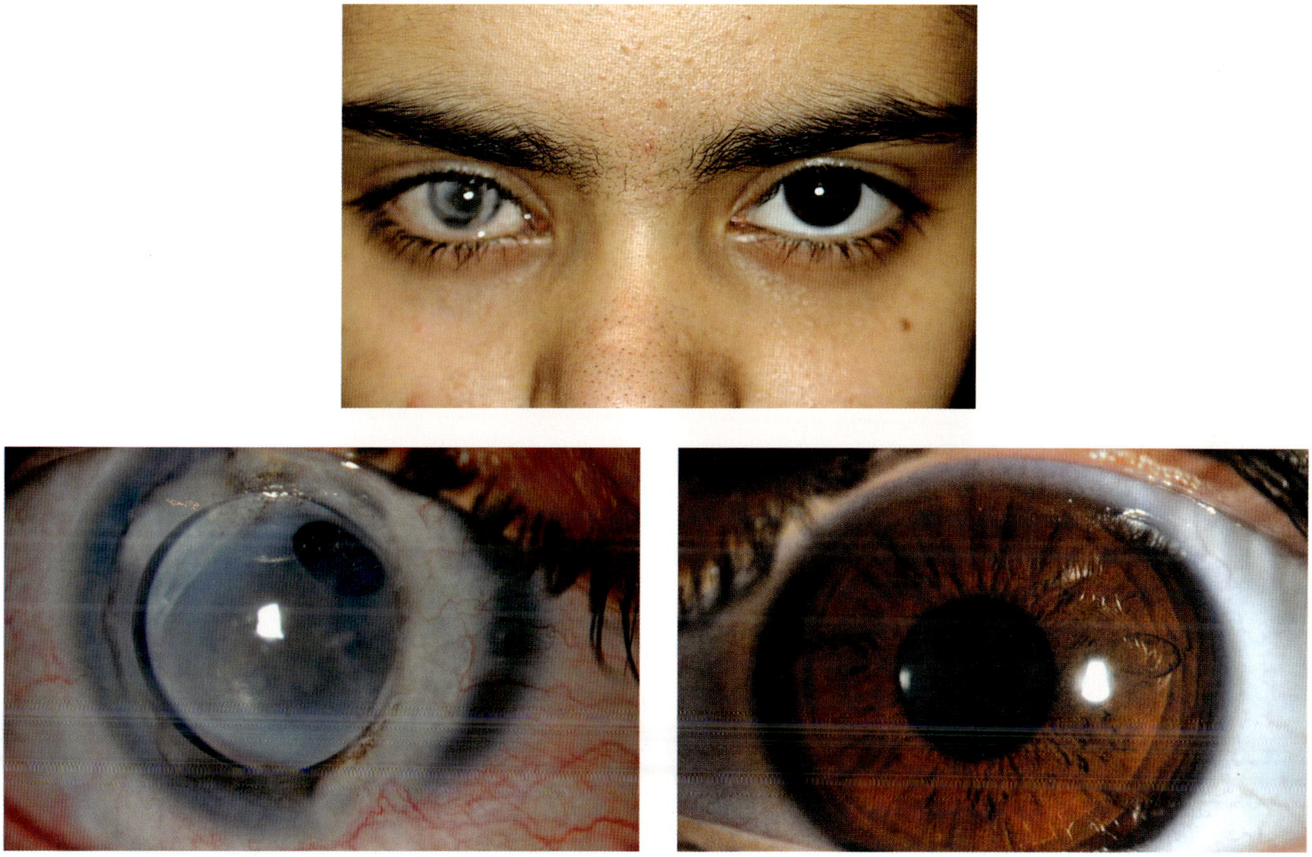

Fig. 10.50: Slit-lamp examination: (Above) Cosmetic appearance of both eyes; (Below) Normal left eye and traumatic right eye

Postoperative Results

Patient was very satisfied, with an excellent appearance and a complete resolution of her band keratopathy (Figure 10.51).

Follow-up and Comments

Good cosmetic result, with a minimal superficial corneal staining in the neovascularized area (Figure 10.52).

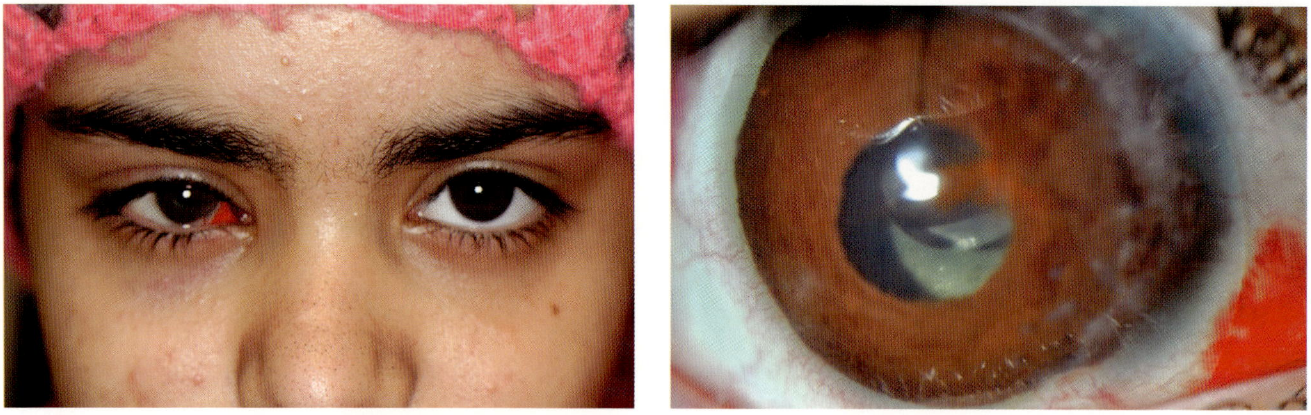

Fig. 10.51: Postoperative results. (Right) Slit-lamp examination after keratopigmentation; (Left) Cosmetic appearance of both eyes

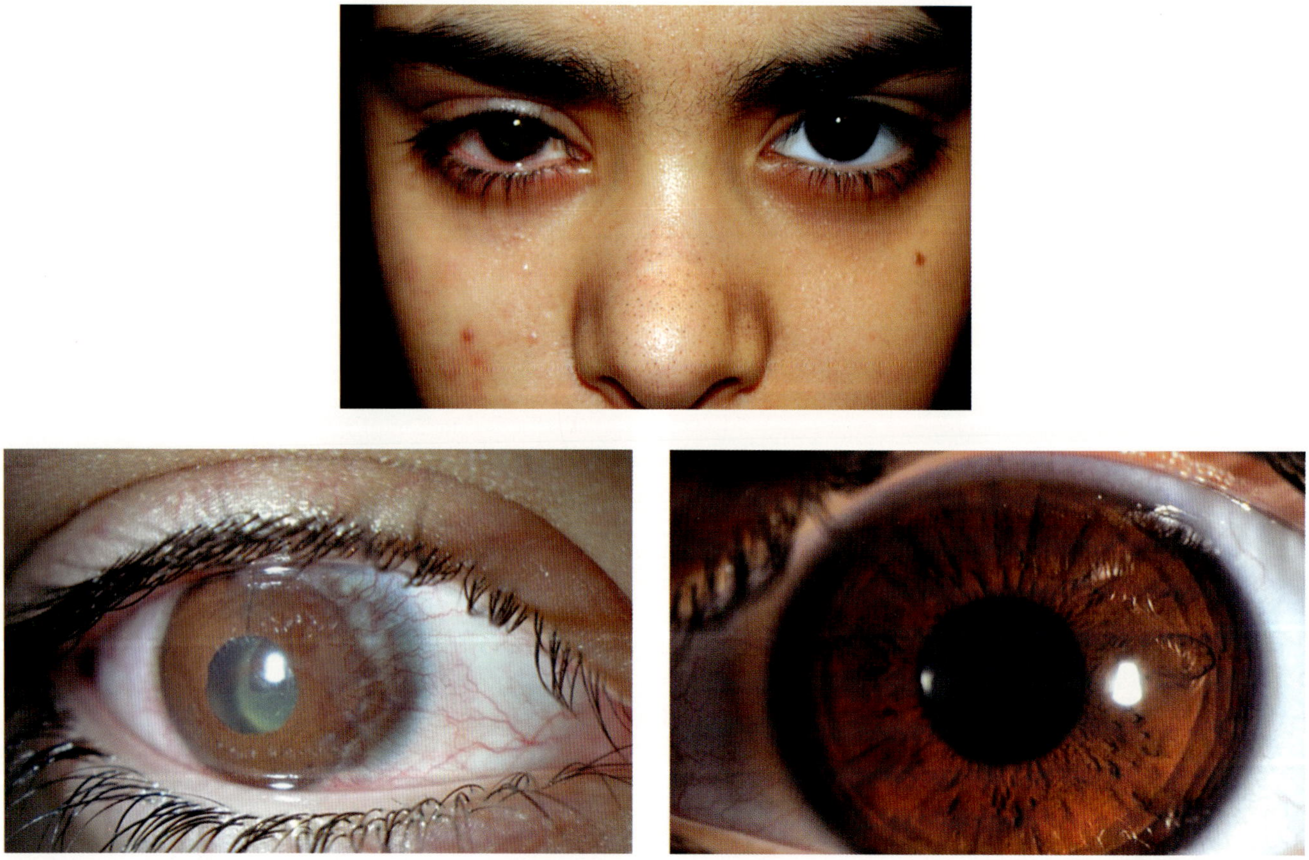

Fig. 10.52: Cosmetic results

CASE 20

Clinical History

A 71-year-old female, underwent cataract surgery and she had a severe blunt trauma a year after this surgery.

Preoperative Data

On examination, she presented with a corneal neovascularized opacity probably related to a previously treated nasal corneal laceration. There was also an almost total traumatic aniridia, aphakia and some vitreous strands in the anterior chamber. Her visual acuity was counting fingers (CF) at 10 cm (Figure 10.53).

Surgical Technique

Anterior segment reconstructions:
- Anterior vitrectomy
- Secondary intraocular lens implant
- Strabismus correction
- Femtosecond-assisted keratopigmentation

The tunnel was created with an external diameter of 9.4 mm and an internal diameter of 4.5 mm, at 300 microns of depth and the incision at 90 degrees, another tunnel was created with the same parameters but at 200 microns of depth and the incision at 270 degrees, then manual intrastromal dissection was performed, using black (VEMP 191) and brown (VEMP 290) pigments.

Postoperative Results

First visit postoperatively: Good results but a repigmentation enhancement might be required (Figure 10.54).

Follow-up and Comments

- Second keratopigmentation surgery was carried out using brown (VEMP 290) pigment, and the pupil was marked with 4 mm of diameter.
- On follow-up, good pigmentation, with no edema but a minimal conjunctival injection and subconjunctival hemorrhage. Some pigment deposits were noticed on the intraocular lens (IOL) (Figure 10.55) but they were resolved. Spontaneously a few months later.

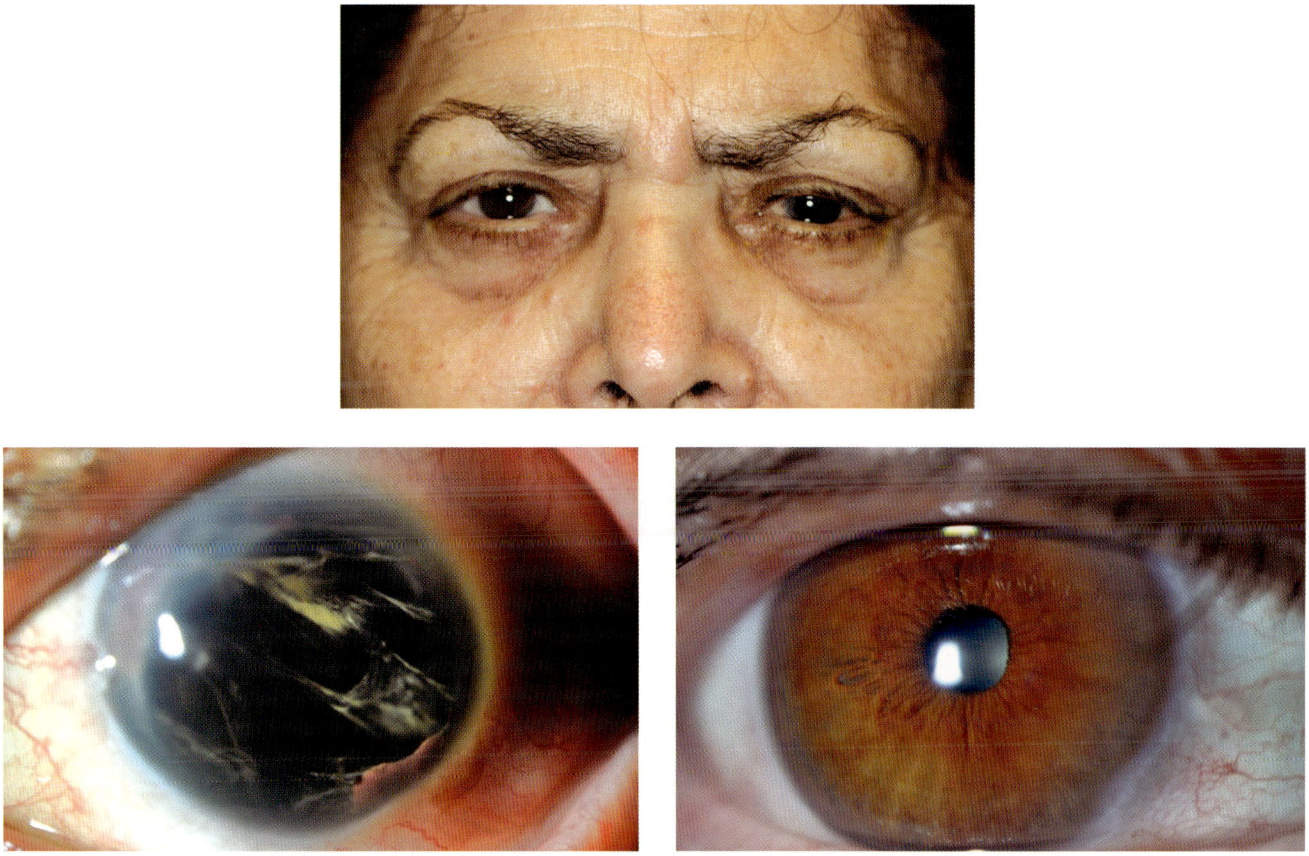

Fig. 10.53: Slit-lamp examination: (Above) Cosmetic appearance of both eyes; (Below) Normal right eye and left traumatic eye

- Six months after the surgery a repigmentation was considered
- A third keratopigmentation was performed and the pupil was marked with 3 mm of diameter using black (VEMP 191) pigment and the iris tone was changed with brown (VEMP 290) pigment
- Final examination demonstrated a uniform and stable pigmentation (Figure 10.56).

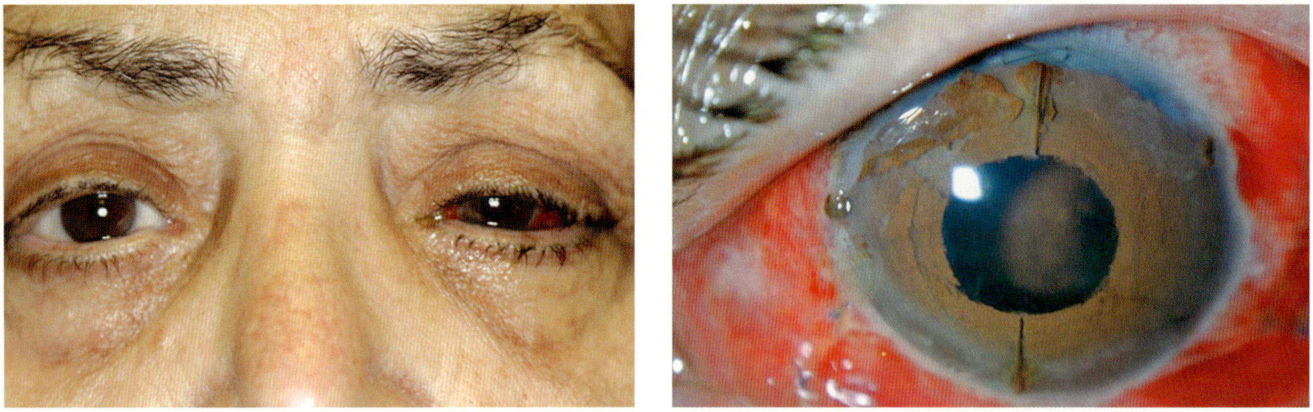

Fig. 10.54: Postoperative results. (Right) Slit-lamp examination after keratopigmentation, (Left) Cosmetic appearance of both eyes

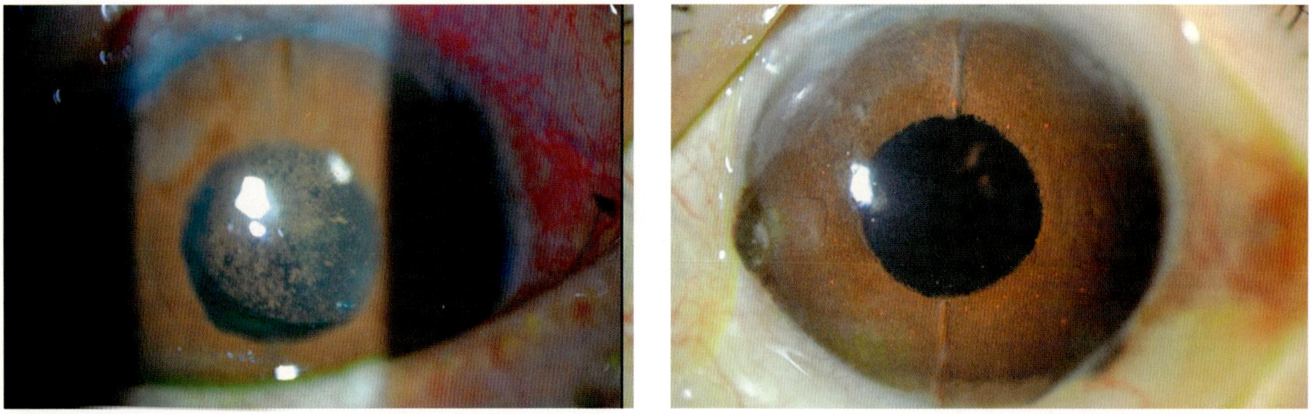

Fig. 10.55: Pigment deposits on IOL on the left, spontaneous resolution of these deposits on the right

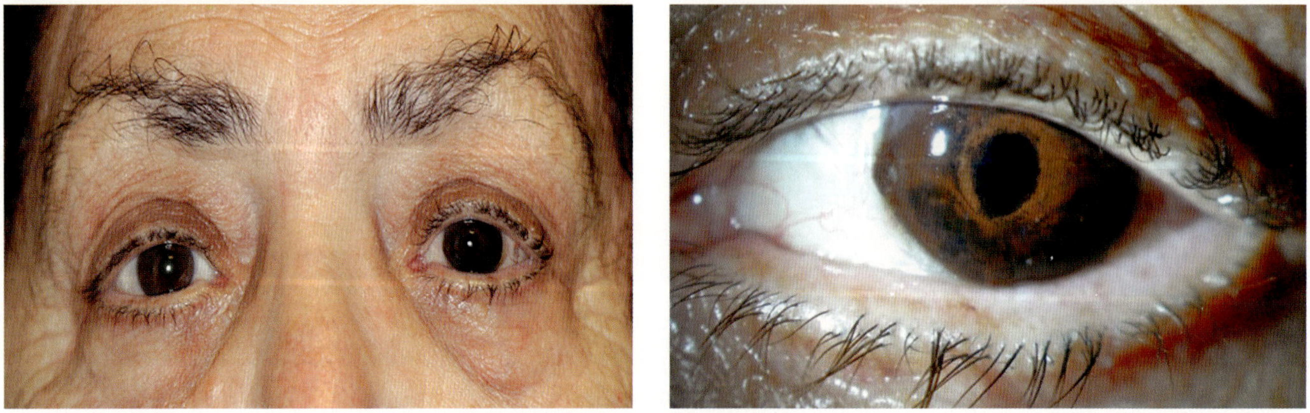

Fig. 10.56: Final results after keratopigmentation

CASE 21

Clinical History

A 35 years female patient, who underwent complicated congenital glaucoma surgery at the age of 3 months, with final visual acuity of no perception of light. She was referred by her consultant for cosmetic solution.

Preoperative Data

On examination: Left eye megalophthalmos with white to white of 14 mm compared to 12 mm in the right eye. Edematous cornea in the left pseudophakic eye with upper conjunctival scarring. She underwent strabismus surgery before keratopigmentation for further improvement of the cosmetic appearance with cyclophotocoagulation in the same setting (Figure 10.57).

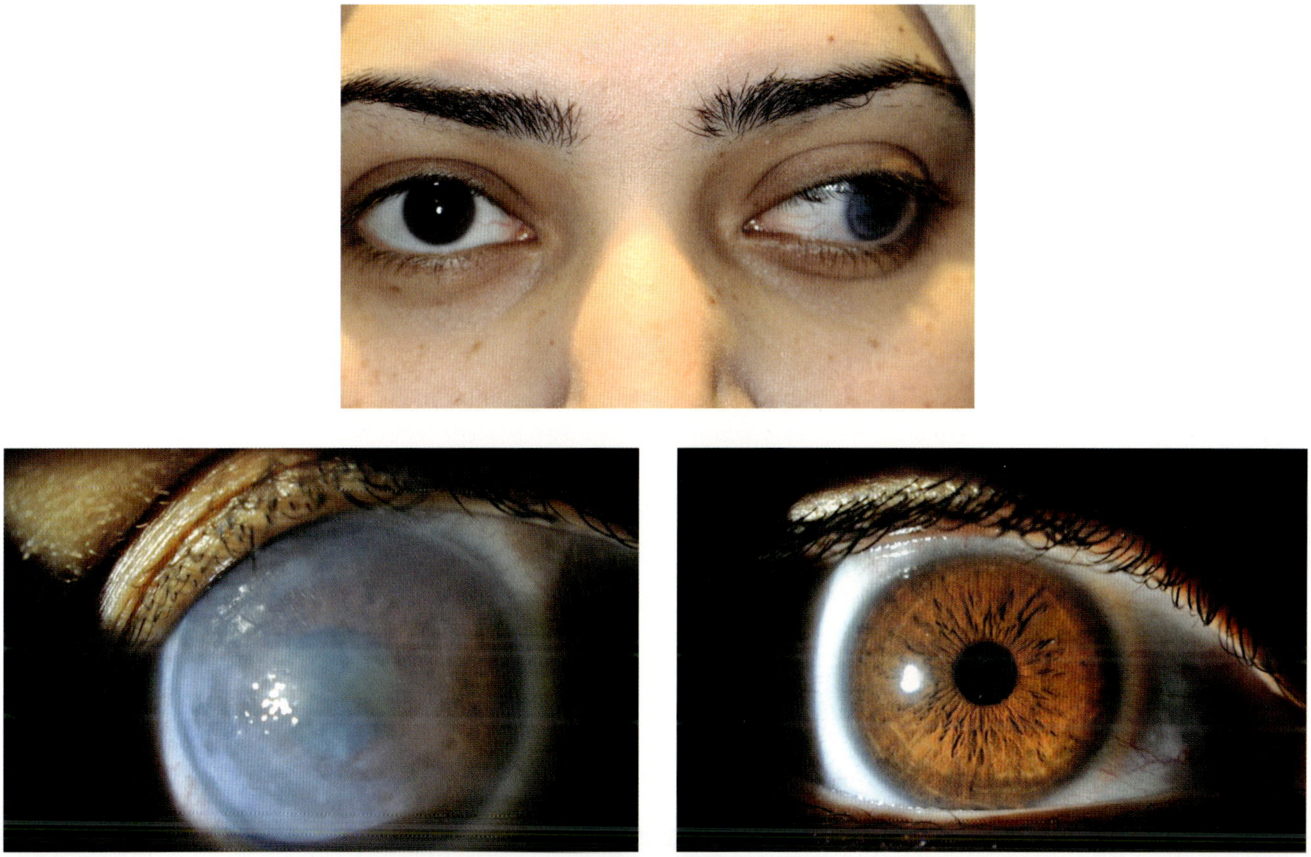

Fig. 10.57: Slit-lamp biomicroscopy: (Above) Cosmetic appearance of both eyes; (Below) Normal right eye and corneal opacification of left eye

Surgical Technique

Femtosecond-assisted Keratopigmentation

- Depth 440 microns with outer and inner limits of 9 mm and 4, 5 mm
- Using dark brown (VEMP 200) pigment for iris and black (VEMP 100) pigment for pupil.

Postoperative Results

Patient satisfied with results with no complications (Figure 10.58)

Follow-up and Comments

On follow-up: Satisfactory cosmetic results with grayish brown appearance due to minimal edema and good limbal staining pattern.

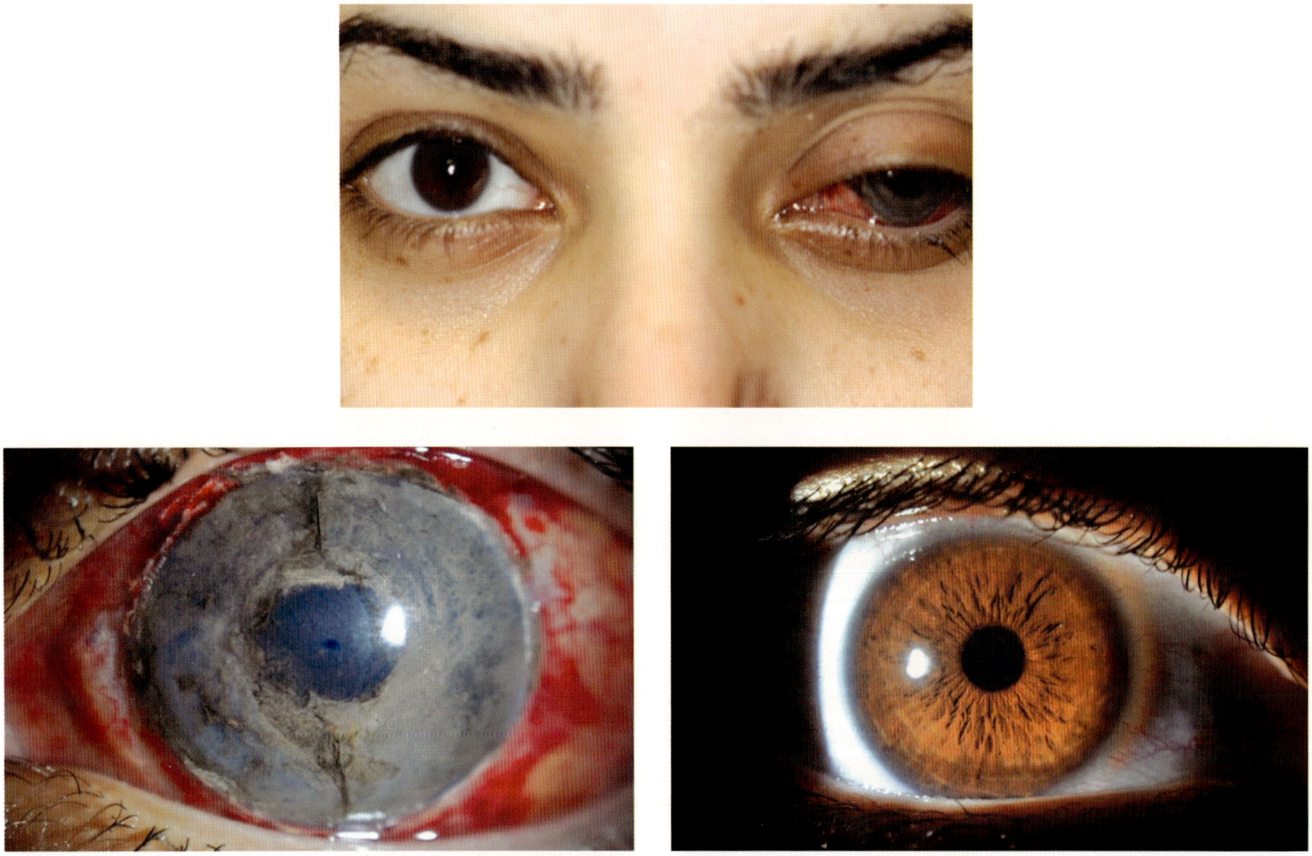

Fig. 10.58: Three weeks follow-up cosmetic results

CASE 22

Clinical History

A 50-year-old male with history of left eye old trauma with a stone at the age of 24.

Preoperative Data

On examination, left corneal opacity, opacified lens (traumatic cataract) with iris rubeosis and optic disc atrophy. His visual acuity was no perception of light on that eye (Figure 10.59).

Surgical Technique

Femtosecond-assisted keratopigmentation combined with intralamellar manual technique, using brown (VEMP 201) pigment for the iris and black (VEMP 100) pigment for the pupil.

Postoperative Results

Excellent appearance and minimal conjunctival injection (Figure 10.60).

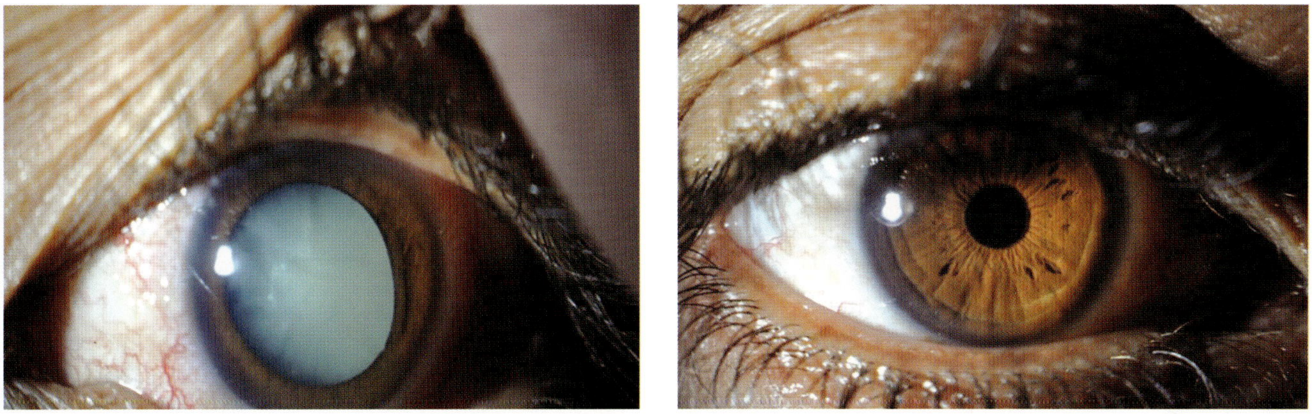

Fig. 10.59: Slit-lamp examination: (Right) Cosmetic appearance of both eyes; (Left) Normal right eye and traumatized left eye

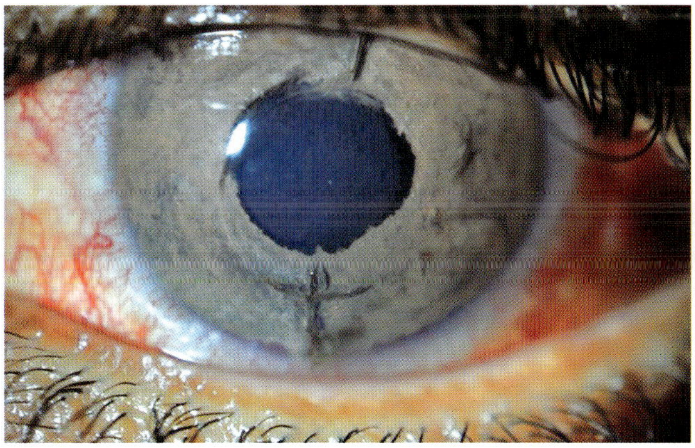

Fig. 10.60: Postoperative result

Follow-up and Comments

Patient was very satisfied with the outcomes, the pigmentation was uniform showing good cosmetic results (Figure 10.61).

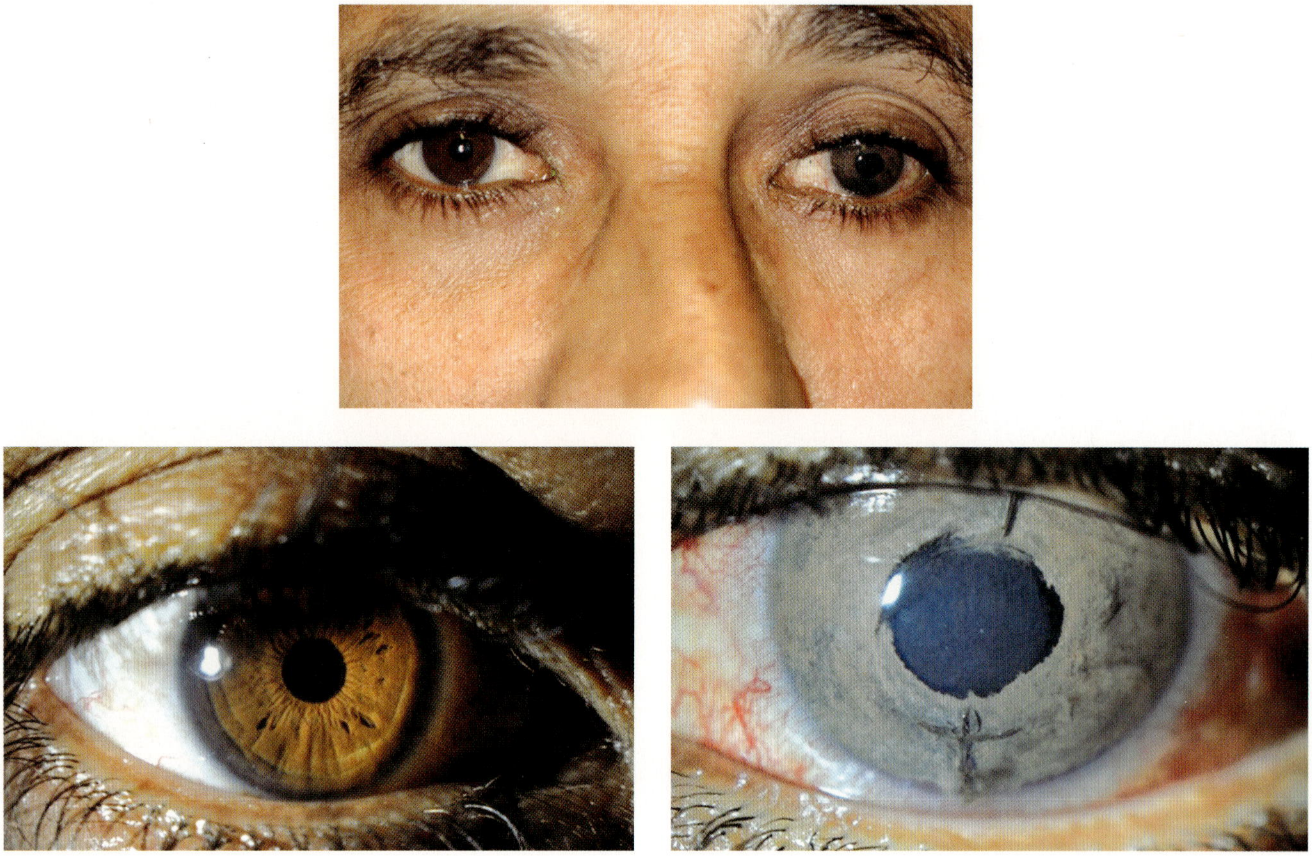

Fig. 10.61: Cosmetic results 3 months after surgery

CASE 23

Clinical History

A 45-year-old male with history of left eye retinal detachment as a child, that required a vitrectomy and later on a cyclodiode-photocoagulation.

Preoperative Data

On examination: Left eye corneal opacity complicated with a white cataract. The visual acuity was 1.0 (decimal) and no perception of light in right and left eyes respectively (Figure 10.62).

Surgical Technique

Femtosecond-assisted keratopigmentation, two tunnels were performed at 250 microns for the pupil area and 350 microns for the iris simulation, completed with manual dissection, using brown (VEMP 290) pigment for the iris and black (VEMP 190) for the pupil.

Postoperative Results

Mild conjunctival injection and very good cosmetic appearance (Figure 10.63).

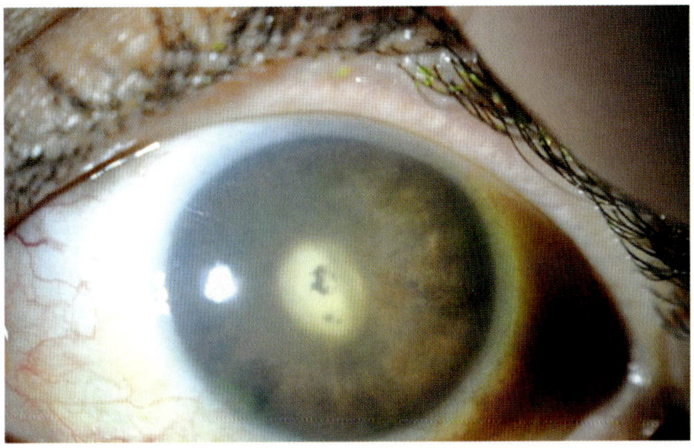

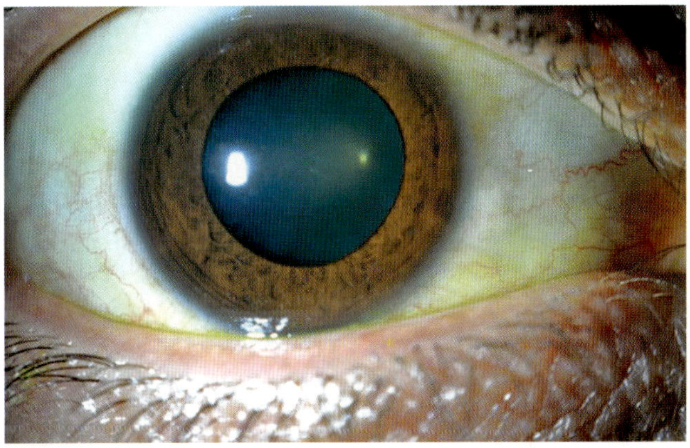

Fig. 10.62: Slit-lamp examination: (Right) Cosmetic appearance of both eyes; (Left) Normal right eye and corneal and lens opacity of left eye

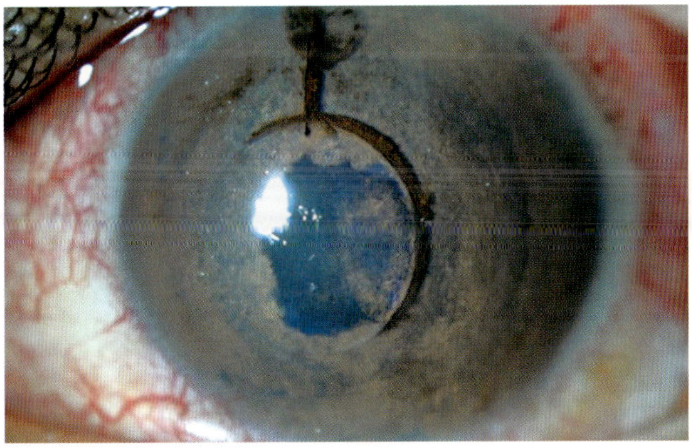

Fig. 10.63: Cosmetic results after surgery

Follow-up and Comments

Stable pigmentation months after the surgery and very high patient satisfaction (Figure 10.64).

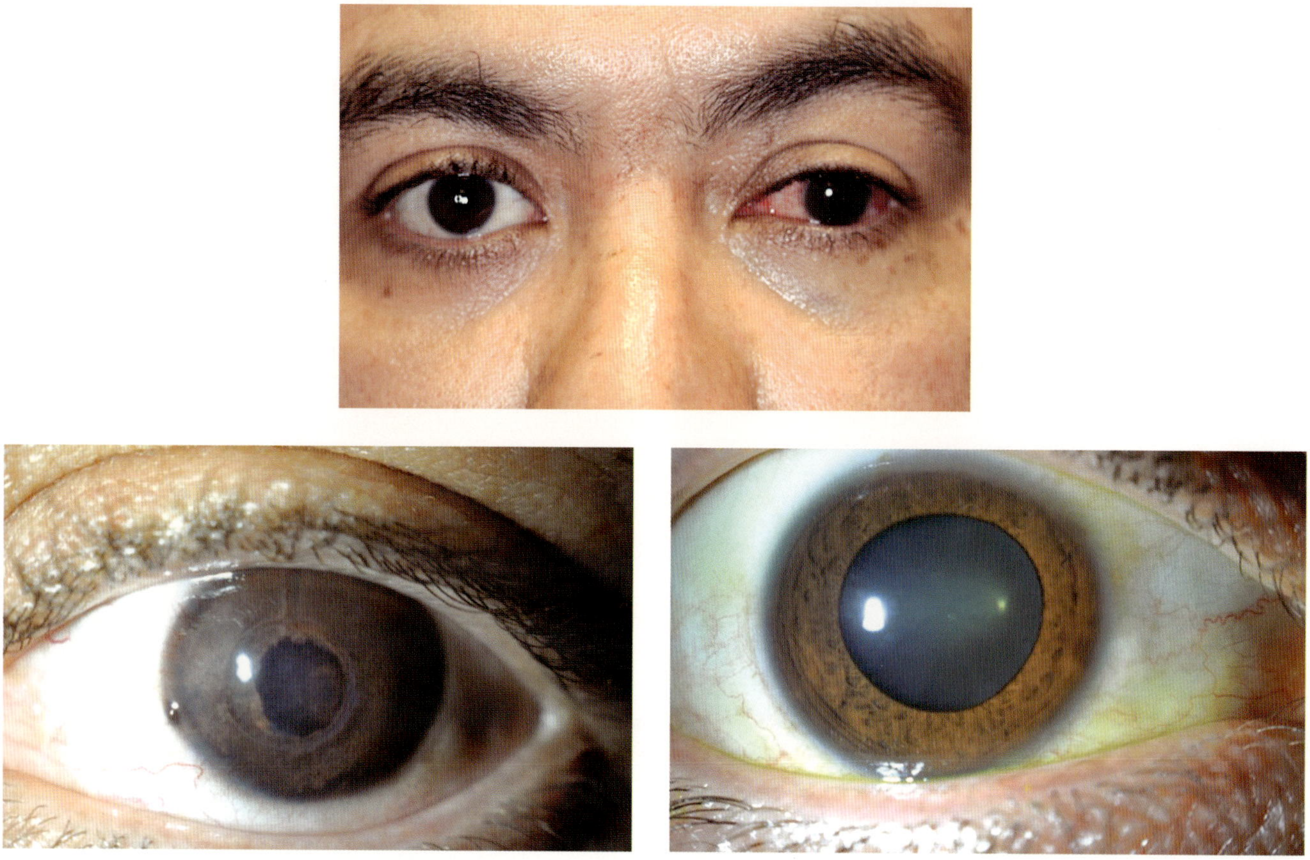

Fig. 10.64: Cosmetic results after keratopigmentation

CASE 24

Clinical History

An 18-year-old male with history of right eye trauma and visual acuity of no perception of light on his right eye and 1.0 (decimal) on his left eye.

Preoperative Data

On examination cornea was clear with traumatic iris and pupil abnormalities. The anterior chamber was filled with silicone and the fundus examination revealed a funnel retinal detachment (Figure 10.65).

Surgical Technique

Femtosecond-assisted keratopigmentation technique. The pupil was marked in the center with 4 mm of diameter and the cornea was pigmented using a black (VEMP 190) pigment for pupil and limbus and a brown (VEMP 290) pigment for the iris.

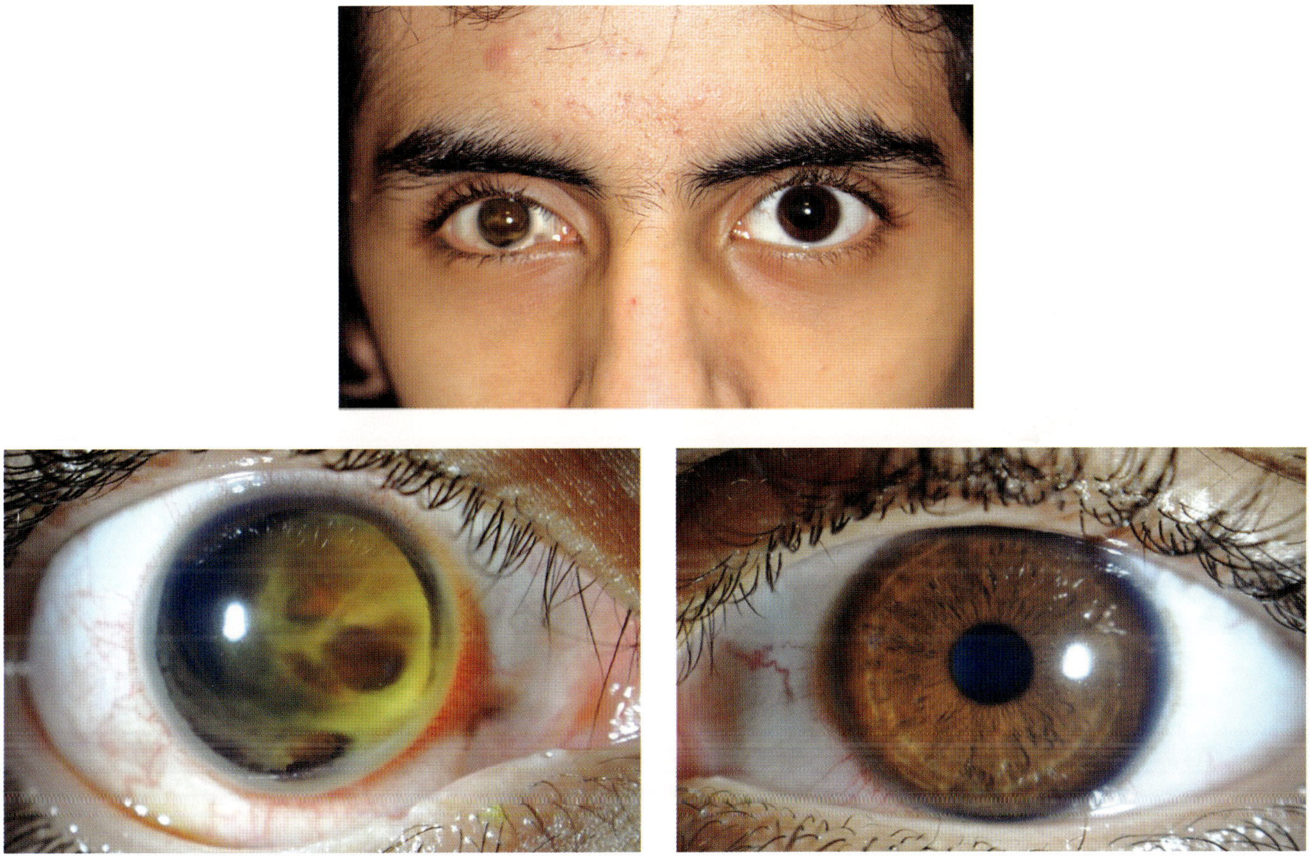

Fig. 10.65: Slit-lamp examination: (Above) Cosmetic appearance of both eyes; (Below) Normal left eye and right traumatic eye

Postoperative Results

First visit postoperatively: Minimal conjunctival injection and subconjunctival hemorrhages, but good cosmetic results and color saturation and high patient satisfaction (Figure 10.66).

Follow-up and Comments

One month after the surgery, the subconjunctival hemorrhage was resolved, with excellent cosmetic outcomes (Figure 10.67).

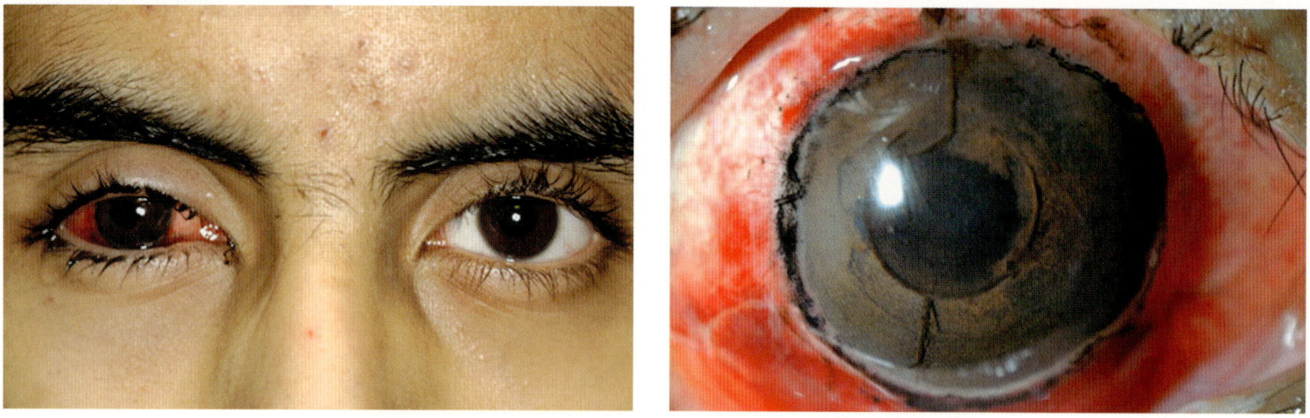

Fig.10.66: Postoperative results. (Right) Slit-lamp examination after keratopigmentation; (Left) Cosmetic appearance of both eyes

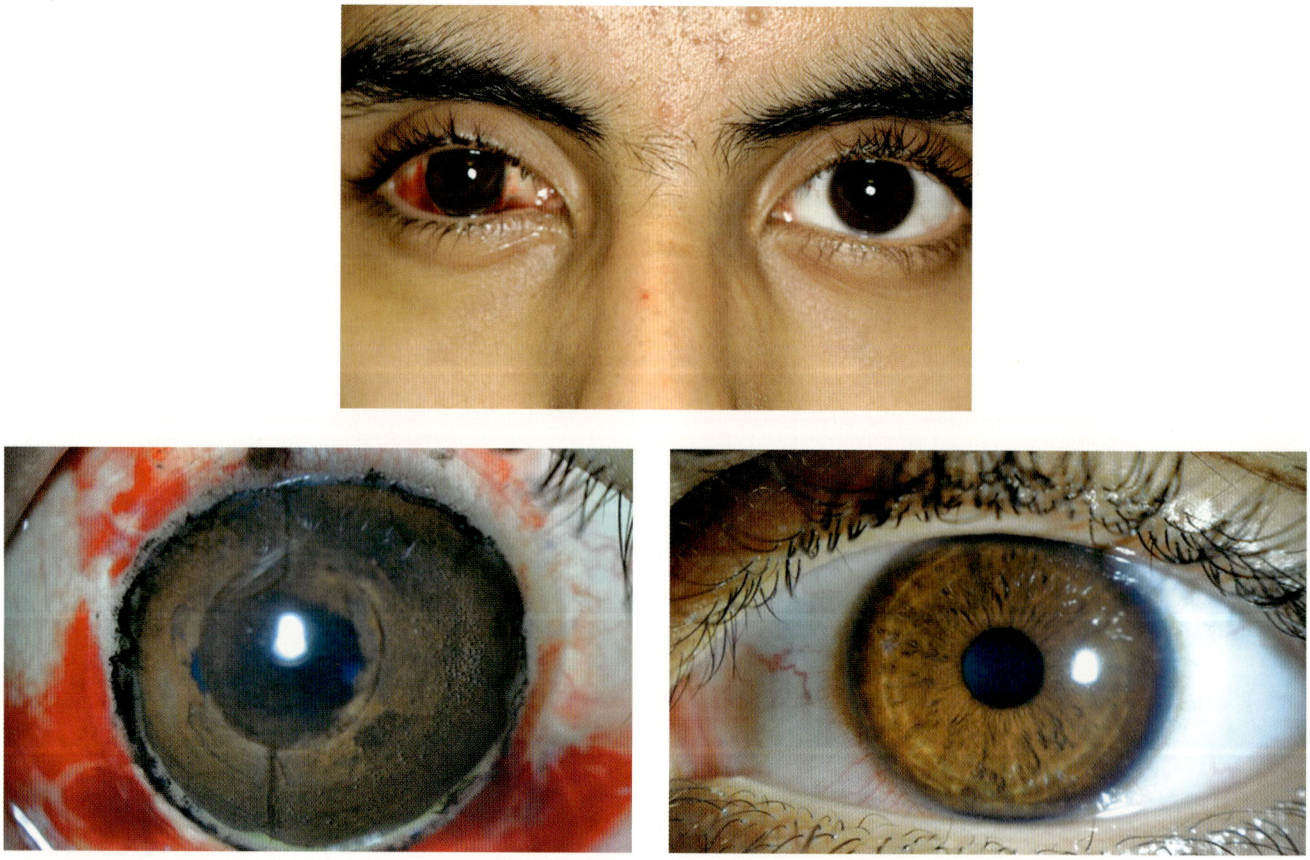

Fig. 10.67: Cosmetic results one month after surgery

CASE 25

Clinical History

A 51-year-old female, with history of left eye formaldehyde chemical burn 25 years ago, presented with a gradual visual loss over the past 12 years secondary to uncontrolled increased intraocular pressures in her left eye.

Preoperative Data

On examination: Severe keratopathy related to the previous corneal chemical burn and epithelial dystrophy, traumatic subluxated lens and traumatic aniridia. Fundus examination revealed a left eye optic nerve atrophy and her visual acuity was no perception of light (Figure 10.68).

Surgical Technique

Femtosecond-assisted keratopigmentation combined with intralamellar manual technique. The tunnel was performed at 466 microns of depth, with an outer and inner diameter of 8.6 mm and 5 mm respectively, completed with manual dissection, using yellow (VEMP 801) with green (VEMP 501) pigments for the iris and black (VEMP 100) for the pupil. Strabismus surgery and cyclodiode-photocoagulation were also performed.

Postoperative Results

Minimal eyelid swelling and upper lid ptosis was noticed postoperatively. The pigmented eye was slightly lighter in color compared to the normal eye (Figure 10.69).

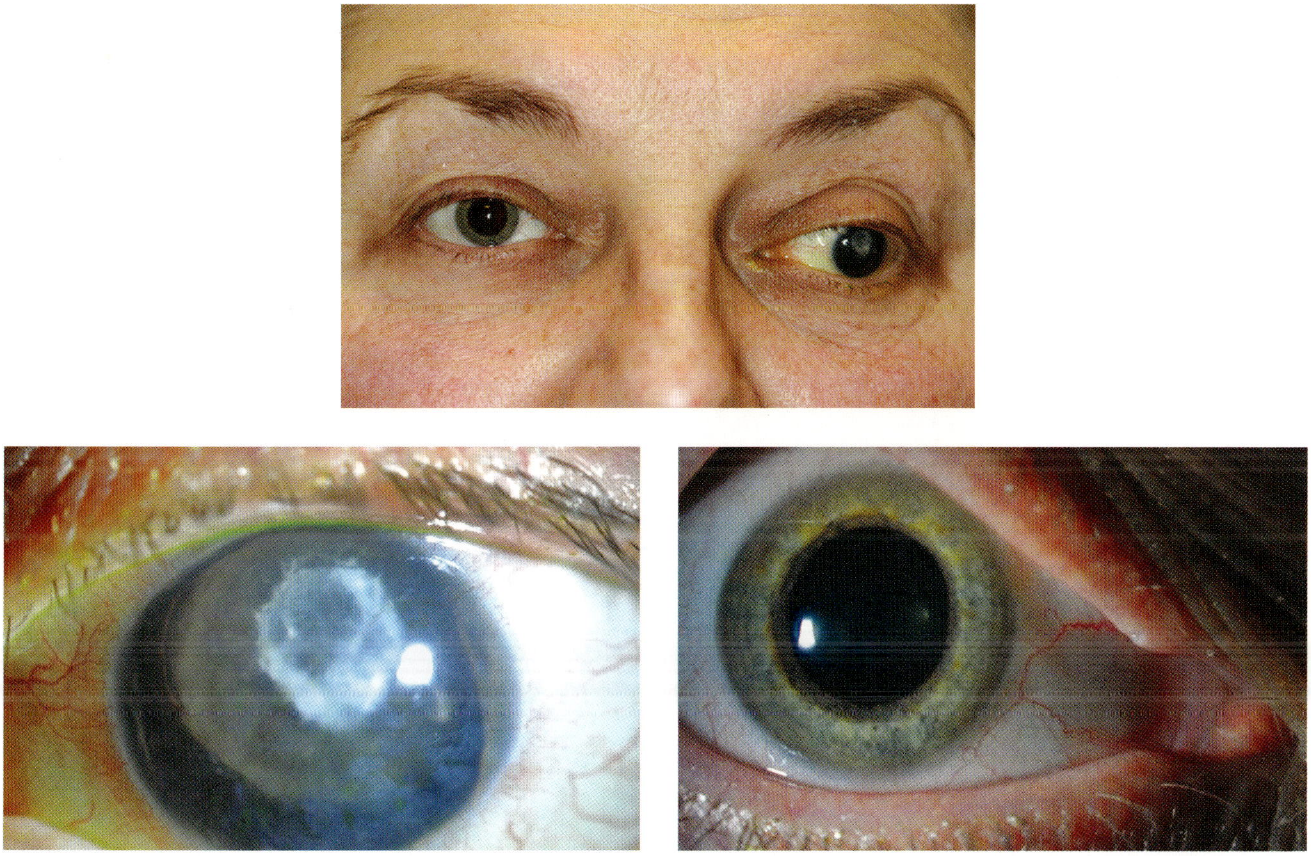

Fig. 10.68: Slit-lamp examination: (Above) Cosmetic appearance of both eyes; (Below) normal right eye and corneal calcification on left eye

Follow-up and Comments

A second keratopigmentation surgery was performed to improve the color using green (VEMP 500) pigment and to simulate the iris of her right eye.

After this second surgery, the patient was very happy except for a minimal degree of foreign body sensation, that settle down spontaneously (Figure 10.70).

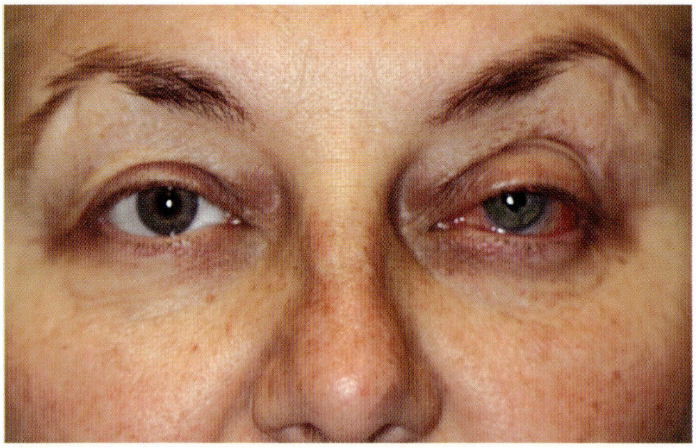

Fig. 10.69: Postoperative results: Cosmetic appearance of both eyes

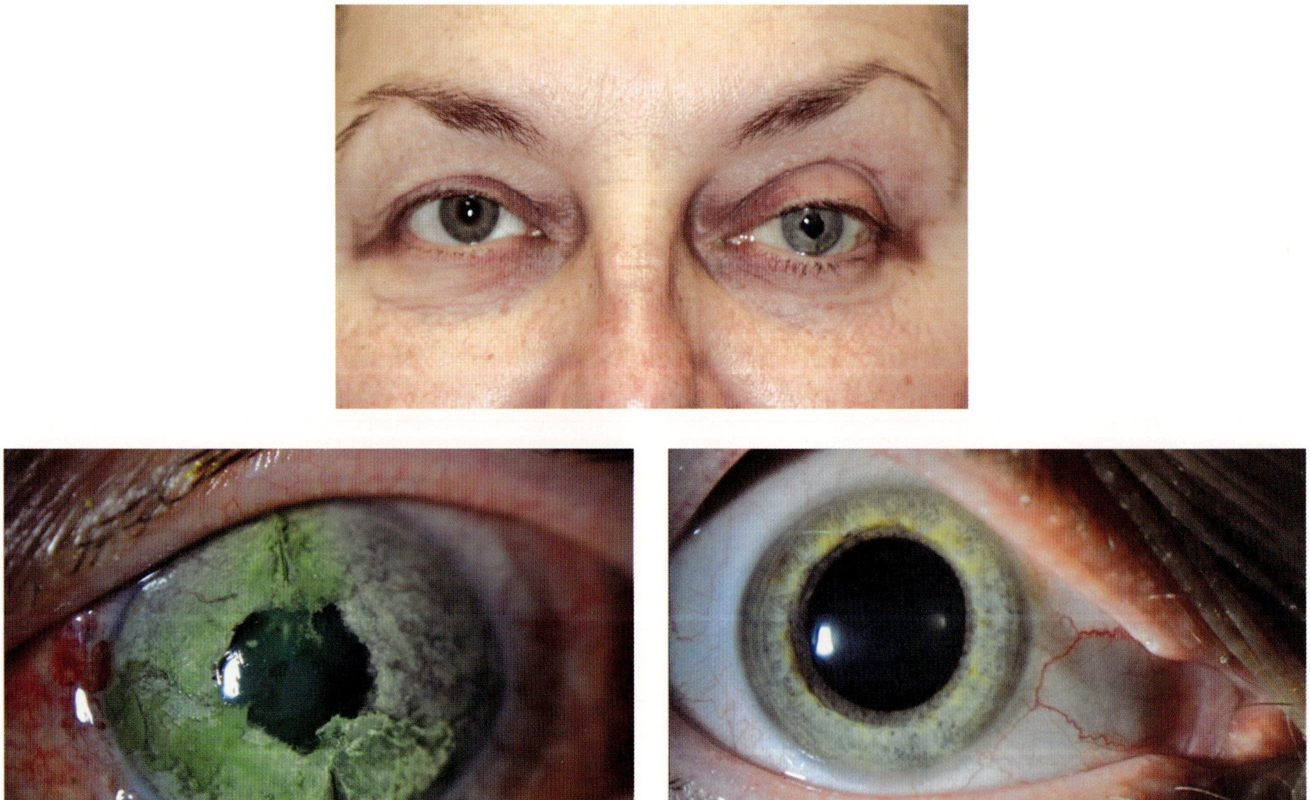

Fig. 10.70: Cosmetic results 6 months after keratopigmentation

CASE 26

Clinical History

A 42-year-old female with right eye previous trauma, underwent a traumatic and complicated cataract surgery. Unfortunately, her visual acuity did not improve after this operation.

Preoperative Data

On examination, corneal scarring and opacification were observed, pupil displacement and increased intraocular pressure under control using Cosopt (IOP 19/14 mm Hg). Her visual acuity was perception of light on the right eye and 1.0 (decimal) on the left eye (Figure 10.71).

Surgical Technique

Right eye femtosecond-assisted keratopigmentation at 350 microns of depth (outer and inner tunnel diameters of 9,2 mm and 4,5 mm) using brown (VEMP 201) pigment for iris and black (VEMP 100) pigment for pupil. A squint surgery was also carried out.

Postoperative Results

Good postoperative results and no signs of complications were observed. The eye pigmented was slightly green compared to the other iris color.

Follow-up and Comments

Patient was happy with the cosmetic results but presented with watery eye and grittiness on that side. The bandage contact lens was removed and the symptoms and signs of postoperative inflammation improved in a few weeks (Figure 10.72).

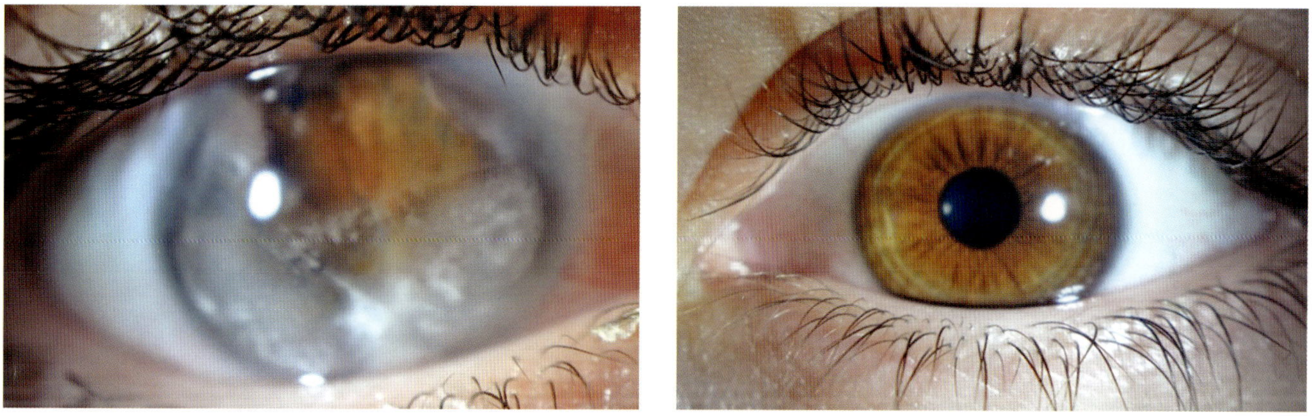

Fig. 10.71: Slit-lamp examination: (Right) Cosmetic appearance of both eyes; (Left) Normal left eye and corneal opacification of right eye

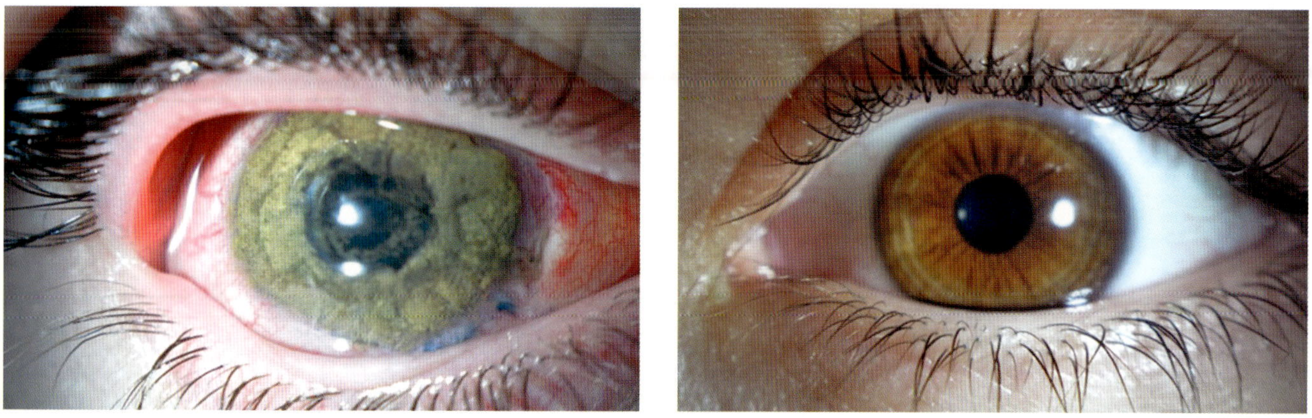

Fig. 10.72: Final cosmetic results

PART II: FUNCTIONAL THERAPEUTIC KERATOPIGMENTATION

SUPERFICIAL AUTOMATED KERATOPIGMENTATION (SAK)

CASE 27

Clinical History

A 50-year-old male with history of right eye perforation, penetrating keratoplasty and extracapsular cataract extraction. Years after the surgery, the corneal graft was decompensated and a second keratoplasty was performed.

Preoperative Data

On examination: Clear corneal graft and mydriatic pupil was noticed on his right eye (Figure 10.73).

Surgical Technique

Superficial keratopigmentation technique, using needle number 3 and brown (VEMP 290) pigment for the iris area. The pupil was marked in the center with 4 mm of diameter.

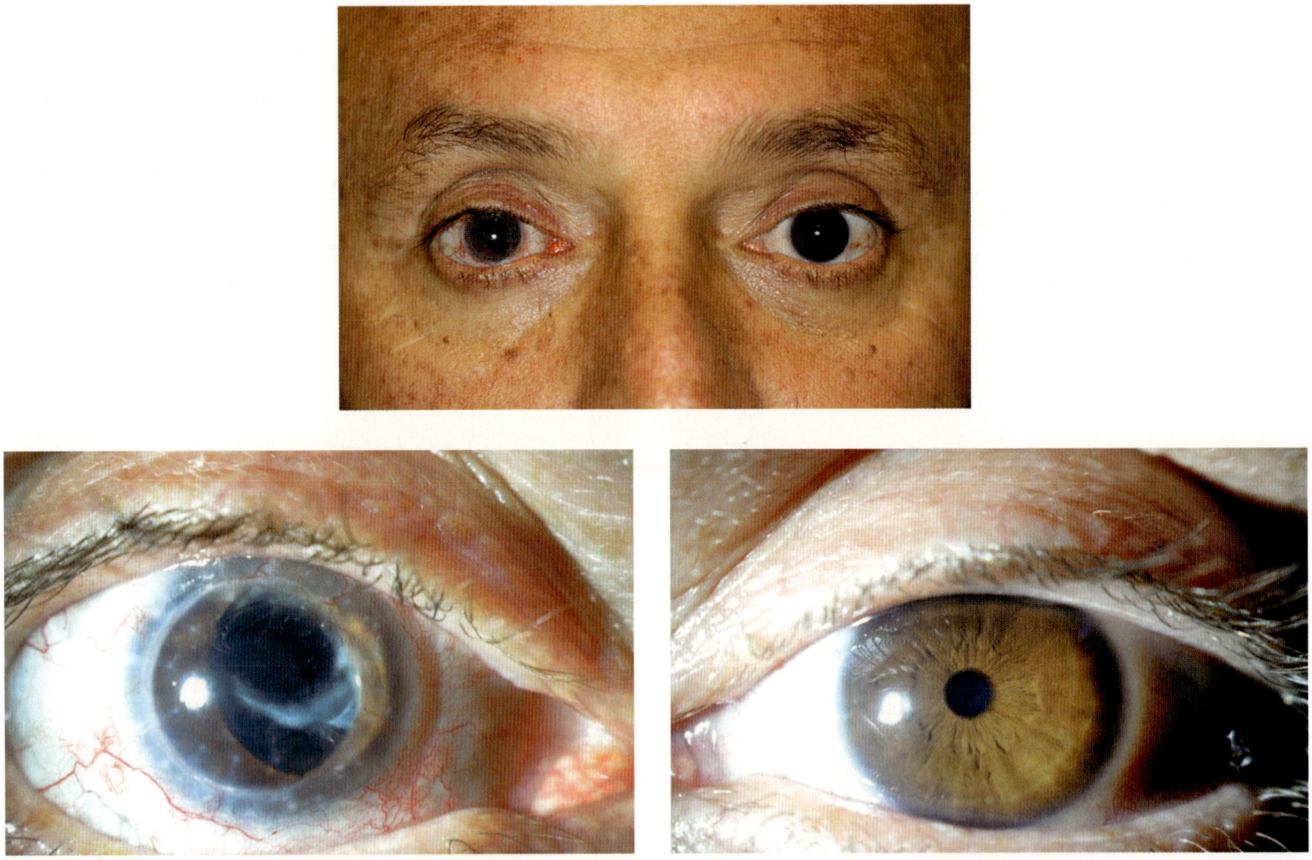

Fig. 10.73: Slit-lamp examination: (Above) Cosmetic appearance of both eyes; (Below) Normal left eye and corneal graft on right eye

Postoperative Results

Minimal conjunctival injection with mild pigment irregularity (Figure 10.74).

Follow-up and Comments

Stable peripheral pigmentation and good cosmetic outcomes, except for a minimal degree of conjunctival injection (Figure 10.75).

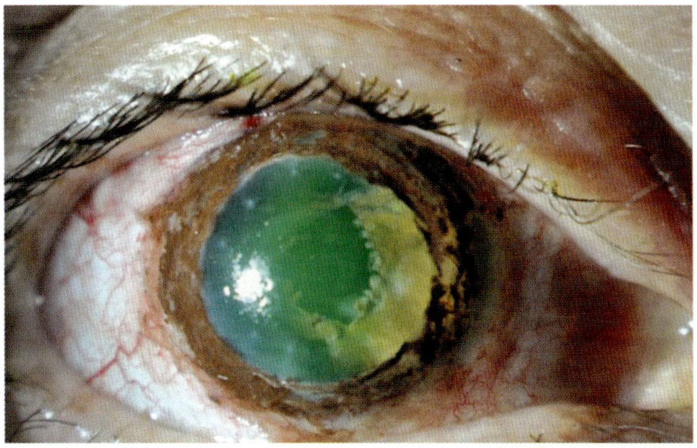

Fig. 10.74: Postoperative results. Slit-lamp examination after keratopigmentation

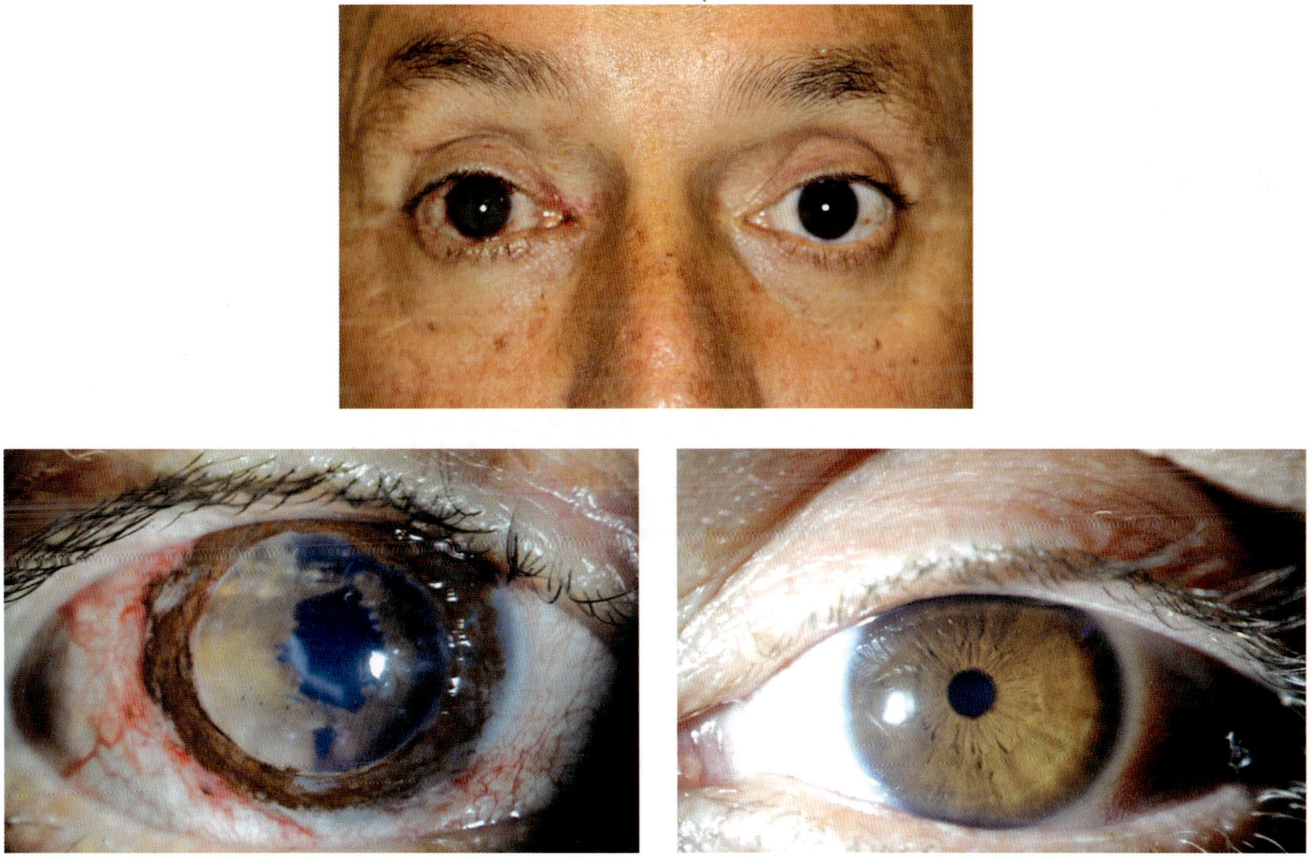

Fig. 10.75: Cosmetic results 6 months after surgery

CASE 28

Clinical History

A 69-year-old female with history of right eye cataract surgery and keratoplasty, resulting in extensive wound healing and scarring, causing some problems to the patient.

Preoperative Data

On examination, patient presented with a clear graft (grade four scar healing), her visual acuity was 0.5 (decimal) and her refraction was -1.25/-0.25 at 105° (Figure 10.76).

Surgical Technique

Superficial keratopigmentation technique, using brown (VEMP 290) pigment and needle number 1.

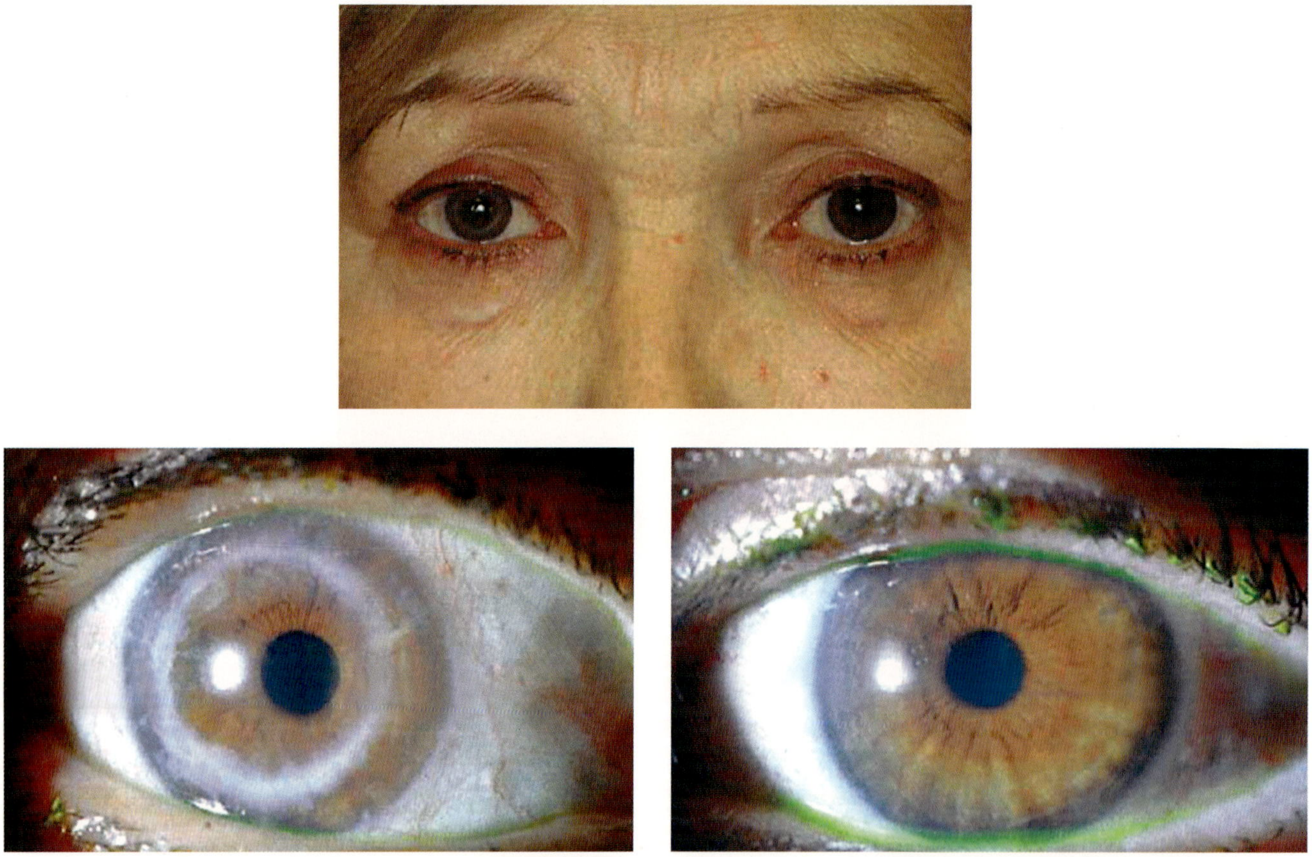

Fig. 10.76: Slit-lamp examination: (Above) Cosmetic appearance of both eyes; (Below) Normal left eye and PK on right eye

Postoperative Results

First visit postoperatively: Very good result with fine superficial pigmentation (Figure 10.77).

Follow-up and Comments

Three months after the surgery, the patient was satisfied, and the final visual acuity was 0.6 (decimal) and her refraction was -1.00/-0.75 at 75° (Figures 10.78 and 10.79).

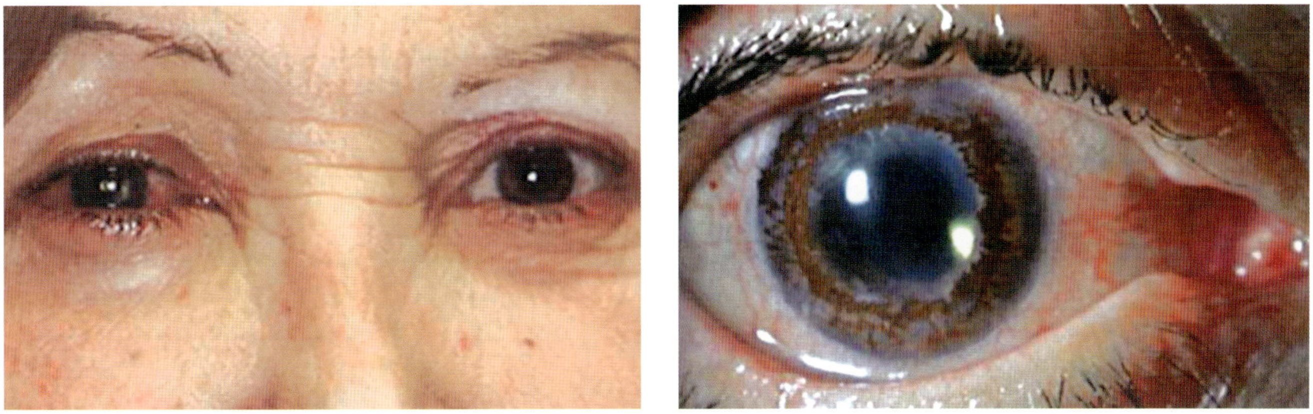

Fig. 10.77: Postoperative results. (Right) Slit-lamp examination after keratopigmentation; (Left) Cosmetic appearance of both eyes

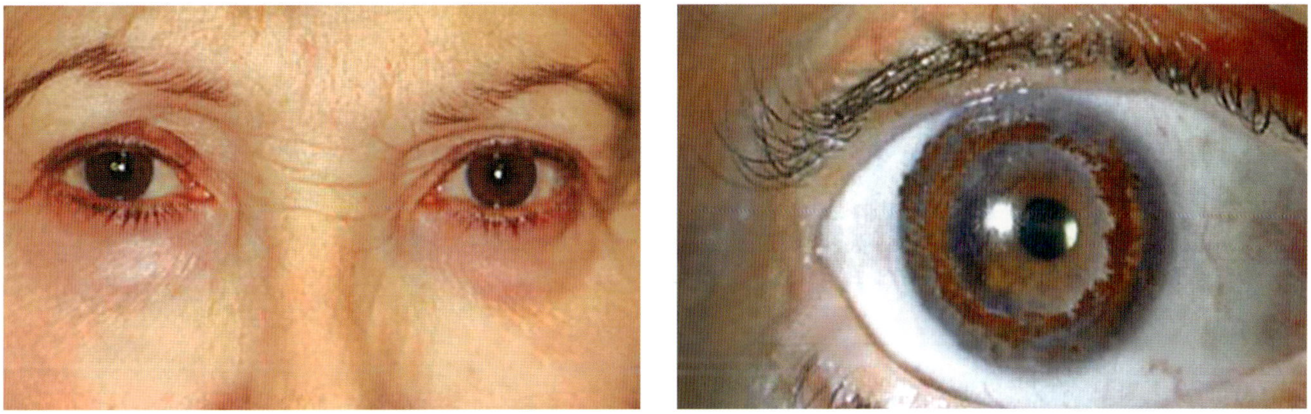

Fig. 10.78: Cosmetic appearance 3 months after keratopigmentation

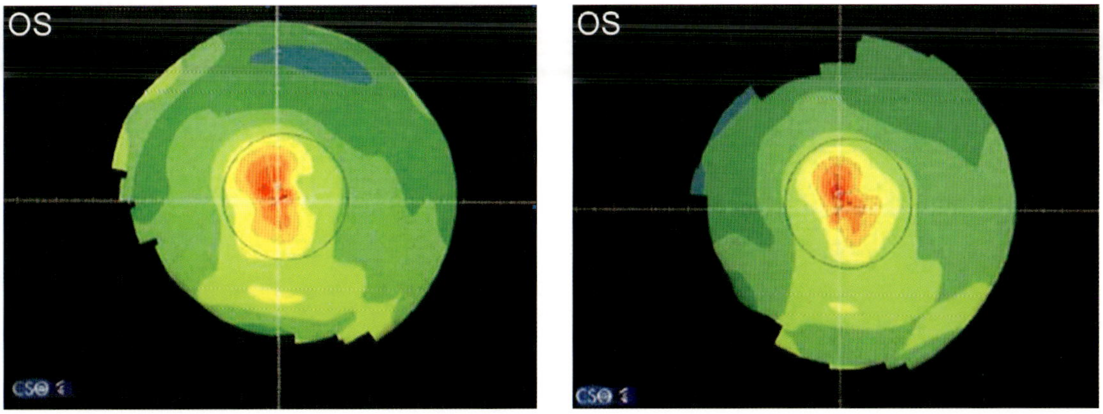

Fig. 10.79: Minimal changes between preoperative topography on the left and postoperative on the right

CASE 29

Clinical History

A 40-year-old female with history of left eye ocular trauma who was interested in a cosmetic solution for her whitish cornea and her squint.

Preoperative Data

Patient presented with an extensive corneal opacity and visual acuity of 0.1 (decimal). The examination of her right eye was unremarkable. She also had history of previous squint surgery in both eyes (Figure 10.80).

Surgical Technique

Superficial keratopigmentation technique, using multiple needles and brown (VEMP 291) pigment for the iris area, and a single needle.

Postoperative Results

First visit postoperatively: Minimal degree of inflammation and some superficial epithelial defects were observed, but excellent cosmetic outcomes and high patient's satisfaction (Figure 10.81).

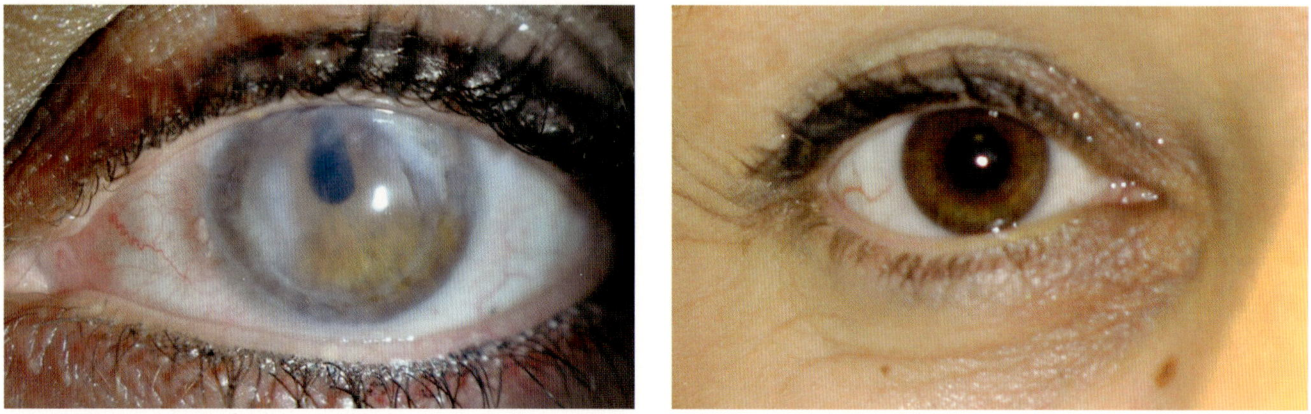

Fig. 10.80: Slit-lamp examination: normal right eye and corneal opacity of left eye

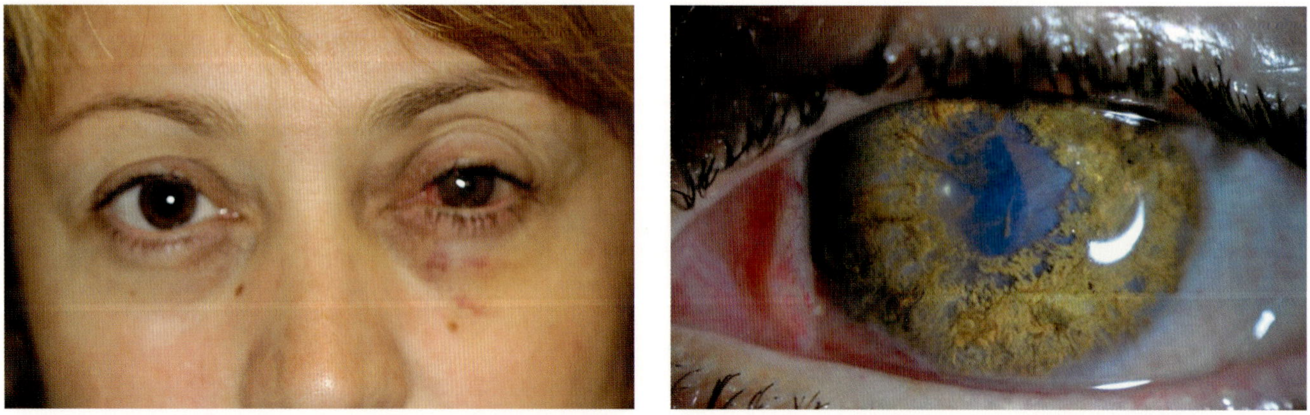

Fig. 10.81: Postoperative results. (Right) Slit-lamp examination after keratopigmentation; (Left) Cosmetic appearance of both eyes

Follow-up and Comments

One month after keratopigmentation, good cosmetic appearance and visual acuity improvement.

Six months after surgery: moderate conjunctival injection.

A second keratopigmentation surgery was carried out using the superficial technique using brown (VEMP 200) pigment and cyclodiode-photocoagulation was also performed.

One year after surgery, good cosmetic results with high patient's satisfaction (Figure 10.82).

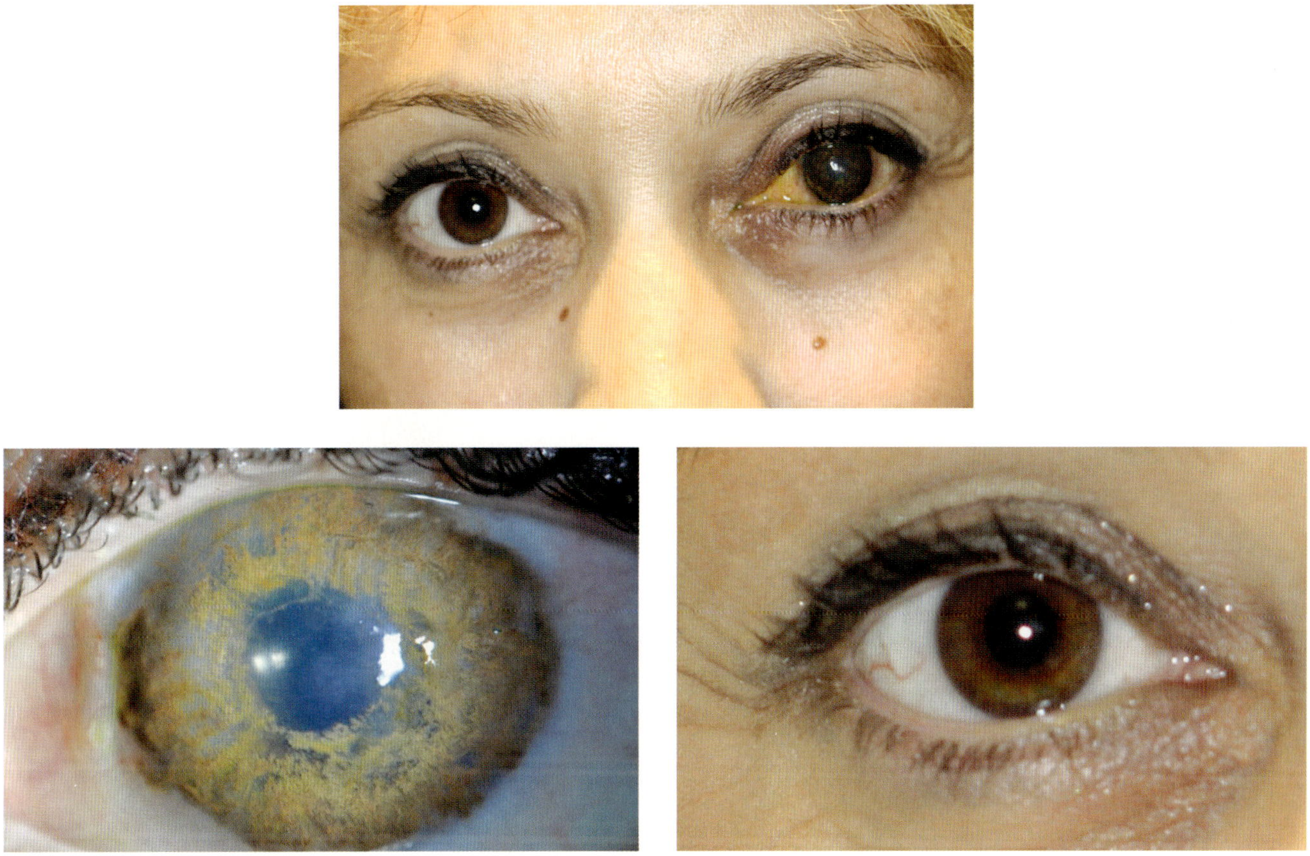

Fig. 10.82: Final results after keratopigmentation

CASE 30

Clinical History

A 50 years old male patient with a history of left eye old corneal trauma at the age of 8, he underwent rupture globe repair and vitrectomy several years after the primary repair, patient represented with neovascularized corneal mass for which he underwent resection biopsy under topical anesthesia, pathology revealed no malignancy and he had triple procedure after that; keratoplasty with intraocular lens implantations and express valve for the control of intraocular pressure, his vision with stable 0.05 and continued on platelet rich plasma treatment to improve healing and corneal surface integrity (Figure 10.83).

Preoperative Data

Patient presented with extensive wound healing at the keratoplasty interface, developing a disfiguring scar for which he was advised the application of cosmetic keratopigmentation to improve the cosmetic appearance (Figure 10.83).

Surgical Technique

Superficial keratopigmentation technique, using light brown (VEMP 410) and blue (VEMP 601) with needle number 3 for the iris pattern and black (VEMP 100) pigment for the pupil margin and limbus, where the pupil was set at 4 mm

Postoperative Results

First visit postoperatively: Patient expressed satisfaction with the cosmetic results with no pain or any other complications, the cosmetic evaluation showed a very good aspect with slight retention of fluorescein dye (Figure 10.84).

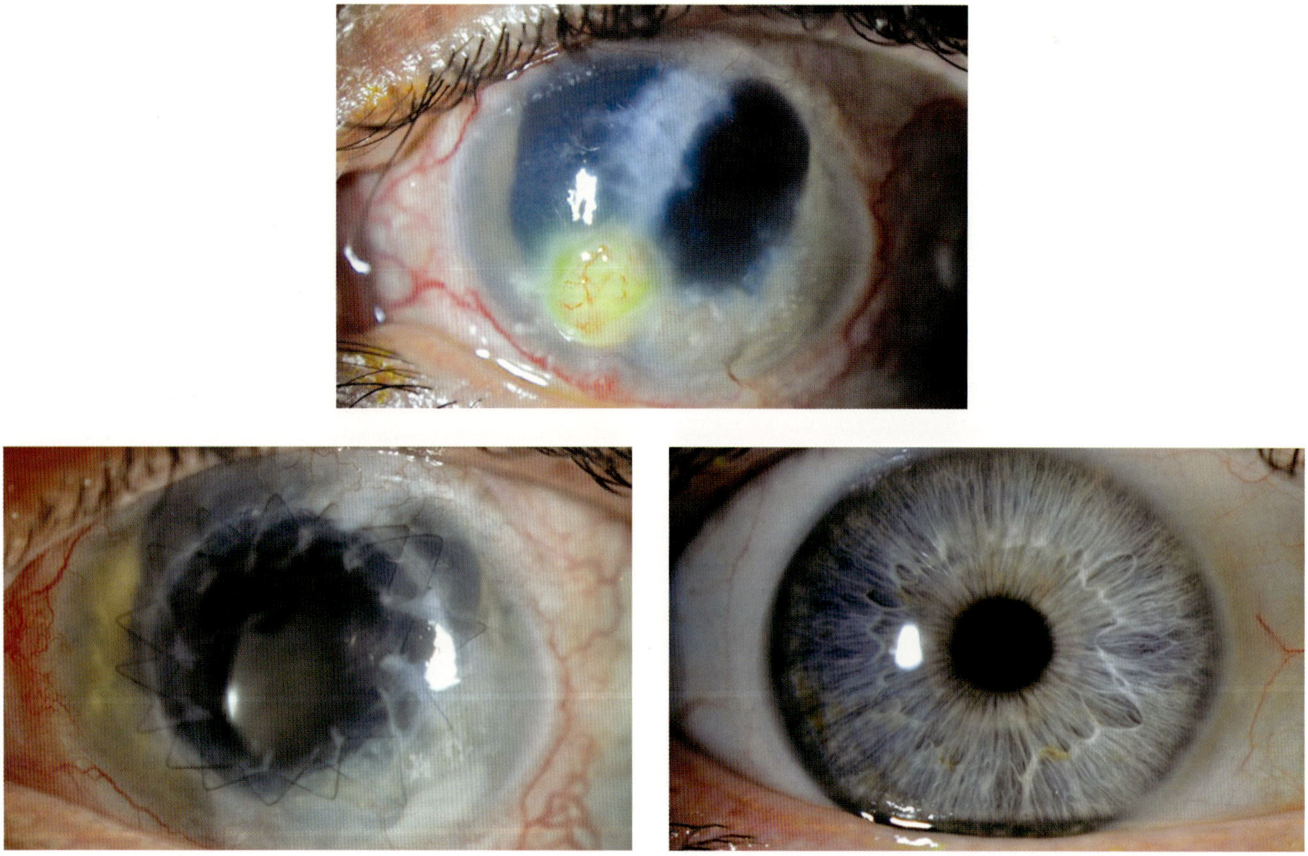

Fig. 10.83: Slit-lamp biomicroscopy: (Above) Corneal mass; (Below) Left eye after keratoplasty and normal eye

Follow-ups and Comments

On 3 months follow-up: Satisfactory results with good profile, except for loss of pigment at the temporal part for which the patient was advice pigment augmentation surgery.

Second surgical enhancement was done with superficial technique using the same settings as the first surgery using customized gray (VEMP 701).

On follow-up: Great improvement in the structure and pigment distribution with good limbal aspect (Figure 10.85).

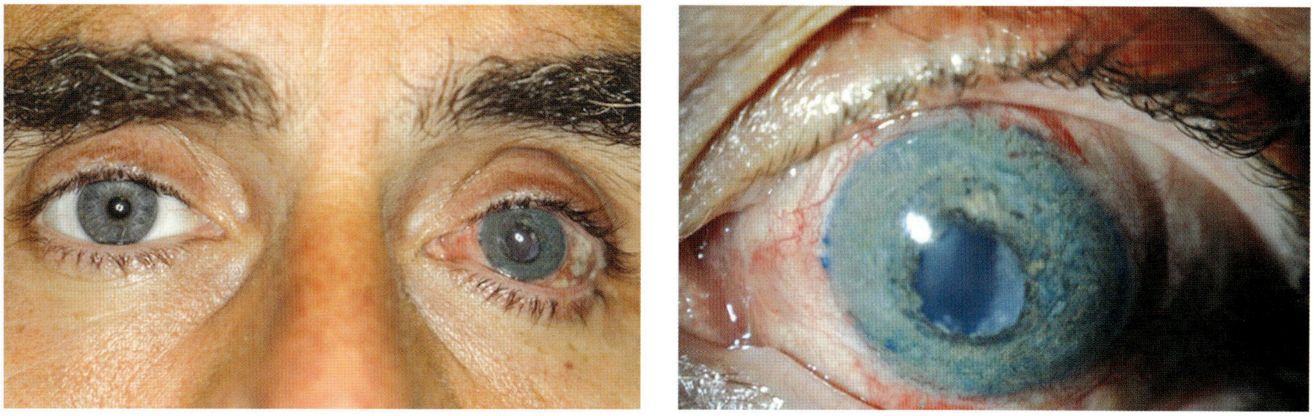

Fig. 10.84: Postoperative results. (Right) Slit-lamp biomicroscopy of keratopigmentation pattern; (Left) Cosmetic appearance of both eyes

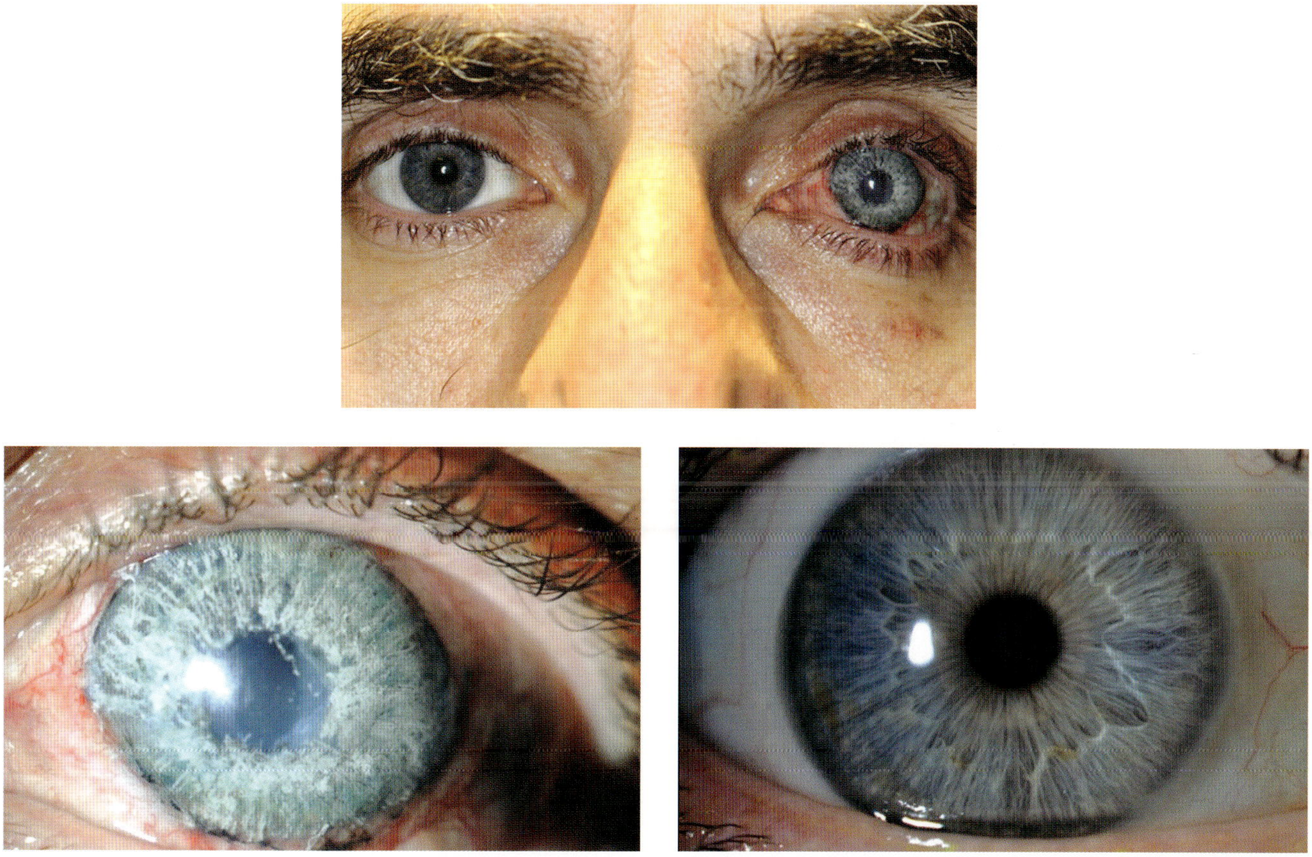

Fig. 10.85: Final follow-up cosmetic results

MANUAL INTRALAMELLAR KERATOPIGMENTATION (MIK)

CASE 31

Clinical History

A 39-year-old female and bilateral pseudophakia presented with a progressive visual loss in her right eye.

Preoperative Data

On examination, there was an inferior iris cyst with a mild pupil irregularity and decreased visual acuity (decimal 0.5) on that eye. Therefore, the iris cyst resection was performed and cosmetic contact lenses were used to cover the iris defect. Unfortunately, the patient could not tolerate them and he was listed for therapeutic keratopigmentation a few months later (Figure 10.86).

Surgical Technique

Manual intrastromal dissection was carried out with the medium brown (VEMP 292) with brown (VEMP 498) pigments and the pupil diameter was marked in the center (approximately 4.25 mm).

Postoperative Results

First visit postoperatively: No pain, conjunctival injection or any complication were observed. The pigmentation was

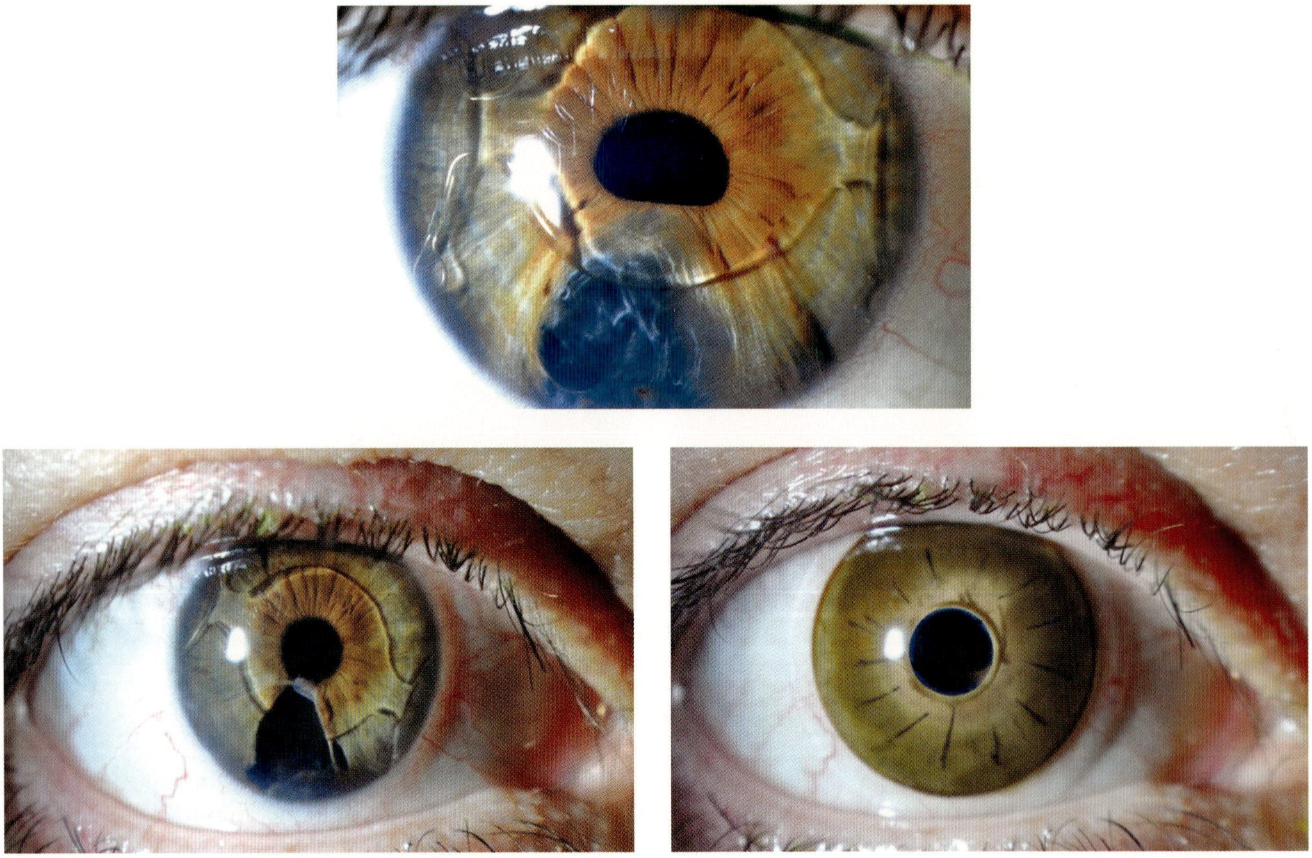

Fig. 10.86: Slit-lamp examination: (Above) Iris cyst; (Below-left) Iris defect after surgery; (Below-right) Patient wearing cosmetic colored contact lens

simulating the natural iris color and the unaided visual acuity was 0.94 (decimal) (Figure 10.87).

Follow-up and Comments

One month after the surgery, the patient presented with a slightly decreased visual acuity (decimal 0.76) and ocular examination revealed a cataract (Figure 10.88), therefore a phacoemulsification and intraocular lens implant was performed. After this surgery, the cosmetic result and the visual outcome were very good showing minimal degree of pigment dispersion superiorly.

One year after the surgery, the pigmentation was stable and the patient was satisfied and her visual acuity was 0.94 (decimal) (Figure 10.89).

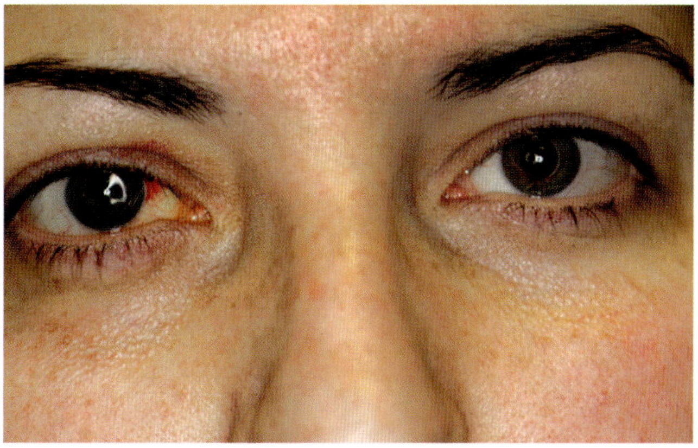

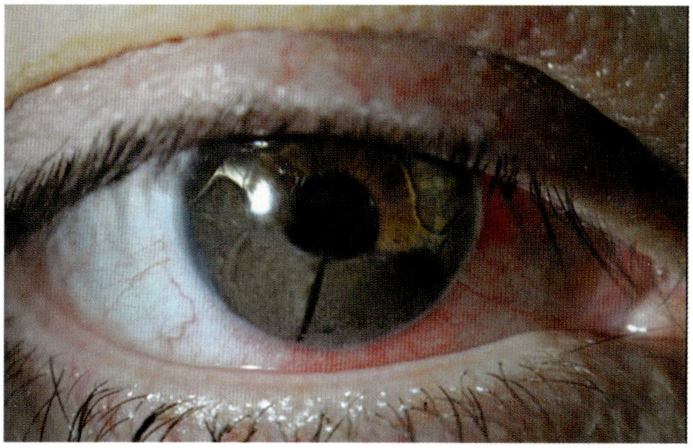

Fig. 10.87: Postoperative results. (Left) Slit-lamp examination after keratopigmentation; (Right) Cosmetic appearance of both eyes

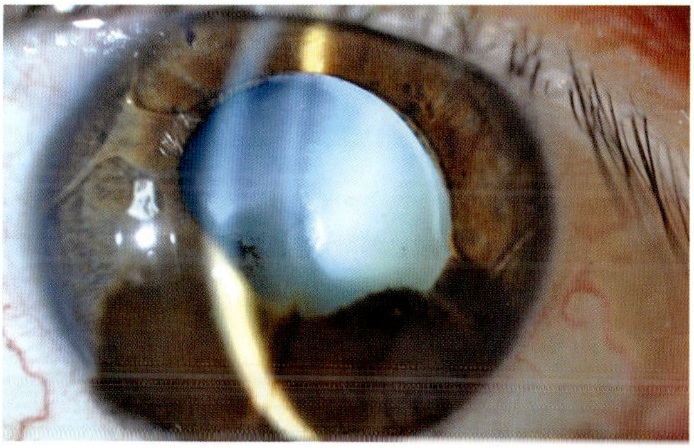

Fig. 10.88: Right eye cataract with stable keratopigmentation pattern

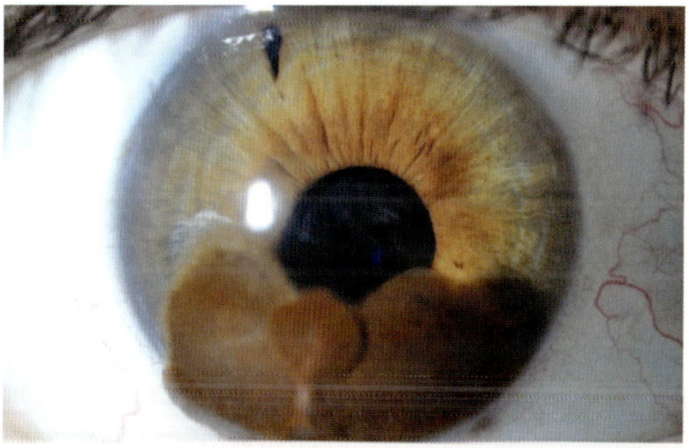

Fig. 10.89: Final result after cataract extraction surgery

CASE 32

Clinical History

A 27-year-old male with history of bilateral phakic intraocular lens implantation and complaining of persistent unilateral diplopia and photophobia.

Preoperative Data

On examination there was a right superior iris coloboma from 10 o'clock to 2 o'clock with an aided visual acuity of 0.98 (decimal). The examination on his left eye was normal and the visual acuity was 1.0 (decimal) (Figure 10.90).

Surgical Technique

Manual intrastromal dissection was performed using brown (VEMP 290) pigment.

Postoperative Results

First visit postoperatively: Great improve on preoperative symptoms (diplopia) and minimal inflammatory reaction. The cosmetic result was excellent after pigmentation, and perfect iris simulation with Purkinje reflect marking matching new pupil centers (Figure 10.91).

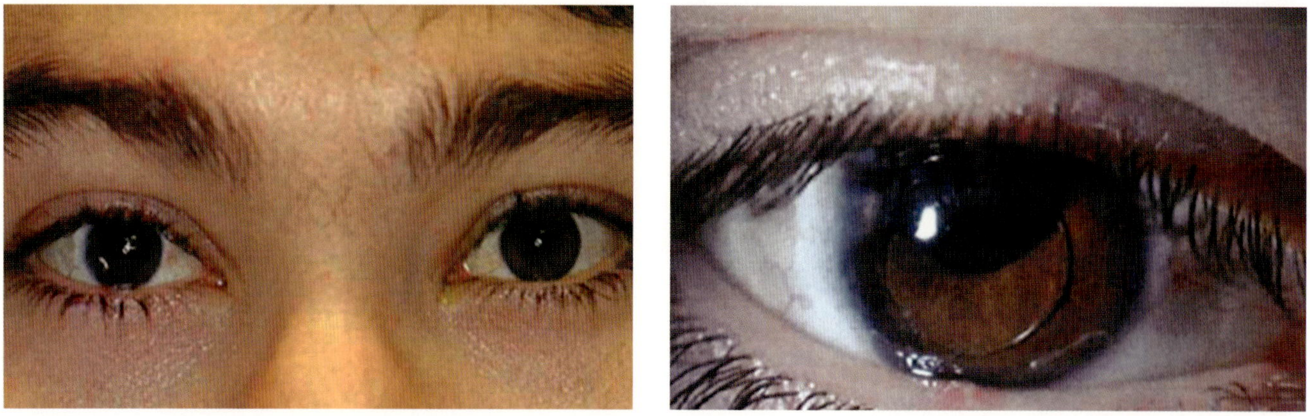

Fig. 10.90: Slit-lamp examination: (Left) Cosmetic appearance of both eyes; (Right) Right iris coloboma

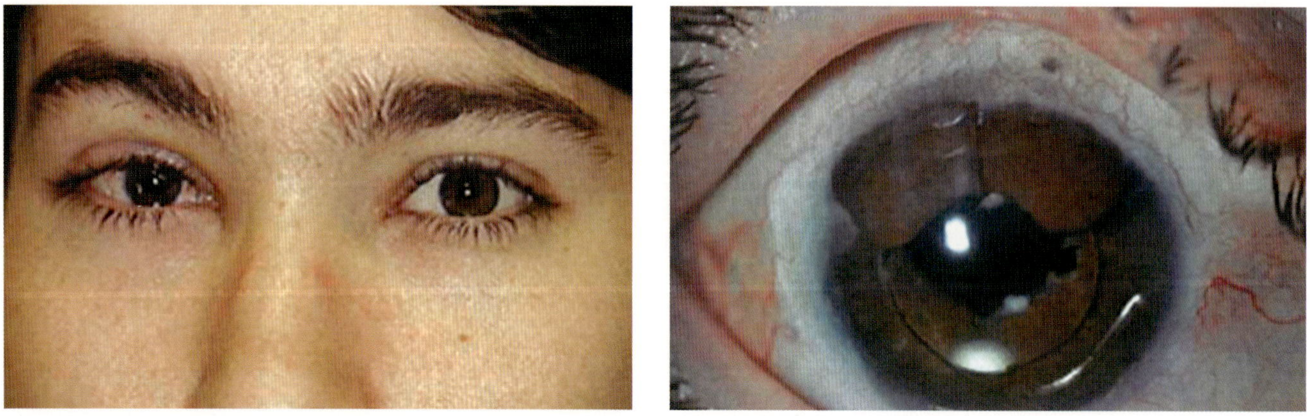

Fig. 10.91: Postoperative results. (Right) Slit-lamp examination after keratopigmentation; (Left) Cosmetic appearance of right eye

Follow-up and Comments

Ten days after surgery: Complete relief of double vision but the visual acuity was 0,56 (decimal) and topography (Figure 10.92) was done to study the surface irregularities that could be causing the unexplained drop of vision.

One month after the surgery, the keratopigmentation pattern showed good cosmetic results with full recovery of vision to 1.0 decimal). One year after the surgery the examination showed constant stability of the pigmented area and vision, with high patient's satisfaction.

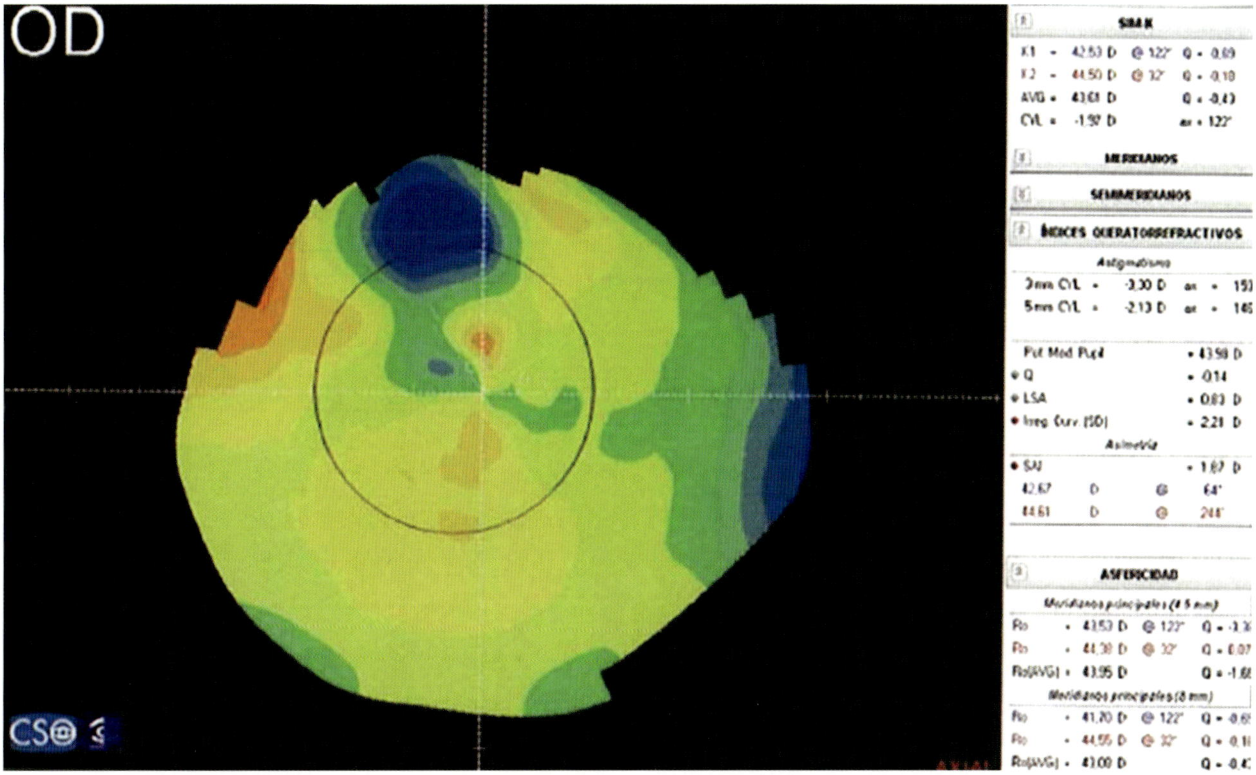

Fig. 10.92: Postoperative topography

CASE 33

Clinical History

A 23-year-old female, with history of left air bag trauma, causing an iris traumatic atrophy and mydriasis. She was complaining of glare and blurred vision most of the time.

Preoperative Data

On examination, her left eye presented with a sectorial inferotemporal iris atrophy with a traumatic anterior subcapsular cataract. The visual acuity was 0.9 (decimal) (Figure 10.93).

Surgical Technique

Manual intrastromal keratopigmentation using the VISSUM micropigmentation dissectors with brown (VEMP 291) pigment was performed.

Postoperative Results

First visit postoperatively: Excellent results and patient was very satisfied with the cosmetic appearance (Figure 10.94).

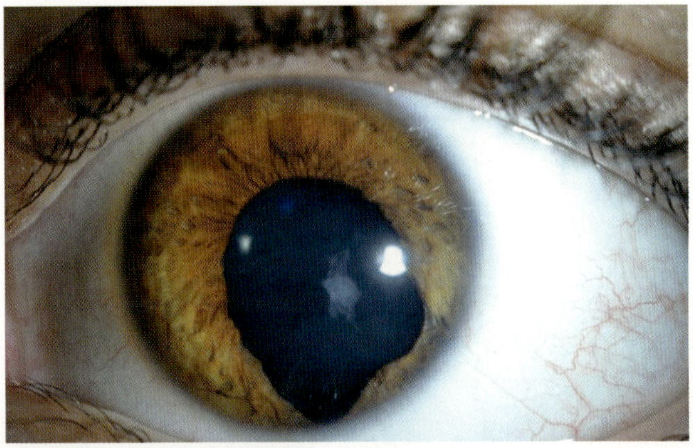

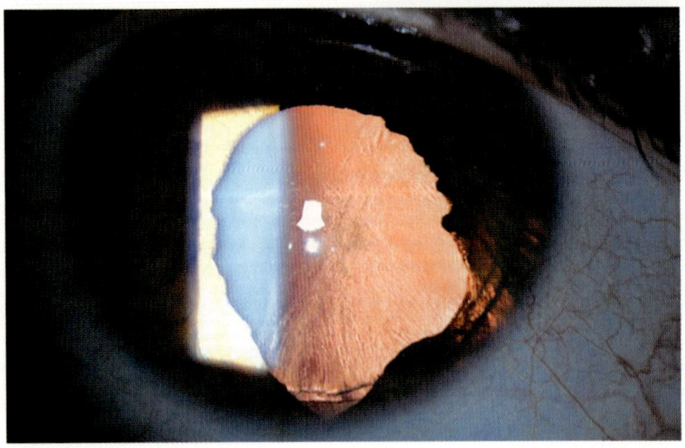

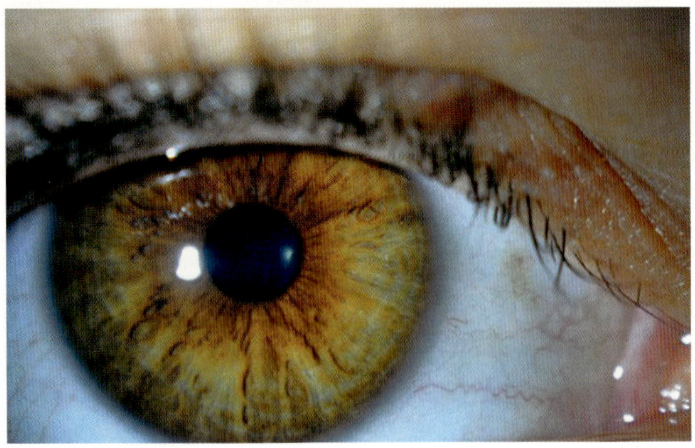

Fig. 10.93: Slit-lamp examination: (Above) Left eye irregular iris with traumatic cataract. (Below) Normal right eye and retroillumination on left eye

Follow-up and Comments

Six months after surgery: Stable pigmentation, but a second keratopigmentation was considered to change the color and to have a more natural look.

One year after keratopigmentation, the patient was satisfied with the results and expressed a complete relief of her visual symptoms (diplopia) (Figure 10.95).

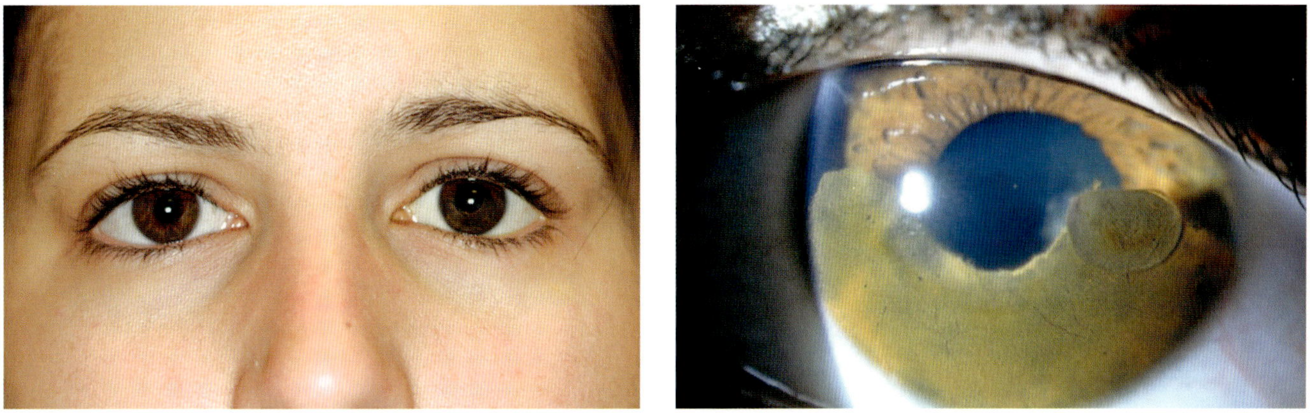

Fig. 10.94: Postoperative results. (Right) Slit-lamp examination after keratopigmentation; (Left) Cosmetic appearance of both eyes

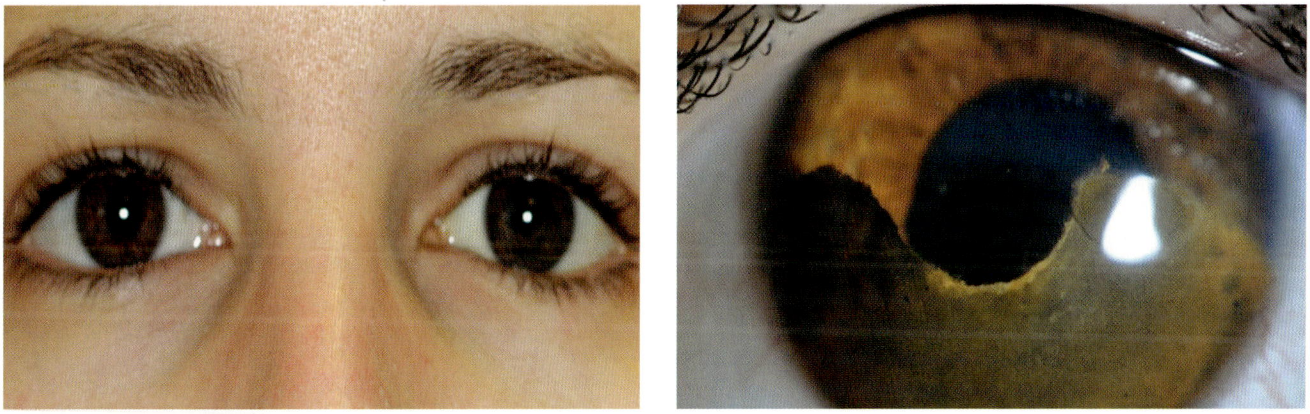

Fig. 10.95: Final cosmetic result

FEMTOSECOND-ASSISTED KERATOPIGMENTATION (FAK)

CASE 34

Clinical History

A 12-year-old female with history of left eye blunt trauma due to an accident, that required surgery and vitrectomy.

Preoperative Data

On examination: She presented with a left eye traumatic aniridia with an iris remanent peripherally and surgical aphakia. Her visual acuity was 1.0 and 0.6 for right and left eyes respectively (decimal) (Figure 10.96).

Surgical Technique

Femtosecond-assisted keratopigmentation technique using brown (VEMP 290) and black (VEMP 190) for the simulated iris area. The pupil was marked in the center with 4 mm of diameter. At the same time, a secondary intraocular lens implant was inserted in sulcus and a squint surgery was also performed.

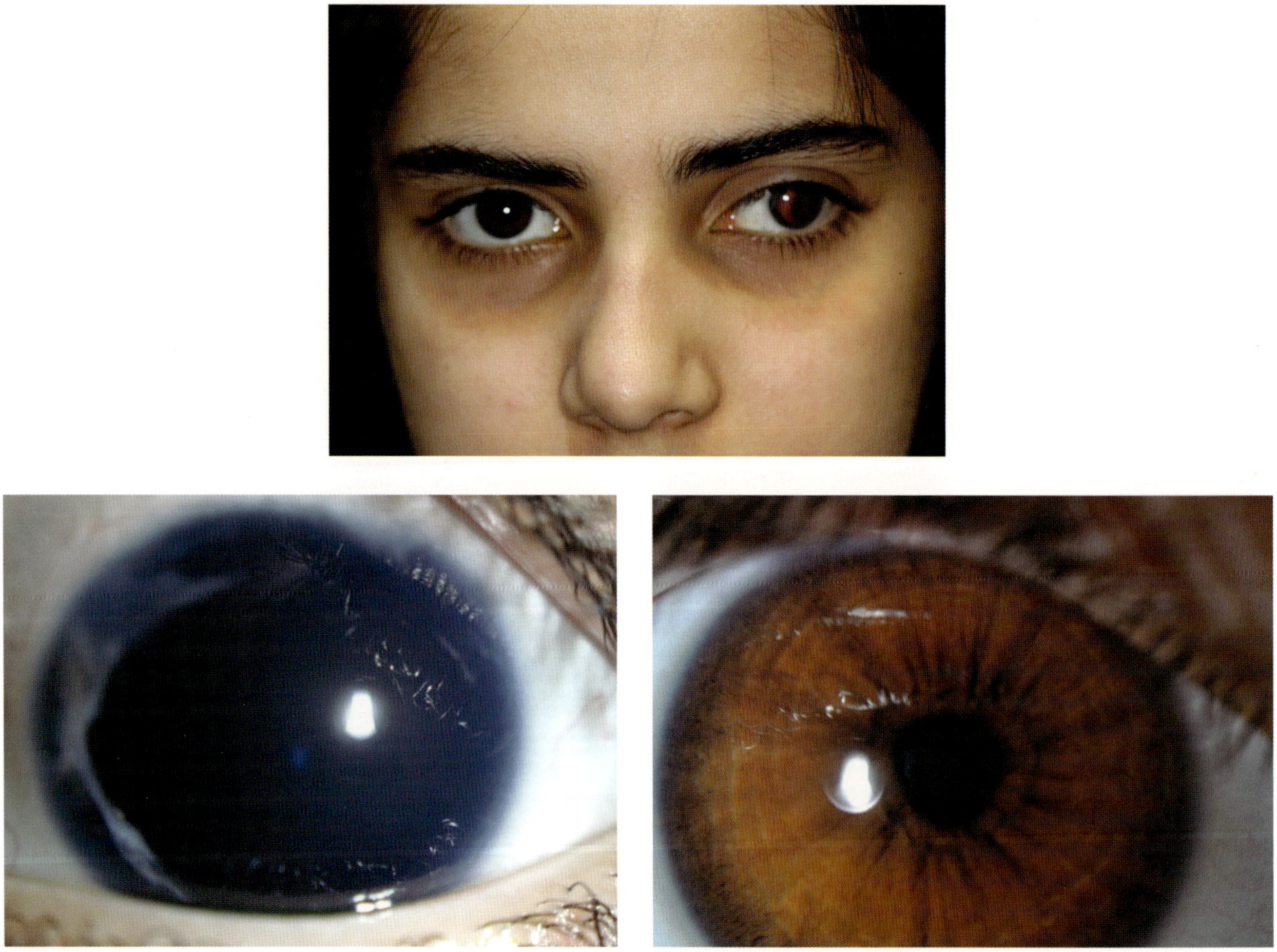

Fig. 10.96: Slit-lamp examination: (Above) Cosmetic appearance of both eyes; (Below) Normal right eye and traumatic aniridia and corneal scar of left eye.

Postoperative Results

On examination, the cornea was clear with minimal conjunctival inflammation and excellent cosmetic result.

Follow-up and Comments

Patient was satisfied with the cosmetic outcomes. The cornea remained clear with a well centered intraocular (Figure 10.97).

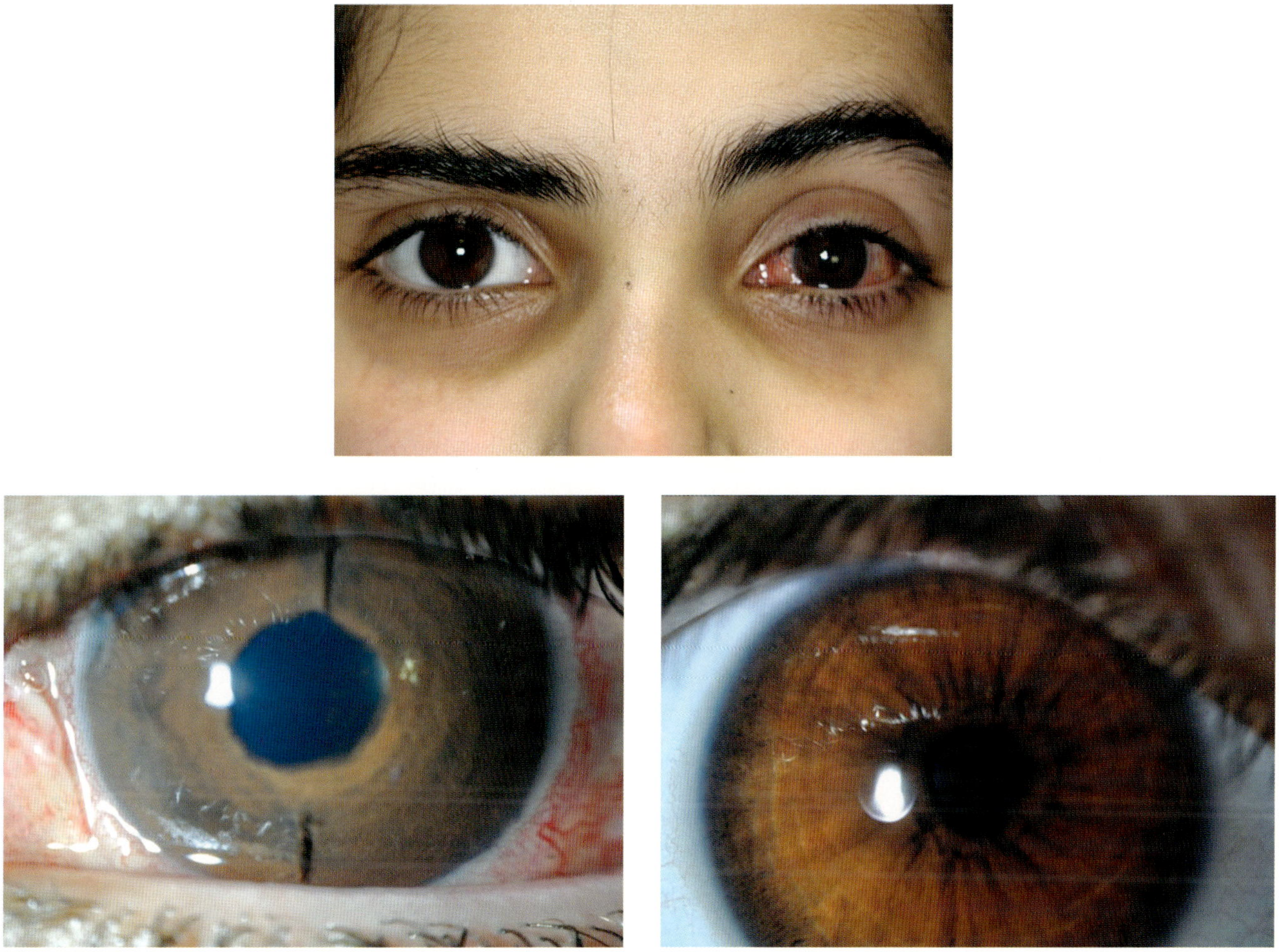

Fig. 10.97: Cosmetic results one month after keratopigmentation

CASE 35

Clinical History

25-year-old female presented with a left eye progressive pupil deformation with an oval shape and photophobia. Her visual acuity was 1.0 and 0.92 for right and left eyes respectively (decimal), and after ocular examination, she was diagnosed with essential iris atrophy.

Preoperative Data

Patient was using cosmetic contact lenses, but they were not well tolerated, because she developed tarsal papillary reaction with conjunctival injection. The essential iris atrophy progressed gradually and developed a total loss of iris in the temporal area (Figure 10.98).

Surgical Technique

Femtosecond-assissted keratopigmentation technique, tunnel depth of 250 microns with an inner diameter of 4 mm and outer diameter of 9.5 mm, using brown (VEMP 290) pigment.

Postoperative Results

First visit postoperatively: The patient presented with watery eye and photophobia but no conjunctival injection was observed. The visual acuity was slightly worse 0.86 (decimal) with an excellent cosmetic appearance except for some atrophic iris defects that were not covered with the pigment and they were evident on transillumination examination. A second surgery was offered to correct (Figure 10.99) and cover these areas and reduce the remanent photophobia.

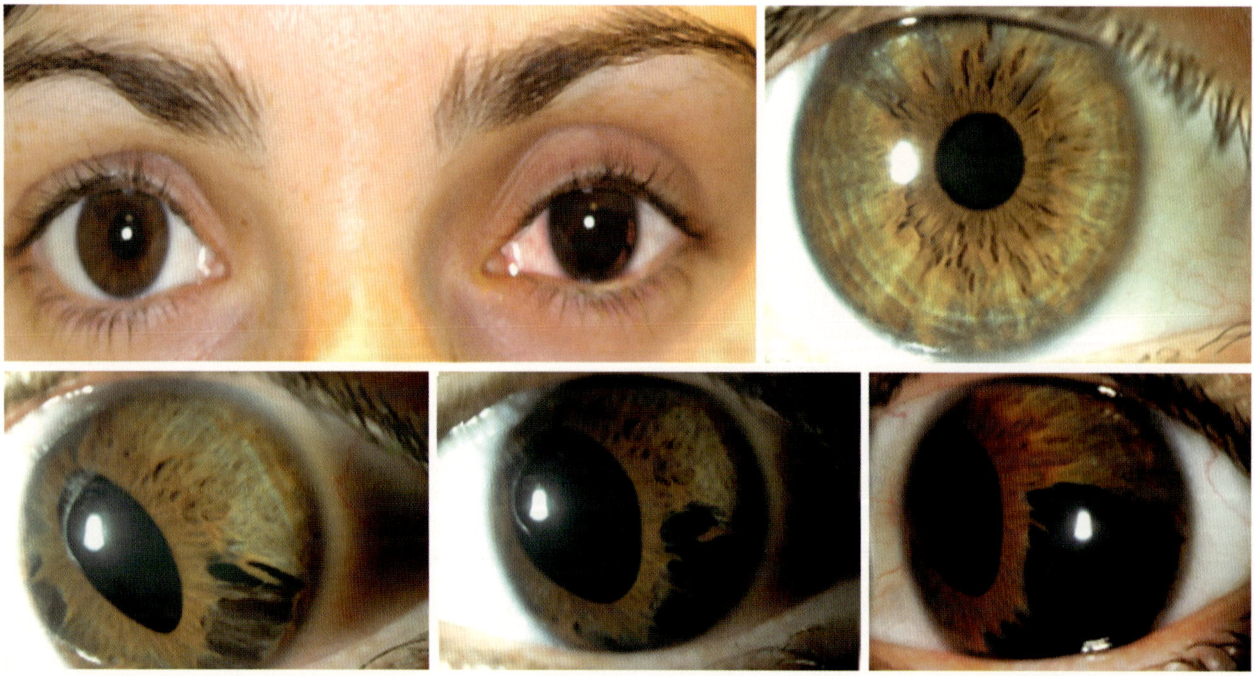

Fig. 10.98: (Above-Right): Slit-lamp examination of normal right eye (Above-Left): Cosmetic appearance of both eyes; (Below) Left eye progressive essential iris atrophy

Follow-up and Comments

A second keratopigmentation was done creating a deeper tunnel at 360 microns of depth and 360 degrees, using black (VEMP 100) pigment.

Three months after surgery, she was very satisfied with both cosmetic and functional results. The visual acuity was better and the photophobia was resolved (Figure 10.100).

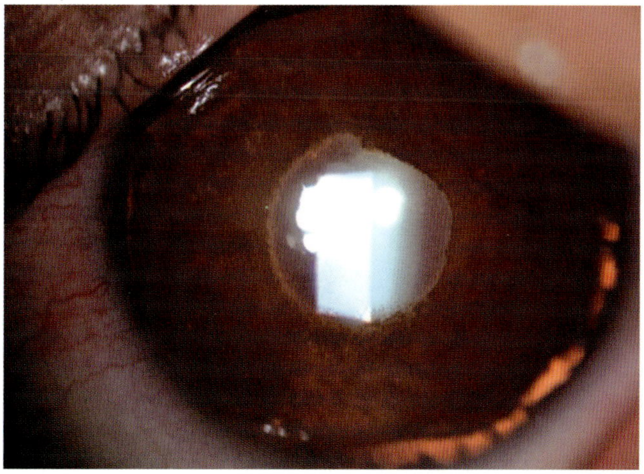

Fig. 10.99: Postoperative results. Slit-lamp examination after keratopigmentation showing transillumination defects

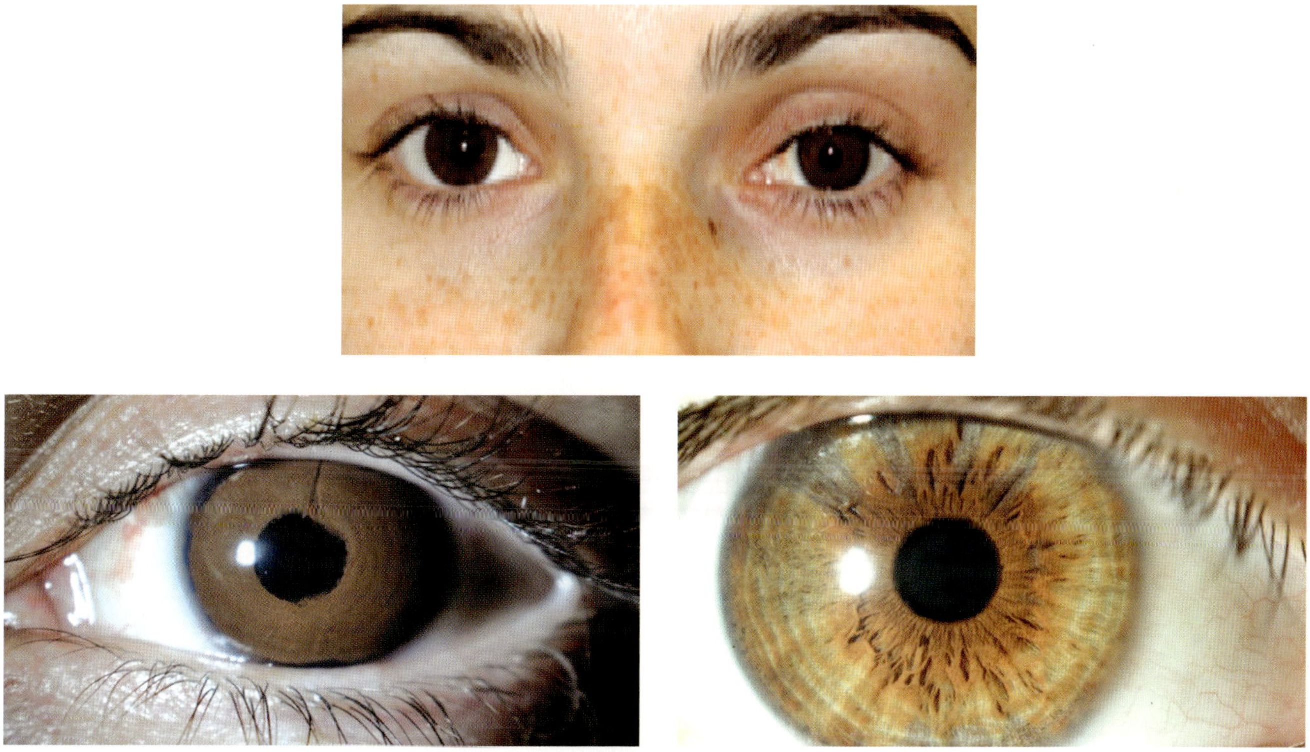

Fig. 10.100: Cosmetic results 3 months after second surgery

CASE 36

Clinical History

A 38-year-old male with history of bilateral bioptics (Phakic IOL and Astigmatic excimer laser photorefractive keratectomy) with postoperative visual acuity of 1.0 in both eyes (decimal). Unfortunately, the patient had a blunt trauma one year after the surgery, which affected his visual acuity with extensive glare and photophobia (decimal visual acuity was 0.1) due to a persistant mydriasis that did not improve with isoptocarpine.

Preoperative Data

A pupiloplasty was performed to repair the dilated and nonreactive pupil, and the discomfort and photophobia improved but the symptoms were not totally resolved (Figure 10.101). On examination, the pupil was irregular with 5-5.4 mm of diameter.

Surgical Technique

Femtosecond-assisted keratopigmentaion technique was performed using greenish brown (VEMP 591) pigment for the iris area and marking the pupil in the center at 6 mm of diameter.

Postoperative Results

Good cosmetic appeerence with major improvement in the visual disability. On cosmetic evaluation both pupil and limbal pigmentation were insufficient specially at 6 o'clock; and the surgeon decided to enhance the cosmetic outcome repeating the keratopigmentation (Figure 10.102).

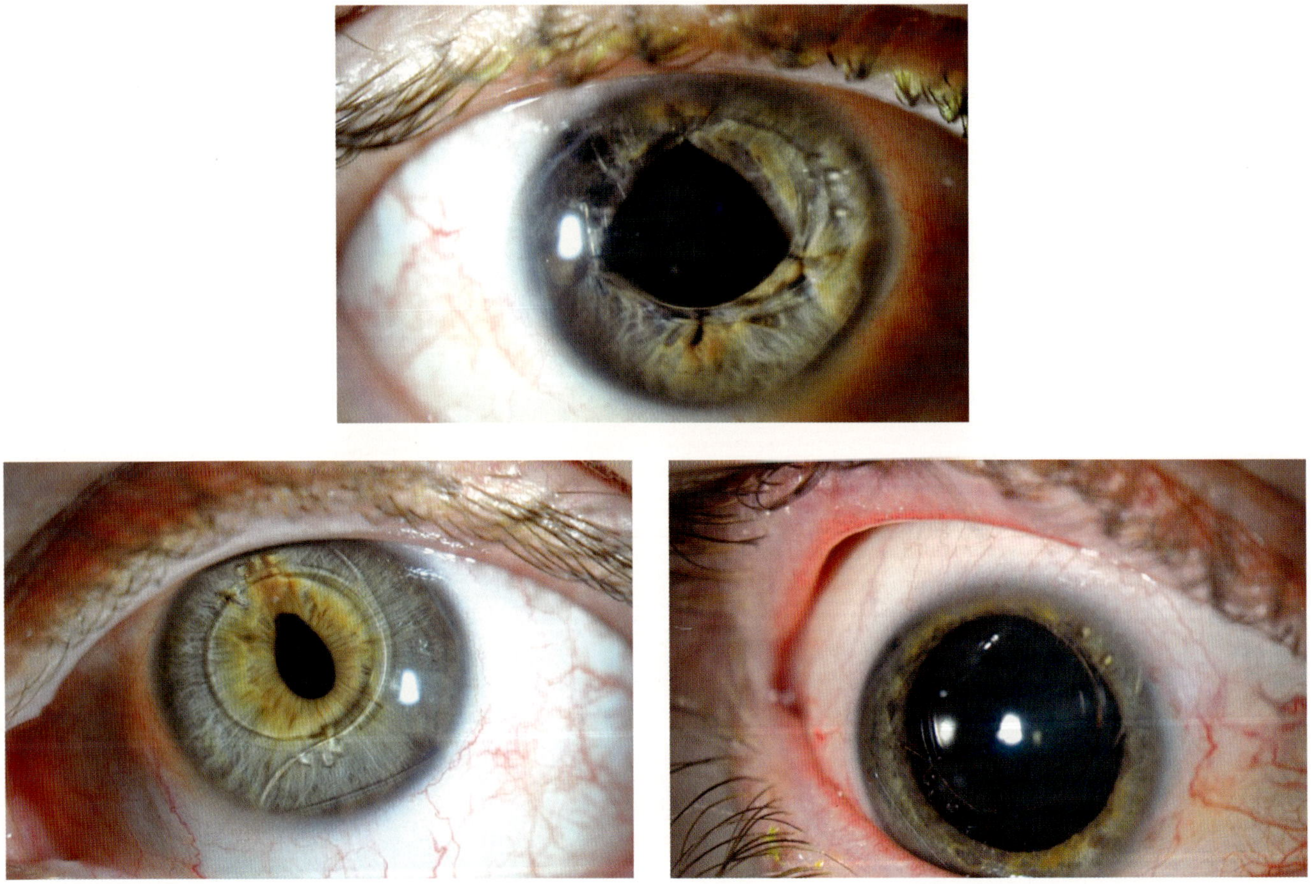

Fig. 10.101: (Above): Traumatic Mydriasis. (Below-right): After pupiloplasty; (Below-left): Normal right eye with intraocular lens

Follow-up and Comments

Second surgical enhancement was done using gray blue (VEMP 791) pigment and completed both limbal and pupil area using a deeper tunnel.

One year after the second surgery, the patient was very satisfied with both cosmetic and visual outcomes, and the cosmetic evaluation showed stable pigmentation with a final visual acuity of 0.96 (decimal) on his left eye (Figure 10.103).

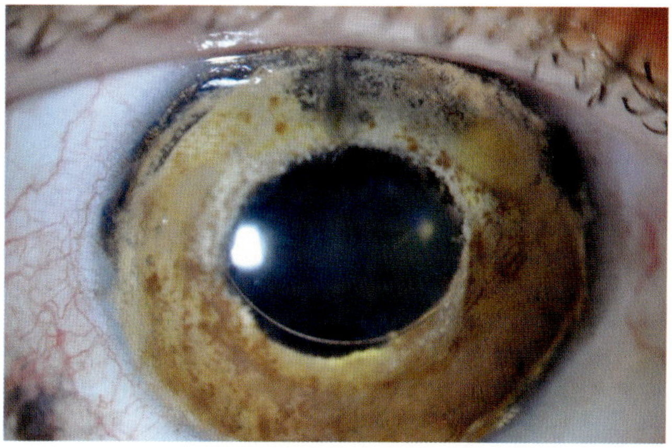

Fig. 10.102: Postoperative results. Slit-lamp examination after first keratopigmentation

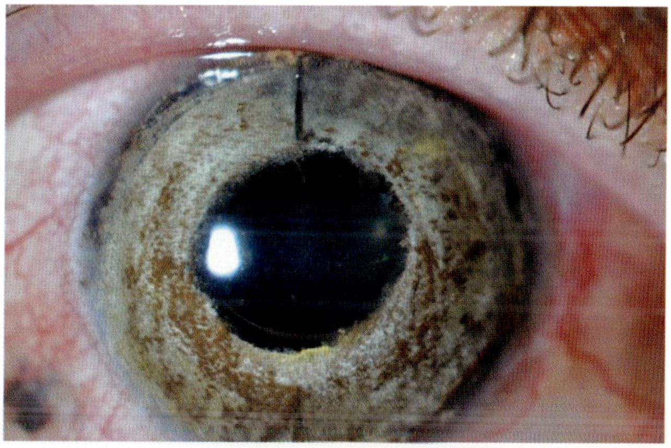

Fig. 10.103: Postoperative results after second keratopigmentation

CASE 37

Clinical History

A 45-year-old female presented with bilateral keratoconus and underwent bilateral keratoplasties. The visual outcome was 0.7 and 0.46 (decimal) for right and left eyes respectively. One year after those surgeries, she had a tennis ball trauma on her left eye, causing a retinal detachment and a traumatic graft dehiscence, that required vitrectomy and resuturing of the corneal graft.

Preoperative Data

On examination her left eye visual acuity was no perception of light and the cosmetic appearance was affected due to extensive scarring of the corneal graft (Figure 10.104).

Surgical Technique

Femtosecond-assisted and superficial keratopigmentation techniques, using light brown (VEMP 200) pigment.

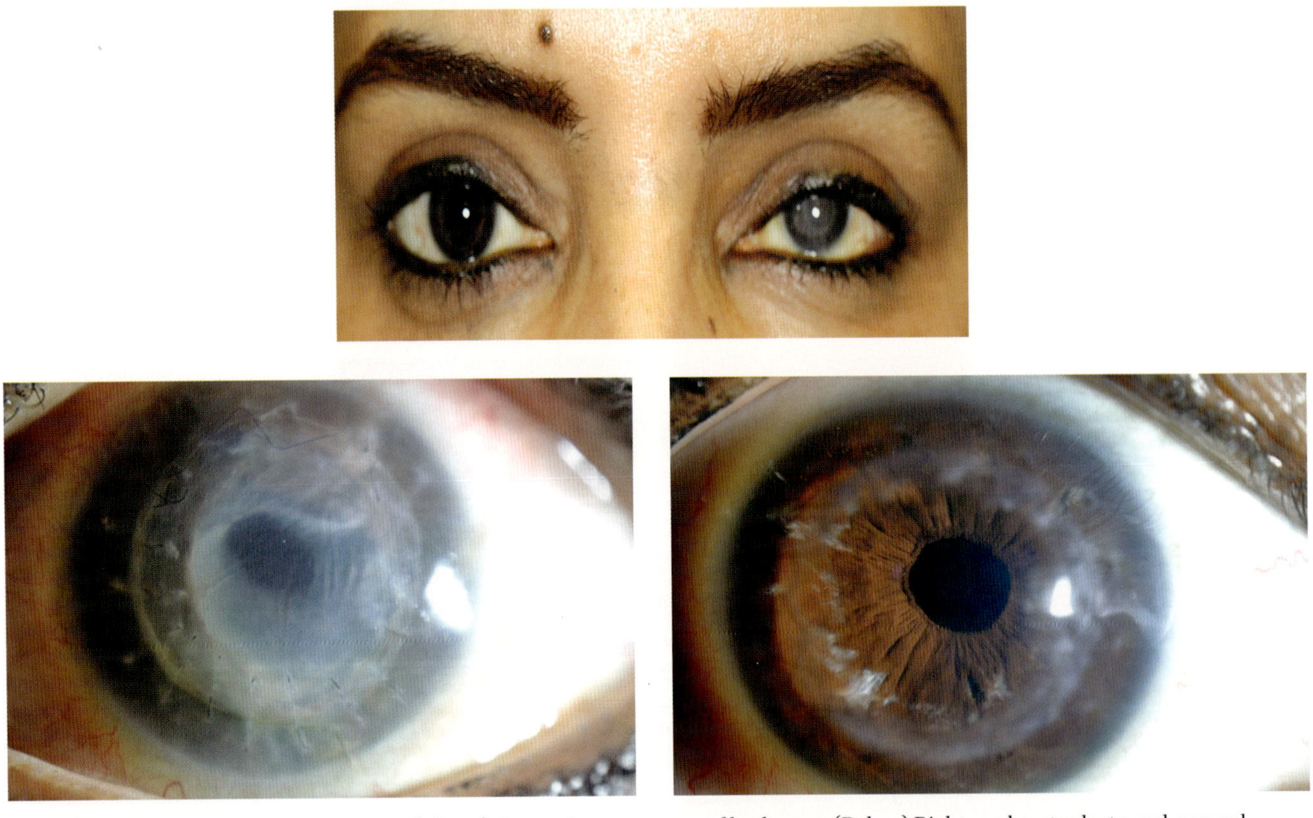

Fig. 10.104: Slit-lamp examination: (Above) Cosmetic appearance of both eyes; (Below) Right eye keratoplasty and corneal opacification on her left corneal graft

Postoperative Results

First visit postoperatively: Excellent cosmetic results and high patient satisfaction (Figure 10.105).

Follow-up and Comments

One year after the surgery, the patient was satisfied and repigmentation was offered to improve the color saturation. A second surgical enhancement was performed and a squint surgery was done at the same time (Figure 10.106).

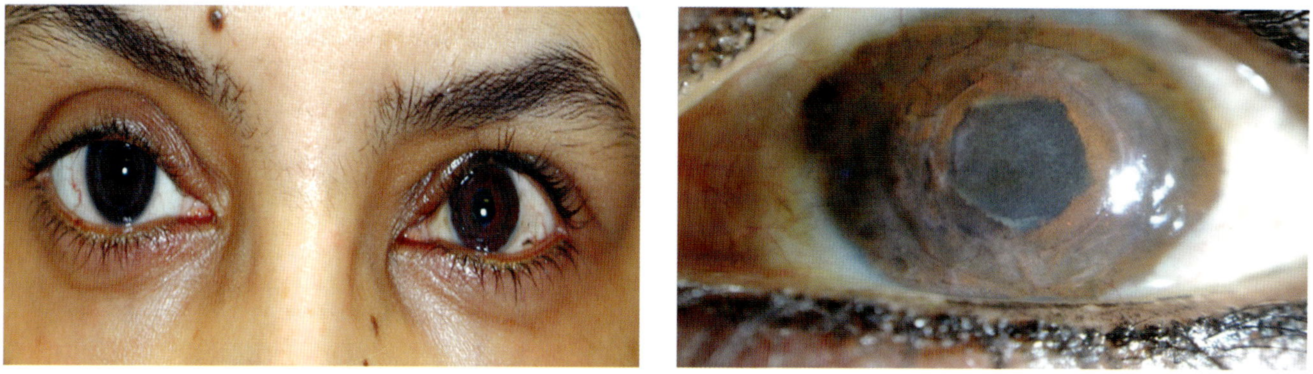

Fig. 10.105: Postoperative results. (Right) Slit-lamp examination after keratopigmentation; (Left) Cosmetic appearance of both eyes

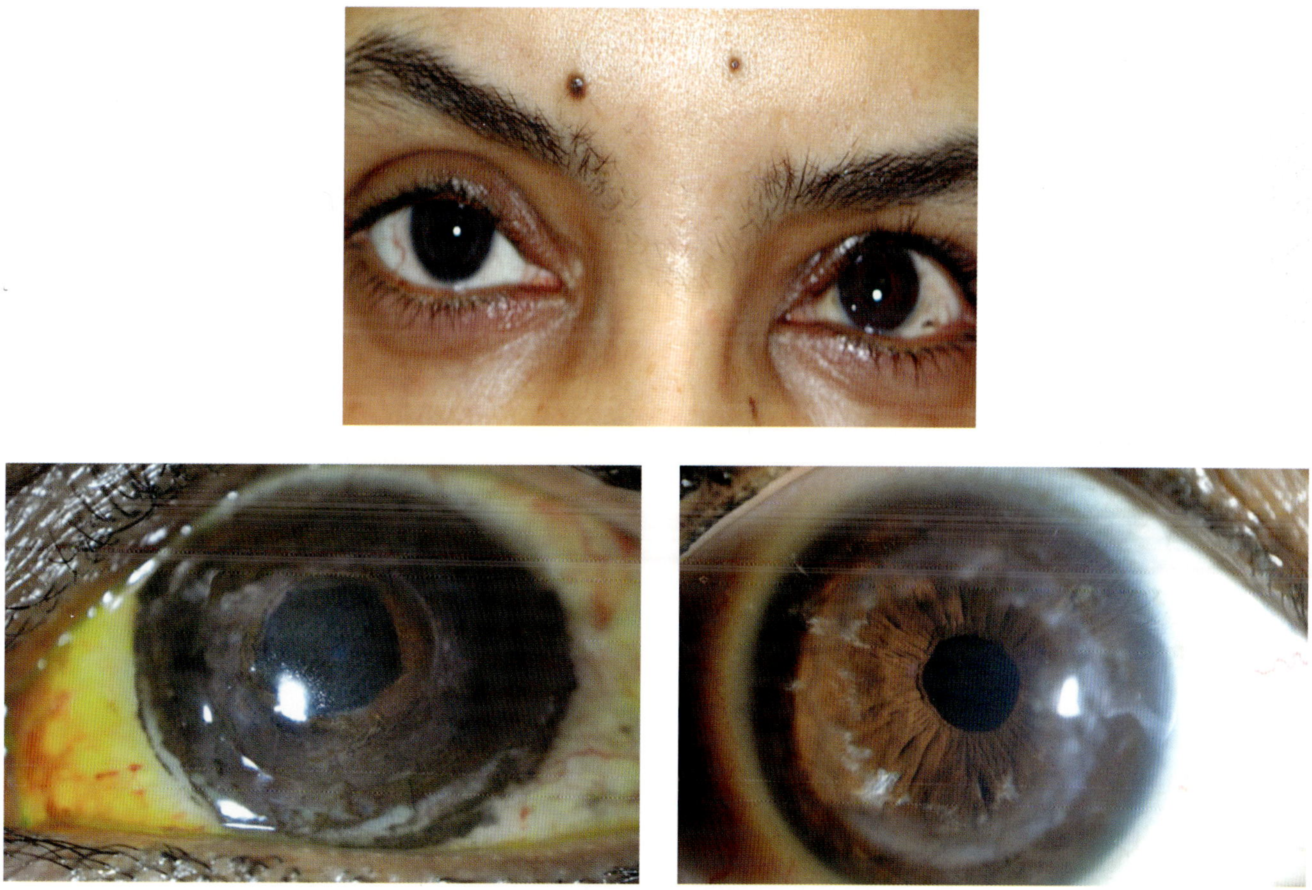

Fig. 10.106: Final cosmetic results

PART III: PURELY COSMETIC KERATOPIGMENTATION

CASE 38

Clinical History

A 46 years old male patient with who is complaining of the different colors of this eyes since his birth and asking for cosmetic solution for this porblem.

Preoperative Data

On examination: Heterochromia in which right eye is light blue with a sector of brown and left eye is brown, aided visual acuity was 1.0 bilaterally, with no history of trauma or surgery. The patient was adviced about the application of purely cosmetic keratopigmentation, as a permenant cosmetic solution, as he agreed to the surgery, and requested to change his right blue eye to brown (Figure 10.107).

Surgical Technique

Femtosecond-assisted keratopigmetation, using a mix of brown (VEMP 201) and black (VEMP 110) pigments and setting pupil at 5,5 mm with the depth of 350 microns.

Postoperative Results

Excellent cosmetic results with high patient satisfaction, no changes in vision or refraction were observed on the six months follow-up after the keratopigmentation procedure (Figure 10.108).

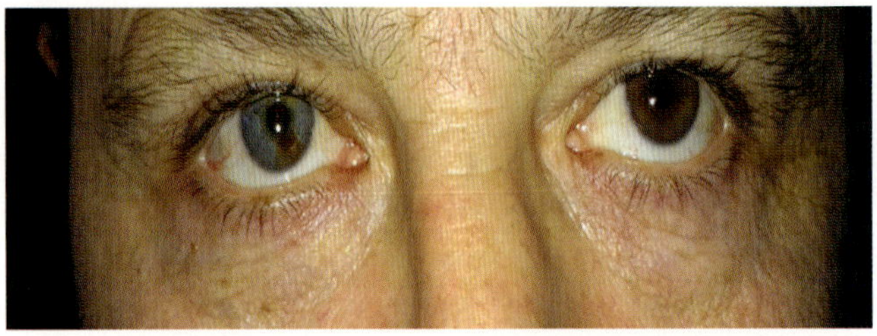

Fig. 10.107: Cosmetic appearance of both eyes

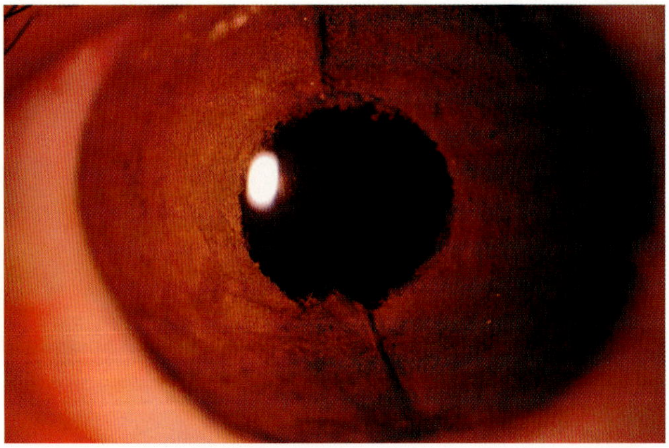

Fig. 10.108: Cosmetic results of right eye

CASE 39

Clinical History

A 30-year-old female who used color cosmetic contact lenses. Due to personal circumstances, she decided to proceed with keratopigmentation to change the color of her eyes.

Preoperative Data

On examination: Both eyes were totally normal and the visual acuity was 1.0 (decimal) bilaterally. There was no history of surgery or trauma. The surgeon discussed the risks and benefits of keratopigmentation as a permanent and purely cosmetic solution. She decided to proceed with this procedure and this case was the first purely cosmetic keratopigmentation surgery (Figure 10.109).

Surgical Technique

Femtosecond-assisted keratopigmentation, the pupil was marked in the center of the cornea with a calliper and 5.5 mm of diameter. The colors used were green mixed with light gray (VEMP 500) pigment.

Postoperative Results

Good cosmetic appearance, but the patient was not completely satisfied and requested a second keratopigmentation procedure to reach the desired color (Figure 10.110).

Follow-up and Comments

A second surgery was performed, customized blue (VEMP 604) pigment were used to recreate the pattern of her contact lenses.

After this surgery, the patient was satisfied with her cosmetic appearance, her visual acuity was normal because the pupil area was clear and it was not affected during the procedure (Figure 10.111).

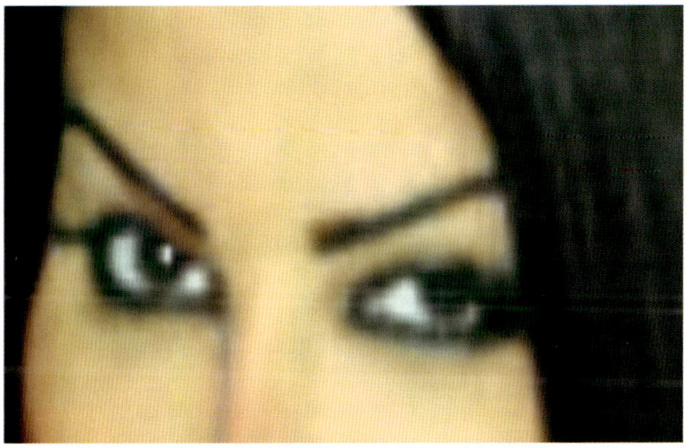

Fig. 10.109: Original dark color of patient's eyes

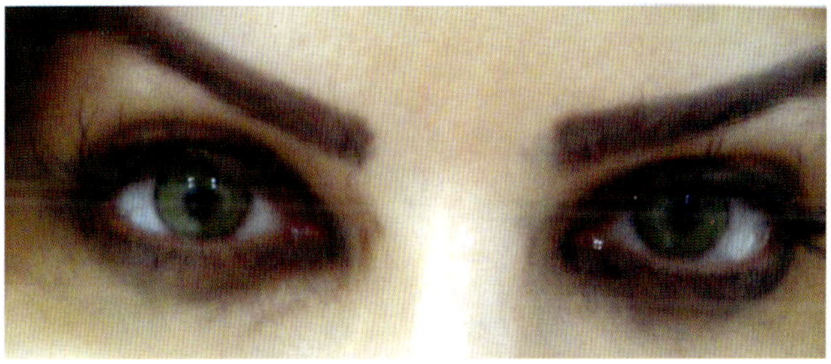

Fig. 10.110: Postoperative result

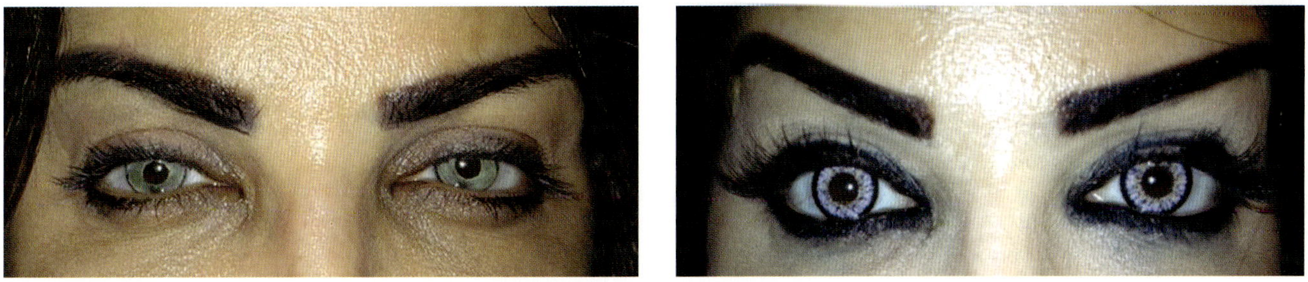

Fig. 10.111: Final cosmetic result (Right) with more natural look than the despired contact lens look (Left) after second keratopigmentation surgery

CASE 40

Clinical History

A 27-year-old female with dark brown eyes who used color cosmetic contact lenses. Due to personal circumstances, she decided to proceed with keratopigmentation to change the color of her eyes.

Preoperative Data

Preoperative examination revealed healthy eyes with no history of surgery or trauma, her visual acuity was 1.0 (decimal) in both eyes (Figure 10.112).

Surgical Technique

Femtosecond-assisted keratopigmentation, using blue (VEMP 605) pigment at a corneal depth of 300 microns. The pupil size was marked in the center with 5.5 mm of diameter, who used color cosmetic contact lenses. Due to personal circumstances she decided to proceed with keratopigmentation to change the color of her eyes.

Postoperative Results

First visit postoperatively: The patient did not have any problem or discomfort after the procedure. The visual acuity was normal in both eyes, and she was satisfied with the cosmetic result. The obtained color was slightly light, causing

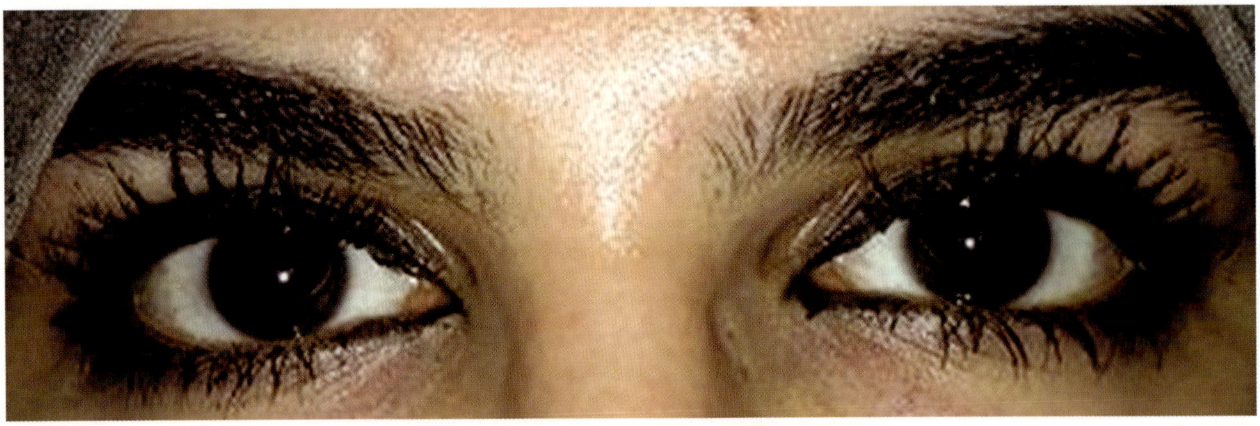

Fig. 10.112: Preoperative cosmetic appearance of both eyes

an artificial look and a second pigmentation was suggested to modify the color and to give her a more natural look (Figure 10.113).

Follow-up and Comments

A second keratopigmentation surgery was performed using the superficial technique and black (VEMP 110) pigment to delineate the pupil and limbus. A personlized gray blue and orange pigments were also injected to modify the iris color.

One year after this procedure, the pigmentation pattern was stable with high patient satisfaction and a very natural look of the simulated iris in both eyes (Figure 10.114 and 10.115).

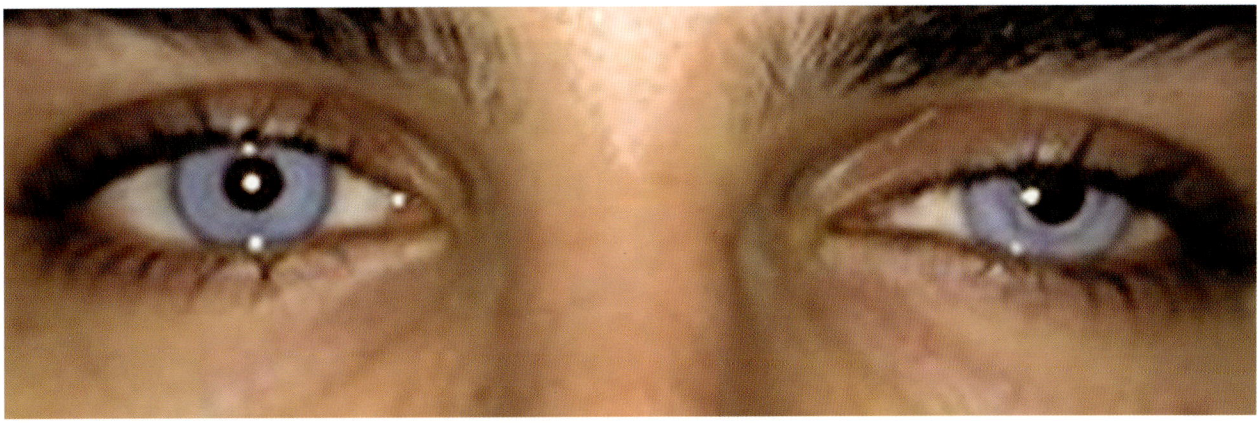

Fig. 10.113: Postoperative results

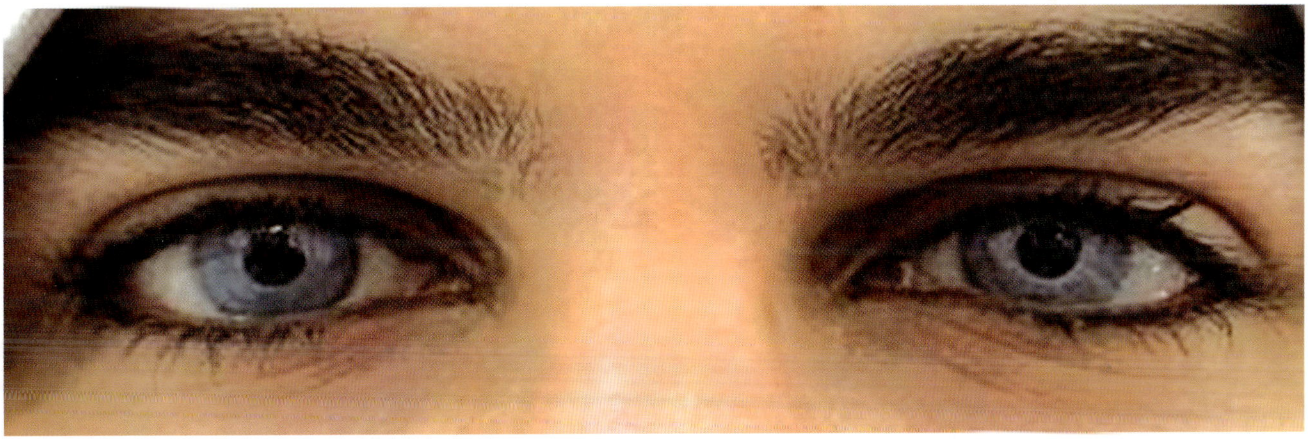

Fig. 10.114: Cosmetic appearance one year after keratopigmentation

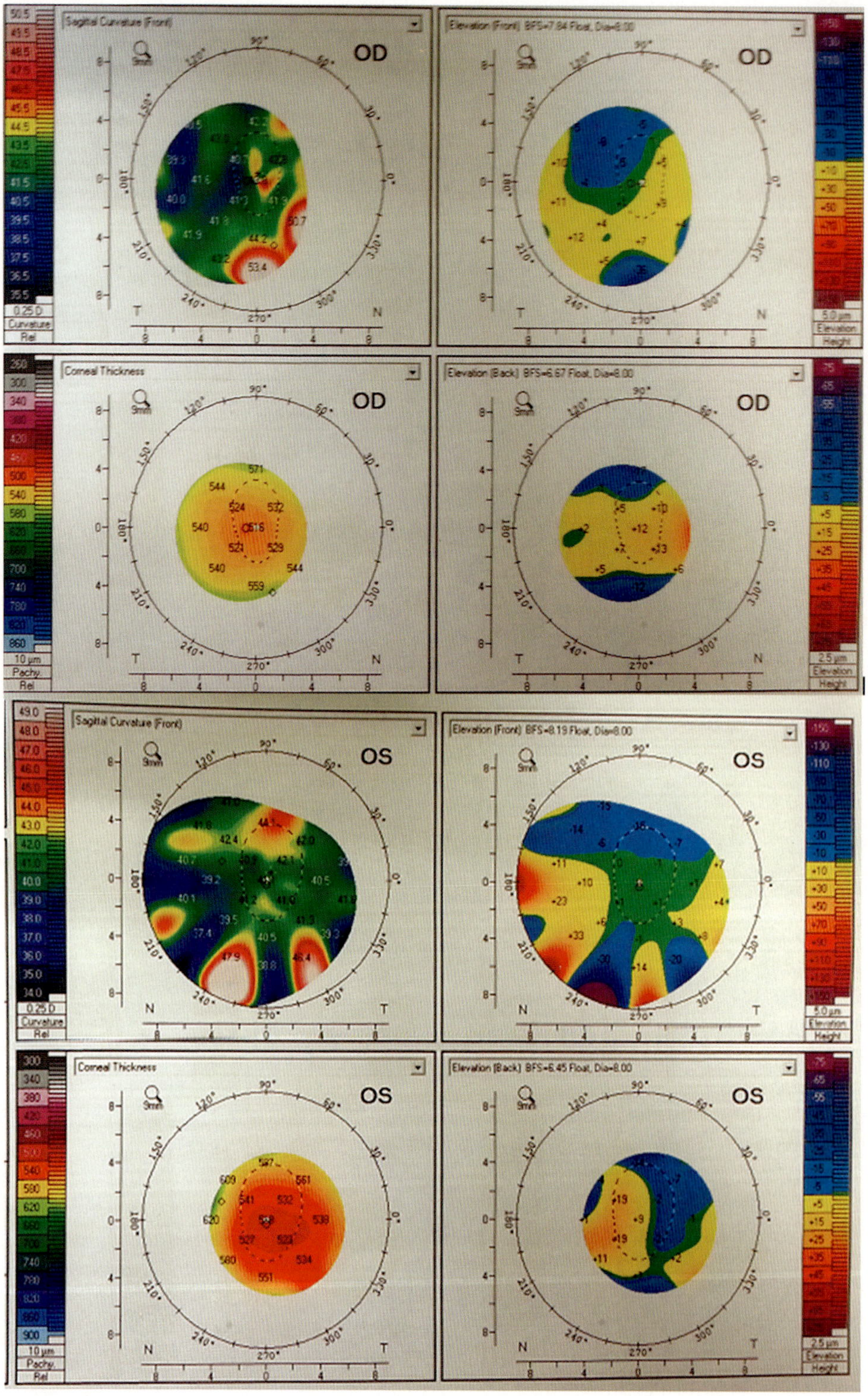

Fig. 10.115: Post-operative topography, showing peripheral blockage by the pigmentation

Appendices

Appendices

APPENDIX 1

Congress	Dates	Form	Title	Authors
85 Congreso de la Sociedad Española de Oftalmogia, Santander	23–26 September 2008	Poster	Queratopigmentación con pigmentos minerales microizados para mejorar la apariencia de ojos con limitaciones visuales	Alió JL, Sirerol B, Walewska-Szafran A
ARVO Annual meeting	3–7 May 2009	Poster	Hen as a new experimental model for keratopigmentation studies	Alió JL, Sirerol B, Walewska-Szafran A
American Academy of Ophthalmology meeting, Orlando	22–25 October 2011	Poster	Keratopigmentation (KTP) for the management of visual disabilities related to iris defects	Alió JL, Toffaha BT, Rodriguez AE
ESCRS Congreso, Vienna	17–21 September 2011	Free Paper	Corneal keratopigmentation for the correction of functional dysfunctions of the eye related to iris defects	Alió JL, Toffaha BT, Rodriguez AE
87 Congreso de la Sociedad Española de Oftalmogia	21–24 September 2011	Free Paper	Queratopigmentación para el tratamiento de las disfunciones visuales relacionadas con defectos del iris	Alió JL, Toffaha BT, Rodriguez AE, El Aswad A
ASCRS-ASOA Congress	20–24 April 2012	Free Paper	Keratopigmentation (KTP) for the management of visual disabilities related to iris defects	Alió JL, Rodriguez AE, Toffaha BT
World Ophthalmology Congreso, Abu Dhabi	16–20 February 2012	E-Poster	Keratopigmentation (KTP) for the management of visual disabilities related to iris defects	Alió JL, Toffaha BT, El Aswad A, Rodriguez AE
ESCRS Congreso, London	13–17 September 2014	E-Poster	Aesthetic Annual Keratopigmenation	Francis Ferrari
ESCRS Congreso, London	13–17 September 2014	E-Poster	Keratopigmentation Outcomes: A five years follow-up	Alió JL, Rodriguez AE, El Bahrawy M
Eucornea Congreso, London	12–13 September 2014	Free Paper	Long term stability of Keratopigmentation	Alió JL, Rodriguez AE, El Bahrawy M
American Academy of Ophthalmology meeting, Chigaco	17–25 October 2014	Poster	Five years follow-up in patients with keratopigmentation	Alió JL, Rodriguez AE, El Bahrawy M
Sircova Congress, Valencia	7–8 November 2014	Case Presentation	Keratopigmentation in a keratoconus patient after keratoplasty	Alió JL, Rodriguez AE, El Bahrawy M
ARVO Egypt meeting, Cairo	13–14 November 2014	Poster	Keratopigmentation: Applications and Outcomes	El Bahrawy M, Alió JL, Rodriguez AE
ASETCIRC, Madrid	14–15 November 2014	Poster	Queratopigmentación: Cinco años de seguimiento	Alió JL, Rodriguez AE, El Bahrawy M

APPENDIX 2

Clinical science

Corneal tattooing (keratopigmentation) with new mineral micronised pigments to restore cosmetic appearance in severely impaired eyes

Jorge L Alio,[1] Belucha Sirerol,[2] Anna Walewska—Szafran,[3] Mauricio Miranda[3]

[1]Instituto Oftalmológico de Alicante, VISSUM Corporación, Miguel Hernandez University, Alicante, Spain [2]Research and Development Department, Instituto Oftalmológico de Alicante, VISSUM Corporación, Alicante, Spain [3]Cataract and Refractive Surgery at Instituto Oftalmológico de Alicante, VISSUM Corporación, Alicante, Spain

Correspondence to
Professor Jorge L Alió, Instituto Oftalmológico de Alicante, VISSUM Corporation, Avda Denia, s/n, (Edificio VISSUM) 03016 Alicante, Spain; jlalio@vissum.com

Accepted 17 July 2009
Published Online First 2009

ABSTRACT

Aim To investigate keratopigmentation (KTP) with new mineral micronised pigments as a surgical alternative to improve cosmetic appearance in severely impaired eyes.
Methods 40 eyes underwent KTP alternatively to invasive cosmetic reconstructive surgery. Corneal staining with mineral micronised pigments was performed using an intralamellar or superficial technique.
Results One year postoperatively, all but two patients (95%) were satisfied. Pigmented eyes were improving patient's appearance. Eight cases needed a second KTP. Two patients with preoperative corneal oedema did not obtain an adequate cosmetic appearance due to progressive pigment clearance observed from 6 months postoperatively. Three eyes with traumatic aniridia observed good cosmetic outcome and a significant reduction in glare.
Conclusions KTP achieves good cosmetic results and is associated with high patient satisfaction, avoiding extensive and mutilating reconstructive surgery.

Our study aims to investigate the potential of corneal tattooing to improve ocular cosmetic appearance using new, micronised mineral pigments in cases of severely impaired eyes; to demonstrate the safety and medium-term durability; and to investigate its potential as an alternative to invasive reconstructive surgery for the cosmetic correction of disabled eyes. To the best of our knowledge, this is the largest modern report on KTP performed for cosmetic purposes in a consecutive group of human eyes, since 1936.[15] This project is also, to the best of our knowledge, the first study in which micronised mineral pigments were used for this purpose.

METHODS

Study design

Prospective, interventional, consecutive, non randomised, non-comparative series of cases.

APPENDIX 3

Binocular Vision & Strabismus Quarterly© A Medical Scientific e-Periodical

Intrastromal Corneal Tattooing As Treatment in a Case of Intractable Strabismic Diplopia (Double Binocular Vision) C. Laria, MD, J.I. Alió, MD, PhD, D.P. Piñero, PhD

Fourth Quarter of 2010 Volume 25 (No.4): Pages 238-242

Case Report

INTRASTROMAL CORNEAL TATTOOING AS TREATMENT IN A CASE OF INTRACTABLE Strabismic DIPLOPIA (Double Binocular Vision)

CARLOS LARIA, M.D., PhD,[1,] JORGE L. ALIÓ, M.D.,PhD[2,3] and DAVID P. PIÑERO, PhD[4]

from (1) Paediatric Ophthalmology & Strabismus Unit. Instituto Oftalmológico de Alicante. VISSUM Corporation, Universidad San Pablo CEU Madrid, (2) Cornea, Cataract, Refractive Surgery and Anterior Segment Surgery Unit. Instituto Oftalmológico de Alicante. VISSUM Corporation. (3) Division of Ophthalmology, Universidad Miguel Hernández, (4) Departamento de Óptica, Farmacología y Anatomía, Universidad de Alicante, Alicante, Spain

ABSTRACT: We present the case of a 29-year old man complaining of intractable diplopia during the last 5 years. He had undergone several surgical procedures for the treatment of his infantile strabismus since age 6 years. After surgery, the patient had been treated on 4 occasions with Botox. He also performed antisuppresion exercises to encourage binocular vision.

On our examination, the patient showed a 20/20 visual acuity in both eyes and a strabismic dysfunction with a slight alphabet pattern, which induced a disturbing constant diplopia. Several treatment options were considered for this patient as occlusion therapy or cosmetic contact lenses, but they were not used because they were not acceptable esthetically or not tolerated.

Finally, an optical penalization was induced by means of a black corneal tattooing placed at the centre of the cornea. The patient was followed for a period of 18 months, showing a complete elimination of diplopia with esthetical acceptance and no inflammatory signs.

APPENDIX 4

Keratopigmentation (corneal tattooing) for the management of visual disabilities of the eye related to iris defects

Jorge L Alio,[1,2] Alejandra E Rodriguez,[3] Bader T Toffaha[1,2]

[1]Cornea and Refractive Surgery Department, VISSUM Corporation, Alicante, Spain
[2]Division of Ophthalmology, Universidad Miguel Hernández, Alicante, Spain
[3]Research & Development Department, VISSUM Corporation, Alicante, Spain

Correspondence to
Professor Jorge L Alio, VISSUM Corporacion Oftalmologica, Avda. de Denia s/n, 03016 Alicante, Spain; jlalio@vissum.com

Accepted 26 June 2011
Published Online First 27 July 2011

ABSTRACT

Aim To investigate the functional and cosmetic outcomes of keratopigmentation (KTP) in cases of moderate to severe visual dysfunctions owing to different iris disorders.
Methods 11 eyes with moderate to severe visual disabilities related to iris defects underwent KTP for functional and cosmetic restoration using micronised mineral pigments and assisted with modern technologies such as femtosecond laser and new automated keratopigmentation instruments for the intrastromal and superficial application of the pigments.
Results Following the KTP surgery, the visual-function-related symptoms improved in all cases, from significant improvement to total elimination. Eight patients were asymptomatic after the surgery. In two patients, minimal non-disabling symptoms remained after surgery. One patient with traumatic aniridia complained of significant residual glare at the 3-month postoperative visit and was reoperated to reduce the simulated pupil to 4 mm. The cosmetic outcomes were analysed and classified as excellent in eight patients and good in three.
Conclusion KTP using new micronised mineral pigments and new surgical protocols has proven in this series to be an effective surgical technique for the management of moderate to severe visual dysfunctions related to iris defects.

highly beneficial in these difficult cases, as it is a less invasive technique than intraocular procedures[11 12] and may provide advantages for the practical surgeon owing to its reduced cost and potential accessibility.

In this study, we report, to the best of our knowledge, the first systematic clinical series of cases with 11 patients affected by different degrees of functional light disabilities caused by moderate to severe iris defects. The purpose of this study is to demonstrate that KTP practised with new micronised mineral pigments and assisted with modern surgical technologies such as femtosecond laser and new automated keratopigmentation instruments for the intrastromal or superficial application of the pigments may be a very effective and relatively simple alternative in the treatment of moderate to severe visual disabilities related to iris defects.

PATIENTS AND METHODS

The purpose of this study is to investigate the functional and cosmetic benefit obtained by KTP in cases of moderate to severe visual dysfunctions owing to different iris disorders. For this purpose, different original micronised mineral pigments and new specific KTP techniques have been used, including manual intralamellar keratopigmentation (MIK), femtosecond assisted keratopigmentation (FAK) and superficial automated keratopigmentation (SAK).

APPENDIX 5

Tolerance and Biocompatibility of Micronized Black Pigment for Keratopigmentation Simulated Pupil Reconstruction

Belucha Sirerol, MSc, Anna Walewska-Szafran, MD,† Jorge L. Alio, MD, PhD,‡ Pawel Klonowski, MD, PhD,* and Alejandra E. Rodriguez, MSc**

Purpose: To study the tolerance and biocompatibility of new mineral micronized pigments for corneal cosmetic pigmentation in an experimental animal model.

Methods: Central corneal intralamellar tattoos were performed with a black iron oxide mineral micronized pigment using an irrigating solution as a control. Animals were examined regularly under a slit lamp to detect any signs of inflammation, pigment diffusion, or color changes and neovascularization. The animals were divided into 2 groups, A and B. These groups were followed up at 1 and 3 months, respectively. At the end of this period, confocal microscopy examination was performed before the animals were killed, and their eyes were processed for histopathological examination to determine the level of pigment diffusion and inflammation and the presence of neovascularization.

Results: Clinical findings included 2 cases of minimal inflammation that resolved within 2 weeks and a severe case of inflammation detected 20 days after the surgery. Confocal microscopy at the end of the follow-up revealed normal corneal structures in all the eyes examined, with a layer of highly reflective material in the mid stroma because of the presence of mineral pigment particles. Histopathological examination corroborated clinical results regarding inflammation. No pigment diffusion or changes in color occurred throughout the study, and there were no cases of corneal neovascularization.

Conclusions: Central keratopigmentation presented good cosmetic appearance without adverse effects. These results suggest the adequacy of mineral micronized pigments for successful keratopigmentation. The hen animal model is a suitable model for assaying the biocompatibility and tolerance of micronized pigments in central keratopigmentation.

Keratopigmentation (KTP) or corneal tattooing has been used for centuries[1,2] to improve the cosmetic appearance of corneas with leukomas.[3–5] Nowadays, this ancient technique has broadened its cosmetic applications to correct opacities after amniotic membrane transplantation[4,6,7] and corneal scars.[8] Corneal tattooing also has a therapeutic effect in patients with symptomatic glare associated with iris loss or trauma,[9–13] cases of vision disabling light scattering,[14] and photophobia in posttraumatic aniridia or iris coloboma.[13] Despite the progress of ocular surface reconstructive surgery and the availability of colored contact lenses, corneal tattooing is a valuable alternative to mutilating surgery in cases of severe cosmetic defects for patients presenting contact lenses intolerance and high risk for penetrating keratoplasty.

The coloring of the cornea can be achieved by reducing metallic salts in situ[5,9,15] or by embedding coloring agents[5,7,14,16,17] into the corneal stroma. The main complications associated with these procedures are toxic reaction to the pigment,[1,17] color fading,[17] color change,[5] and over- or underpigmentation.

The aim of this study was to investigate the tolerance, biocompatibility, and suitability of a micronized black-colored iron oxide–based mineral pigment in central tattoos in hen corneas. The smaller particle size of micronized mineral pigments reduces the foreign body sensation and inflammatory response because of the imbedded pigment. Although corneal tattooing has previously been used in animals,[18] to our knowledge, this is the first study in which an animal experimental model is used for investigating the tolerance and toxicity of mineral micronized pigments specially formulated to its application in corneal pigmentation.

APPENDIX 6

TECHNIQUE

Femtosecond-assisted keratopigmentation for functional and cosmetic restoration in essential iris atrophy

Jorge L. Alió, MD, PhD, Alejandra E. Rodriguez, MSc, Bader T. Toffaha, MD, David P. Piñero, PhD, Luis J. Moreno, MSc

We describe a new surgical technique of femtosecond-assisted keratopigmentation (KTP) in a 23-year-old woman with severe visual dysfunction secondary to unilateral essential iris atrophy due to the presence of iridocorneal endothelial syndrome in her left eye. The patient presented with complaints of photophobia and monocular diplopia in the affected eye. Femtosecond-assisted KTP surgery was performed in this eye. Following the procedure, the patient reported complete elimination of photophobia and diplopia, with an excellent cosmetic result. Follow-up of 12 months was unremarkable. To our knowledge, this is the first report of a severe visual function disability caused by essential iris atrophy that was corrected by a new KTP technique.

Financial Disclosure: No author has a financial or proprietary interest in any material or method mentioned.

J Cataract Refract Surg 2011; 37:1744–1747 © 2011 ASCRS and ESCRS

Online Video

APPENDIX 7

CASE REPORT

Femtosecond-Assisted Keratopigmentation Double Tunnel Technique in the Management of a Case of Urrets-Zavalia Syndrome

Jorge L. Alio, MD, PhD,† Alejandra E. Rodriguez, MSc,‡ Bader T. Toffaha, MD,*† and A. El Aswad, MD, MSc*†*

Purpose: To describe the successful use of a double intrastromal tunnel femtosecond-assisted keratopigmentation technique to manage a case of unilateral Urrets-Zavalia syndrome.

Methods: A 33-year-old man was referred with a history of trauma in his right eye due to a labor-related accident. Because of myopic anisometropia, he had been previously implanted with an angle-supported phakic intraocular lens. The patient presented iris atrophy and a fixed dilated pupil. He complained of severe and incapacitating photophobia, glare, and decreased vision. To obtain a complete iris replica, the surgery involved creation of double keratopigmented intrastromal tunnels using femtosecond laser and micronized mineral pigments. The deepest layer was stained black first and then the superficial layer was stained with a contoured greenish blue-gray color, which matched the contralateral eye.

Results: In the immediate postoperative period, the patient reported a complete elimination of photophobia associated with the corrected distance visual acuity improvement. A very adequate cosmetic outcome was also achieved. Stability was observed during the 12-month follow-up.

Conclusion: A femtosecond-assisted keratopigmentation technique using 2 pigmented intrastromal tunnels to achieve an intracorneal pigmented replica of the iris was effective in improving the patient's severe visual function disability and cosmetic appearance. To the best of our knowledge, this is the first report of severe visual function disability caused by atrophic iris and a fixed dilated pupil treated with double intrastromal layers of keratopigmentation by means of femtosecond-created tunnels.

Key Words: femtosecond, keratopigmentation, Urrets-Zavalia syndrome, corneal tatooing

(*Cornea* 2012;31:1071–1074)

Keratopigmentation (KTP) or corneal tattooing has been used in the past to cosmetically restore severely impaired eyes.[1,2] Recently, KTP has also been reported to restore functional visual symptoms related to iris defects[3–6] and even intractable diplopia.[7]

Dilated and areflexic pupils with an atrophic iris are serious conditions with irritating and even incapacitating photophobia for young patients. The alternatives to solve these problems are limited to cosmetic contact lenses or intraocular surgery with or without lensectomy such as artificial iris prosthesis, intraocular diaphragm lens, or iris repair.[8,9]

We report an encouraging experience using KTP in a patient with a fixed dilated pupil (Urrets-Zavalia syndrome), an atrophic iris consecutive to an ocular trauma, and a phakic intraocular lens (IOL). The patient complained about severe incapacitating photophobia and glare. The patient was successfully treated with a femtosecond-assisted double tunnel and double-pigmented layer KTP technique. To the best of our knowledge, this is the first report to show the successful application of a double tunnel layer femtosecond-assisted KTP approach.

APPENDIX 8

BJO Online First, published on September 26, 2014 as 10.1136/bjophthalmol-2014-305611

Corneal tolerance to micronised mineral pigments for keratopigmentation

Maria A Amesty,[1] Jorge L Alio,[2] Alejandra E Rodriguez[2]

[1]Department of Ophthalmology, Nottingham University Hospitals, Nottingham, UK
[2]Vissum Corporación Oftalmológica, Alicante, Spain

Correspondence to
Professor Jorge L Alio, Vissum Corporación Oftalmológica, Avenida de Denia s/n, Alicante 03016, Spain; jlalio@vissum.com

Received 4 June 2014
Revised 8 August 2014
Accepted 7 September 2014

ABSTRACT

Purpose To study the tolerance and biocompatibility of micronised mineral pigments for corneal cosmetic pigmentation in an experimental animal model.

Methods Corneal intralamellar keratopigmentation was performed in 28 New Zealand white rabbits using micronised mineral pigments. Prophylactic actions using intraoperative antibiotic prophylaxis and gamma radiation of the pigment mixtures were performed to avoid infection. Animals were examined regularly by slit lamp to detect any sign of inflammation, pigment diffusion, colour changes or neovascularisation. Histopathological examination was performed to determine the level of pigment diffusion, the level of inflammation and the presence of neovascularisation.

Results No pigment diffusion or changes in colour, inflammation or neovascularisation were detected in the eyes treated. Histopathological examination corroborated clinical results regarding inflammation. Pigmented corneas showed a good cosmetic appearance without signs of ocular toxicity.

Conclusions Micronised mineral pigments could be a valid alternative treatment for cosmetic keratopigmentation. The intralamellar keratopigmentation technique presented good cosmetic appearance without adverse effects in the eyes treated.

Cosmetic contact lenses, enucleation or evisceration are the most frequently used methods to improve aesthetic appearance in cosmetically unacceptable, disabled eyes.[18–20] However, there is enough evidence of the excellent outcomes using KTP to achieve good cosmetic results and high patient satisfaction, avoiding extensive and mutilating reconstructive surgery.[1]

After reviewing the tolerance and biocompatibility of micronised mineral pigments for KTP,[1 12 13 16 17] the aim of our study is to investigate in an experimental animal model the potential of corneal tattooing using these pigments for cosmetic reasons. We also sought to demonstrate the safety, tolerance and medium-term durability of this procedure. The smaller particle size of micronised mineral pigments reduces the foreign body sensation and inflammatory response because of the imbedded pigment.

This work addresses the need of non-toxic and biocompatible pigments which may have fewer side effects. A variety of pigment colours to mimic different types of iris is also reported in this study. The poor practice and experience in corneal tattooing lies in the fact that reliable commercial products are unavailable. This is probably related to the lack of studies demonstrating the corneal biocompatibility of these pigments.

APPENDIX 9

www.coloreyetattoo.com

A Screen shot of our update website www.coloreyetattoo.com, a great tool for both patient and professional education.

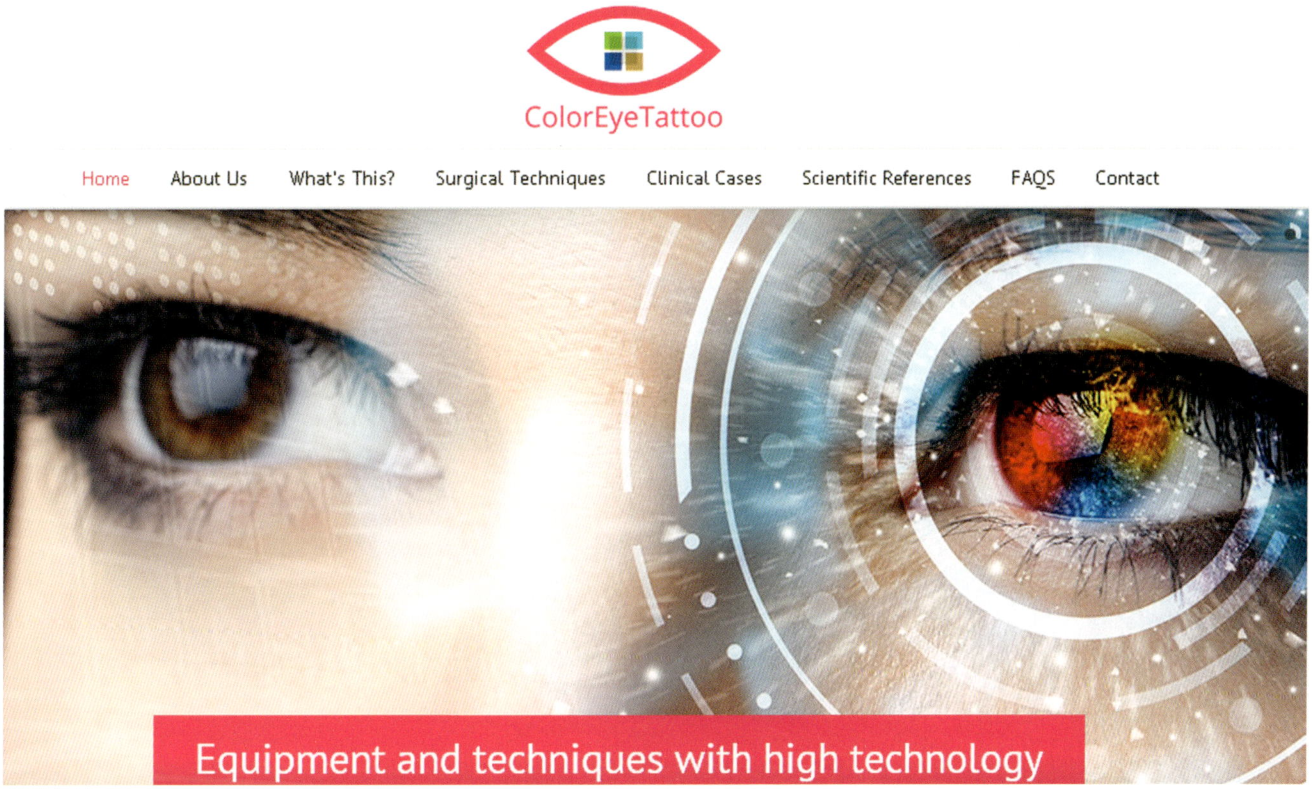

Index

Page numbers followed by *f* refer to figure